The Substance Abuse Problems

Sidney Cohen has degrees in Pharmacy and Medicine and was awarded a Doctor of Sciences degree from Columbia University in 1976.

Dr. Cohen has researched LSD for the past 20 years and marihuana for the past 5. He has published over 250 articles and 4 books in the areas of psychopharmacology and drug abuse. He is editor of the *Drug Abuse and Alcoholism Review* and the *Drug Abuse and Alcoholism Newsletter* and is on the editorial board of *Psychosomatics,* the *International Journal of Addictions, Drug Dependence,* the *American Journal of Drug and Alcohol Abuse,* the *Journal of Psychedelic Drugs,* and *Substance and Alcohol Misuse.*

Dr. Cohen served as Director of the Division of Narcotic Addiction and Drug Abuse, NIMH, from 1968 to 1970. He is now a Clinical Professor of Psychiatry at the Neuropsychiatric Institute, UCLA. He has spoken on all aspects of the drug problem in the United States and abroad.

The

Substance Abuse

Problems

Sidney Cohen, M.D.

 The Haworth Press, New York

The Haworth Press, 149 Fifth Avenue, New York, New York 10010

Earlier versions of most of the chapters in this book were published in the Vista Hill Foundation's *Drug Abuse & Alcoholism Newsletter,* volumes 1-8, 1972-1979.

Library of Congress Cataloging in Publication Data

Cohen, Sidney, 1910-
  The substance abuse problems.

  Earlier versions of most of the chapters in this book were published in the Vista Hill Foundation's Drug abuse & alcoholism newsletter, v. 1-8, 1972-79.
  Includes bibliographic references and index.
  1. Drug abuse. 2. Drugs—Psychological aspects.
3. Drugs—Physiological effect. 4. Drug abuse—Treatment.
I. Vista Hill Foundation. II. Title. (DNLM: 1. Drug abuse. WM270 C678s)
RC564.C63   362.2'9   80-21280
ISBN 0-917724-18-6
ISBN 0-917724-22-4 (pbk.)

Printed in the United States of America

CONTENTS

FOREWORD

It was nearly a decade ago that I first heard Sidney Cohen speak. He and I were on the same program at the National Naval Medical Center in Bethesda, Maryland. As I waited anxiously for my turn to speak, I listened, at first casually, and then with increasingly rapt attention to what I concluded was the best overview I had ever heard of the various drug abuse treatments. It was comprehensive, balanced, and easy to understand. At that time, even more than today, the drug abuse treatment field was filled with single-minded advocates of one or another of the particular treatment modalities. Few of the experts bothered to learn much about what their colleagues were up to. I had, over the preceding years, found that speeches made by representatives of the National Institute of Mental Health were even more narrow and opinionated than those by the clinicians themselves. And yet, to my utter surprise, here was a gray-haired guru from NIMH who could comprehend the whole field and present it directly, even simply.

I went up to Sidney Cohen after that talk to tell him I thought it was magnificent. His reaction, as I recall, was, "Oh, that was nothing really; I was just stating the obvious things that everyone already knows." He said this without arrogance (I have never known him to exhibit arrogance) but with modesty for his own contributions and with respect for his colleagues and his audience.

Over the next ten years, I came to know Sidney Cohen well. My admiration for him has grown beyond that auspicious beginning. When I was Director of the National Institute on Drug Abuse (an independent HEW Institute which grew out of the smaller NIMH office which Sidney headed when he gave that 1970 talk), I often felt besieged and confused. Every few months, without calling ahead for an appointment, Sid would appear at my door, having first shaken the hands of his many friends at NIDA as he walked down the hall and through the outer office. I greeted him with open arms. I was always ready to talk and to listen because I knew I would learn something new about drug abuse prevention. After an hour, Sid would leave and I would return to the hurley-burley of administering a large government program. He was particularly helpful to me on complex and controversial issues. His wide range of knowledge and his open and respectful mind never failed to orient and educate me. When he left I felt not only better informed, but wiser.

Now it is my pleasure not only to honor a respected colleague, but to introduce readers, new and old, to a rare treat. Since 1972, Cohen has published for the Vista Hill Foundation unique short essays. His instincts—better to call it what it is, his restless curiosity—have led him to the most important and difficult issues in the field of drug abuse and alcoholism prevention. His wisdom shines from eage page of this new book, which presents these essays in updated and revised anthology form. His writing is the best in the field. I know of no other person who can take so much complex research, administrative, and even "political" material, and digest it so it *seems* simple.

The publication of this new work, *The Substance Abuse Problems,* is a landmark in the field of drug abuse prevention. It introduces the novice to the issues, as well as offering the jaded expert a fresh and readable overview. It is the first time the general reader has had the opportunity to glimpse the scope and skill of a great man in the drug abuse field who has no peer.

Robert L. DuPont, M.D.
Founding Director,
National Institute on Drug Abuse (1973-1978)
Currently President,
American Council on Marijuana

INTRODUCTION

It is quite possible that long before humans planted crops, they already had a good working knowledge of the local plants that could alter their consciousness. It appears that not only were pain-relieving and sleep-procuring herbs known, but also, in some regions, dissociating or hallucinogenic drugs were identified and held in high esteem. In places where they did not exist, long treks were made to acquire such items. Peyote pilgrimages extended from Canada down to Texas or northern Mexico. Pituri trails running for hundreds of miles can still be made out in central Australia. The search for botanicals that could drive people beside themselves (*ec stasis*) is no latter-day quest. Some anthropologists have called it a universal drive, for where such plants were not to be found, physical techniques of sensory deprivation, whirling, meditation, and other rituals were developed.

Sometimes these precarious mind-shaking practises were used as rites of passage, into manhood, for example. Often they were employed to achieve a prophetic experience or to heal a sick member of the tribe. Sometimes only the shaman was allowed to have these out-of-the-body experiences. When others participated, it was only after careful preparation, a far cry from the casual acid-dropping of recent years.

The search for mind-altering roots, leaves, and cacti continues, but it is overshadowed these days by the sterochemist's computerized scanning of potentially consciousness-altering molecular configurations. It is now almost possible to predict from the atomic arrangements and electrical charges of the compound whether it will allay distress, procure pleasure, achieve self-transcendence, or simply intoxicate. Such knowledge is, of course, a finely honed, double-edged sword that can cut for good or ill. We know of psychedelic chemists who keep one molecule ahead of the law by bringing forth compounds not yet covered by legislation.

We live in a time of rapid change, turmoil and uncertainty, and an erosion of established values and beliefs. Therefore, it is also a time of unease, frustration, anxiety, and depression. Nor have we learned how to endure psychological pain and stress with fortitude. On the contrary, many of us have come to expect instant relief from noxious feelings, and, in fact, to look for instant pleasure, chemically procured, if necessary. The cultural taboos against drugs for enjoyment and fun have been broached by more citizens than ever before. Add to this the enhanced precision of synthetic compounds that will do it better, and we have a situation that is not about to go away.

On the contrary, the drug scene of the past twenty years has been changing—but not improving. The twisting, turning, psychochemical fashions are worth following and understanding. These essays on the current problems of substance misuse are attempts to inform the reader of the dimensions and the directions of the issues—sometimes to try to look into their future. They were written during the 1970s and brought up to date as necessary. Most of the essays were published in the Vista Hill Foundation *Newsletter*. One of the *Newsletter* essays ("Drug X: Another Point of View," by Dr. Robert Moore) was printed originally as a response by my earlier effort on the subject. Dr. Richard Phillipson contributed an original essay ("Problem Drinking in Adolescents") for this book. All the remaining essays were written by me.

The book has been divided into five main chapters. The first, and largest, describes the abuse of many legal and illegal drugs and details the effects of that abuse. The second chapter analyzes the trends in drug abuse and relates the global nature of the problem. Chapters III and IV describe, respectively, the various diagnoses and treatments of certain abuse problems. Chapter V concludes with a discussion of special situations and special groups involved in the abuse of drugs.

Throughout the book I have consistently used the masculine pronouns in situations that could refer to both men and women. I have done that, not to deny women their place in the sorry story of drug abuse, but rather for convenience and for (I hope) easier reading.

Perhaps a personal note will be permitted since it may explain some of my attitudes and reflect upon the changing times. At an age that would seriously violate today's child labor laws, I worked as a delivery and cleanup boy for Lascoff's Pharmacy in the Yorkville section of Manhattan. My many duties included pounding blue mass (a mercury concoction) with an iron pestle and mortar. I had the privilege of crushing asafedita so that it could be made into an emulsion for nervous people. Since the odor was outrageous, it effectively provided the patient with a respite from all human interactions. I remember dusting long rows of dark brown bottles with Parke-Davis labels, all containing fluidextracts and tinctures with exotic-sounding Latin names. One of them was Fluidextractum Cannabis

Indica. I never saw it used except on one occasion. The year's supply of corn remover was being made, and a few drops of the Cannabis were added to color the remedy green. What a disappointment after having read about hashish in the *Thousand and One Arabian Nights*! We even had a bottle of leeches. The apothecary was a fascinating place, and it doubtlessly instilled a lifelong interest in drugs and their effects. It lead to pharmacy college, medical school, and decades of research in psychopharmacology, including marihuana, the same drug whose bottle I had dusted more than a half century earlier.

Much more impressive than the personal account is the indication of vast changes in therapeutics from what was essentially a medieval *materia medica* to the fairly scientific pharmacology of today.

Writing these brief commentaries on the drugs and drug issues of the day was a great pleasure. I thank you for looking at them.

Sidney Cohen, M.D.
Westwood, California

ACKNOWLEDGMENTS

The Vista Hill Foundation and its Board supported the writing and publishing of these articles and gave permission for them to be printed in book form. They also provided very helpful critiques of the substance of these essays. I am also grateful to Drs. Richard A. Phillipson and Robert A. Moore for having contributed two pertinent papers to this volume. Dorothy Cohen and Virginia Everett have provided considerable editorial support, and it is greatly appreciated.

I
DRUGS: LEGAL AND ILLEGAL

1. Pharmacology of Drugs of Abuse*

This essay is revised from a paper read at the International Conference on Drug Dependence, May 5-7, 1976, Rome, Italy.

Why are certain drugs abused? Why should one drug be preferred over another although both belong to the same pharmacologic class? What kinds of emotional experiences are sought by abusers of drugs?

All substances of abuse alter consciousness and mood. Consciousness is either raised or lowered. The varieties of changes in awareness range from a complete obliteration of consciousness, such as large doses of central nervous system (CNS) depressants can bring, to a vast intensification of awareness as experienced in the LSD state.

However, psychochemicals also exist that induce markedly altered states of awareness and yet they are never—or rarely—sought out for this purpose. No one seems to relish the diminution of consciousness that accompanies ingestion of the neuroleptics. The author has never met a chlorpromazine addict although he has read case reports of one or two. Street dealers do not stock the phenothiazines, the butyrophenones or the thioxanthines. If they did, few of their customers would be interested. Why not? Perhaps because they have unpleasant side effects, but more important, because they do not produce euphoria.

Just because a drug has unpleasant properties does not mean that it will not be abused. Some may be deterred by a vile tasting or smelling concoction, or one which produces a gastrointestinal upheaval, but others will indulge. *Datura strammonium*, also known as Jimson Weed, is singularly unpleasant but it has a few devotees. Nutmeg and mace (*myristica fragrans*) are difficult to swallow in intoxicating doses but some manage it.

The fly agaric (*amanita muscaria*) has noxious autonomic effects, and the peyote cactus (*lophophora Williamsii*) is far from enjoyable going down or coming back up. Nevertheless, they are sought after. For that matter, the first cigar or the first injection of an opiate can be associated with considerable gastrointestinal turmoil but people persist and acquire tolerance to these side effects.

Another reason why one drug may be preferred over another, similar drug is its rapidity of action. Secobarbital is preferred to phenobarbital for that reason, and cocaine preferred to amphetamines. Rapid onset of euphoric action, the "rush," is also why the intravenous or inhaled route are preferred to oral intake.

EUPHORIA

The feeling tone called euphoria, or "high," is perennially sought after. This sense of physical and emotional well-being has been searched for since the ascent of man and woman. Almost every society has its culturally acceptable euphoriant. We even have accumulating evidence that other animal species are inclined to use agents that will intoxicate them.

The long search for euphoria has some puzzling aspects. Not only stimulants but depressants also evoke the condition called "high." Apparently, it is the distancing from harsh reality that counts—the reduction in ego controls and the feeling of being "stoned." Certain people seem to have no particular need to be other than sober, while others do. The search for euphoria is for many really a flight from dysphoria, or from what is more painful, aphoria.

It is difficult to describe euphoria. Its pharmacology is far from clearly understood. It is not only the elimination of physical and psychological pain. There is a positive aspect to it which may be described as a feeling of rightness with oneself and with existence.

The more intense euphoric states of elation and ecstasy resemble those in which a stimulation of the reward centers of the posterior hypothalamus has occurred. There are clusters of noradrenergic neurones, and their electrical stimulation or microinjections of norepineophrine produces similar intense emotions. It is likely that cocaine and large doses of amphetamines act over such mechanisms.

A second road to euphoria is via tension and drive reduction and the associated drowsy, reverie state. When feelings of psychic emptiness and hunger are relieved, when disturbing sexual drives are set aside, and when a relaxed quietude intervenes, this is experienced as euphoric. The narcotics, working over serotonergic mechanisms, elicit such responses.

The hypnosedatives, the anxiolytics, alcohol and the volatile inhalants provide still another pathway to euphoria. These chemicals depress CNS function. First, they depress the inhibitory controls over affect and behavior, releasing mental functioning from its usual internal double-checking system. The monitors over mood and behavior are attenuated. This is felt as enjoyable and releasing by most people. In larger doses, the depression extends to other mental functions including memory, judgment and rational thought. These impairments also may be experienced as euphoric.

TOLERANCE

Abusable drugs have other important pharmacologic properties. Tolerance and abstinence effects are often, but not invariably, observed (Table I.-1) Cocaine, for example, does not produce tolerance, nor has a cocaine withdrawal syndrome been described. It is not precisely known why this should be so. Admittedly, it is quickly metabolized, and therefore has a brief duration of action. Perhaps, the rate of degradation of cocaine cannot be increased even with frequent administration, and metabolic tolerance cannot develop, except perhaps in enormous doses.

At the opposite end of the tolerance spectrum, as few as three or four daily doses of LSD will result in a complete refractoriness to a challenge dose of the drug. Responsiveness to LSD is regained after two or three days of abstinence. The alleged lack of tolerance or even the reverse tolerance to cannabis is simply due to the use of weak material. When large amounts of potent cannabis or THC are employed, tolerance will develop within a few days.

CROSS TOLERANCE

Cross tolerance between the sedative-hypnotics, the minor tranquilizers, alcohol and the anesthetics has been generally recognized. This means that the organism tolerant to one of these agents is tolerant to all. It also means that detoxification can proceed with any member of any class of depressants for all others. This is cross dependence. Cross tolerance and cross de-

Table I-1: Some Pharmacologic Properties of Abused Drugs

Drug Class	Example	Euphoria	Psychological Dependence	Tolerance	Withdrawal Syndrome
Narcotics	Heroin	+ + +	+ + +	+ + +	+ + +
Sedatives	Barbiturates	+ +	+ + +	+ +	+ + +
Anesthetics	Alcohol	+ +	+ + +	+ +	+ + +
	Toluene	+ +	+ +	+	(+)
Anxiolytics	Diazepam	+ +	+ +	+	+
	Meprobamate	+ +	+	+ +	+ +
Hallucinogens	LSD	+ +	+	+ + +	−
	THC	+ +	+ +	+ +	(+)
Stimulants	Amphetamines	+ + +	+ + +	+ +	+
	Cocaine	+ + +	+ + +	−	−
Ganglionic Stimulants	Tobacco	(+)	+ +	+ +	+

4

pendence between all narcotics exists, and also between hallucinogens like LSD, mescaline and psilocybin, but not to THC.

WITHDRAWAL

The phenomenon of withdrawal is similarly variable. Narcotic and sedative withdrawal syndromes can be intense, in fact, life endangering when high quality material has been used frequently over long periods of time. Sudden stoppage of alcohol and sleeping pills in a tolerant person results in a dramatic series of neuropsychiatric events (Table I.-2) This is the depressant withdrawal syndrome and is readily distinguished from the narcotic withdrawal syndrome except when they occur in a person simultaneously.

The stimulant withdrawal syndrome, I am convinced, is worthy of that designation. The long period of sleep after discontinuing high dose amphetamine intake, the enormous intake of food, the profound, sometimes suicidal depression, fatigue and generalized achiness—these constitute a fairly characteristic abstinence picture, which was identified by studying the "speedfreak crash" of a half dozen years ago.

In general, the higher the level of tolerance, the more pronounced the severity of the untreated withdrawal effects. The exception to this is observed with convulsions. Seizures appear to depend more upon duration of administration of the drug than the level of tolerance that develops. Tolerance also develops more rapidly with successive re-exposures to the drug or to drugs of the same general class.

Hallucinogens, except for cannabis, do not produce withdrawal symptoms. Whether cannabis does induce a full-fledged withdrawal pattern remains a matter for discussion. Certainly nausea, anorexia, jitteriness and insomnia are recorded after discontinuance of large amounts. Whether major symptoms of withdrawal-like convulsions or delirium can occur remains in dispute.

Although clinically, withdrawal symptoms appear to subside after detoxification, and the patient may feel well, a number of physiological indices remain abnormal. In the instance of the detoxified narcotic dependent person, slight elevations of body temperature, blood pressure and respiratory rate can be measured. A slight dilation of pupils is detectable after months of abstinence. Still later, a secondary abstinence phase has been described in which the above signs are reversed.

Even after more than a year of abstinence, previously addicted laboratory animals and man react to a single injection of morphine aberrantly. Altered reactivity can be found in the computer analyzed EEG, in an analysis of REM sleep after injection, and in accelerated tolerance devel-

Table I-2: Withdrawal Syndromes

	Narcotic* Withdrawal	Depressant** Withdrawal	Stimulant*** Withdrawal
Piloerection	X		
Lacrimination	X		
Rhinorrhea	X		
Diarrhea	X		
Muscle Spasm	X		
Muscle Pain	X		X
Nausea, Vomiting	X	X	
Delirium, Hallucinations	X	X	
Convulsions	X	X	
Insomnia	X	X	
Sweating	X	X	
Tremors		X	
Psychic Depression			X
Hyperphagia			X
Hypersomnia			X

  * opium derivatives and synthetic narcotics
 ** hypnotics, sedatives, anxiolytics, alcohol
*** amphetamines, anorectics, cocaine

opment to subsequent doses of morphine. It is postulated by some investigators that these long-persisting effects play a role in late relapse. Certainly, conditioning factors, which develop during addiction and withdrawal, can be the basis for relapse before they are eventually extinguished.

DEPENDENCE

The question of psychological dependence is not a profound one intrinsic in some basic drug mechanism. Instead, it derives from the desire to re-experience the euphoric or stress-relieving effects of the drug. With respect to dependence on tobacco, the psychomotor conditioning plays an important part in the approach behavior. The ritual of smoking is anxiety reducing and reinforcing, and the pharmacologic effects of nicotine are, perhaps, less significant. No doubt the ritual of cannabis smoking also contributes to the desired effects of that plant.

Physical dependence is simply the buildup of tolerance, the withdrawal syndrome on sudden discontinuance, and the desire to avoid withdrawal sickness. The craving is as much a desire to avoid the symptoms of withdrawal as a desire to experience the "high." Narcotic addiction, for example, demands a "fix" every eight hours or less, otherwise early withdrawal effects are noticed. The same is true of alcohol dependence, with the morning shakiness and hangover representing early withdrawal reactions.

SUMMARY

Although drugs of abuse have certain pharmacologic similarities, they also manifest distinct differences. They all may produce euphoria, but euphoria is many things. Tolerance, a withdrawal syndrome, and psychological dependence often occur, but some of these agents do not produce these phenomena. Perhaps a culture would be best advised to seek out the safest euphoriant and teach its members to avoid all others.

2. Marihuana: Recent Research

After alcohol, marihuana is the most widely used mind-altering substance. In this country 25% of the population have tried it at least once. Between three to five million are daily users. It is not only a recreational drug, it is an anti-establishment symbol. Many heated discussions are heard on its merits and hazards. Penalties for simple possession are being reduced with vociferous proponents of "pot" advocating legalization. For a drug that has been around for millenia, reliable information is surprisingly scanty. Aside from a few earlier studies, the scientific investigation of this plant is only a half dozen years old. A report of the recent research findings seems worthwhile in order to develop an informed opinion about the social and medical issues involved.

THE PLANT

Cannabis sativa will grow wild or cultivated in temperate or tropical climates. It is now assumed that only one species exists with two major varieties. The fibre variety is exemplified by the material that grows wild in the United States and Canada. It is low in delta-9-tetrahydrocannabinol (THC) and high in cannabidiol (CBD) content. The drug type is represented by Mexican, Vietnamese, Indian, and Nepalese material. It is high in

THC and low in CBD content. THC is the active constituent, and CBD may be its precursor. Much of the THC and CBD exists as acids. These are decarboxylated by heat or enzymes. Perhaps the threefold potency of marihuana that is smoked over that ingested is accounted for by the conversion of the THC acid to THC. Fibre and drug type seeds grown under identical conditions will contain the same THC-CBD ratio as the parent plants. After fertilization THC levels are reduced, and increasing amounts of cannabinol can be detected. When cannabis is kept at room temperature or exposed to light, the THC slowly changes to cannabinol which is thought to be the end metabolite in the plant. In animals the first metabolite is 17–hydroxy–THC. It is biologically active.

Some typical TCH values for various materials follow:

Street THC	0.0%	THC
Fibre type cannabis	0.05%	THC
Drug type cannabis	1.0–4.0%	THC
Hashish (resin)	10.0%	THC
Red oil (cannabis distillate)	20.0%	THC

The flowering tops and bracts contain the highest percentage of THC, leaves have a lesser amount, and seeds, stems and roots contain negligible quantities. Contrary to the ancient lore, the male plant is as potent as the female. It is removed from cultivated areas to prevent fertilization and loss of THC.

PHARMACOLOGY

THC is insoluble in water, but soluble in certain organic solvents and lipids. Its half life in humans is 28–56 hours. Studies with labelled THC show that the brain receives no more than that anticipated on the basis of body weight. The bulk of the radioactivity is detected over the liver and intestines. The acute toxicity of THC is low with the effective dose far below the lethal dose.

The most reliable physiologic changes accompanying ordinary amounts of marihuana are an increased heart rate and a dilation of the conjunctival blood vessels. The conjunctival injection is not due to the smoke. It also occurs when marihuana or THC are taken by mouth. Other physiologic measures are either unaffected or variably altered. The long held belief that pupillary dilation is a constant finding has not been confirmed in careful studies. Another widely held but incorrect assumption is that hypoglycemia accounts for the hunger feeling that many people report. A consistent lowering of blood sugar does not occur.

The most constantly found neurophysiological alterations are an overestimation of the time interval, some muscle weakness, decreased hand steadiness and an impaired complex reaction time. The increased alpha rhythm of the EEG is consistent with the drowsiness that is mentioned.

Tolerance and withdrawal symptoms with marihuana do not develop. This is a low dose effect since tolerance to THC and nonspecific withdrawal symptoms following heavy, chronic hashish use are known. The often mentioned "reverse tolerance" is an artifact representing an improved smoking technique, and learning to identify the subjective symptoms more readily. A first time user may notice nothing from active material. The novice is somewhat more susceptible to adverse reactions. The experienced user can "maintain," that is, titrate his inhalations to achieve a desired level of intoxication. However, his ability to distinguish between active marihuana and a placebo cigarette is far from accurate.

No conclusive evidence exists for organ damage due to cannabis. A chronic bronchitis is noted in some regular users. Tars are present in the plant. The mechanics of smoking marihuana (deep inhalation, a modified Valsalva maneuver, retention of smoke as long as possible) are such that a proper research question involves its possible pulmonary carcinogenicity. Animal studies using smoking machines and aerosols are now being carried out. The cytogenetic studies that have been reported are equivocal, and more work is being done.

The effects of ordinary amounts of marihuana consist of waxing and waning feelings of relaxation, drowsiness, occasionally hunger particularly for sweets, intensified or dreamlike sensory perceptions, and emotional lability usually in the direction of euphoria. In larger doses illusions, hallucinations, paranoid delusions, ideas of reference, depersonalization, and confusion are possible.

In one study, driving skills under marihuana were impaired less than under alcohol. However, the amounts given were not equivalent. In measures of alertness and attention, both alcohol and marihuana produced significant decrements.

A number of studies have reported on the impairment of immediate recall, or temporal disorganization as it has been called. Among consistent users this loss of recent memory is one aspect of the "spaced out" syndrome. It accounts for the blocking of speech because the speaker has forgotten what he had just said.

ADVERSE EFFECTS

These are infrequent and consist of anxiety reactions, toxic psychoses, and "flashbacks." The anxiety states are seen in novices more often than in experienced users. Panicky feelings, dysphoria, and restlessness dominate the clinical picture. The toxic psychoses are a delirium lasting for up to a day. They may represent an idiosyncratic reaction or an overdose. In-gested material may produce adverse effects more often than smoked ma-terial. The "flashbacks" are spontaneous recurrences of the marihuana state without having taken the drug. Another sort of "flashback" may oc-cur when a person takes marihuana some time after having used LSD. The marihuana experience may be much more intense, and it represents the LSD "flashback."

CHRONIC

The precipitation of a prolonged psychotic decompensation has been documented, but it does not happen too often. Generally, predisposed in-dividuals are involved, and a schizophrenic reaction may be triggered. A specific cannabis psychosis is almost unknown in this country. As in other lands, the heavy, regular use of cannabis has lead to loss of interest in all activities except drug use. This is the amotivational syndrome. Such indi-viduals may make their loss of drive a virtue, and their dropout a social protest of this life. In fact, this behavior and the magical thinking which accompanies it, may be a pharmacologic action of the drug on the central nervous system.

THERAPEUTIC POSSIBILITIES

The folk uses of cannabis are innumerable: tetanus, hydrophobia, neuralgia, uterine hemorrhage, diarrhea, and various skin conditions be-ing only a few of the conditions for which it has been recommended. The pharmacology of the plant indicates that certain of the cannabinoids or modifications of these compounds should be examined for their antianxie-ty, antidepressant, anticonvulsive, appetite enhancing, and muscle relax-ant potential. Analgesic and antibacterial compounds might be derived. Some of this work is being performed, more should be initiated.

QUESTIONS FREQUENTLY ASKED

Is it addictive? No. Psychological dependence can occur.
Does it lead to crime? Not commonly, although law enforcement agen-cies report a large increase in petty theft, shop-lifting and burglary as a means of providing the user of drugs, including marihuana, with funds necessary to maintain their supply. Rarely will a user lose his controls and result to violence. Since its possession, especially for sale, is a crime, the question is circular.

Does it lead to sexual depravity? No.

Is it a stepping stone to heroin? Only "potheads" (heavy users) seem in- clined to progress to narcotics. About 10% of heavy users in one study tried heroin with some becoming addicted. Experimenters or social users of marihuana do not seem to be predisposed to graduate in heroin.

Does it enhance creativity? No.

Does it lead to psychosis? It may, but the old statistics on this point are surely too high.

Should it be legalized? Until such studies are complete, there is insuffi- cient information to establish that marihuana is not a major health hazard.

RECOMMENDED READING

1. *Cannabis.* Report on the Advisory Committee on Drug De- pendence. Her Majesty's Stationary Office, London, 1968.

2. *Marihuana and Health.* A report to the Congress from the Secre- tary, Health, Education and Welfare. U. S. Government Printing Office, March, 1971.

3. *Interim Report of the Commission of Inquiry into the Non-Medi- cal Use of Drugs.* Queen's Printer, Ottawa, 1970.

3. Marihuana: Some Questions and Answers

HOW MUCH THC IS NEEDED TO PRODUCE INTOXICATION?

A marihuana cigarette contains about 500 mg of plant material. Fairly good marihuana contains about 1 percent delta-9-tetrahydrocannabinol (THC), therefore 5 mg of THC is available to the smoker. Half of the THC is destroyed by burning, 20 percent remains in the "roach," and 10 percent is lost in the sidestream smoke. This leaves about 20 percent or 1 mg of THC in the mainstream smoke inhaled. Of that amount the brain does not receive more than its share by weight, or about 0.015 mg. Within the brain the distribution reveals higher concentrations in the frontal and visual cortex, the cerebellum and the limbic system. THC must be con- sidered a powerful hallucinogen, 10 times weaker than LSD and 400 times stronger than mescaline by weight.

DOES MARIHUANA PRODUCE HANGOVERS?

Headache is the symptom most frequently mentioned following intoxication with marihuana. The classic alcoholic hangover syndrome does not seem to occur.

WHAT ARE THE KNOWN PHYSICAL EFFECTS OF SMOKING MARIHUANA?

Some of the acute and subacute complaints following relatively heavy smoking include rhinitis, pharyngitis, asthma, and bronchitis.(2) Continuing use leads to a chronic bronchitis with some impairment of pulmonary function. Swelling of the uvula has been mentioned.

Acne has been described, but it may reflect careless hygiene rather than a specific effect of cannabis. Diarrhea is noted by some people, and this is drug specific. The sinus tachycardia and "red eye" are routinely found.

WHAT SORTS OF MARIHUANA PREPARATIONS ARE USED IN THE U.S.

The following materials can be identified on the black market:

Marihuana (Pot)
This is the leaves, flowering tops, stems and seeds. It is the most commonly used substance. Manicuring removes the stems and seeds. It is sometimes adulterated with oregano, grass or other inactive, leafy plants. In some specimens phencyclidine (PCP) has been identified to enhance potency. Opium, heroin, and other substances have been allegedly added to street marihuana, but this has not been confirmed. The strength varies from practically no THC in wild, American marihuana to 4 to 5 percent in Nepalese or some Vietnamese material.

Hashish (Hash)
The resin collected from the flowers and upper leaves of high grade cannabis. It contains about 10 percent THC when unadulterated with sugar to increase the weight. It is the material used in Europe and is becoming increasingly popular here.

Superpot (Hash Oil)
Minor entrepreneurs are distilling marihuana to produce a preparation of higher potency. The amount of THC is variable depending upon the solvent and method, but it may be stronger than hashish.

THC

At present the material sold as THC is PCP, LSD, or other available hallucinogens. THC has not been identified in black market material, possibly because of difficulty in manufacture and storage. Some day a synthesis of THC by black market chemists will be accomplished. At that time we can anticipate that the psychological complications that accompany casual LSD taking will be duplicated with THC.

CAN MARIHUANA BE DETECTED?

A commercial method of detecting THC in body fluids is not available at present. A variety of research laboratory methods are used including thin layer chromatography, gas liquid chromatography, and immune assay techniques. The plant material has been identified by the above analytical methods plus the older color tests such as those of Duquenois-Levine and Beam.

DOES MARIHUANA IMPAIR MEMORY?

Only immediate recall appears to be reduced. The lack of capability to concentrate and to rehearse data retards and worsens the laying down of information as memory. This is reflected in marihuana speech which is "blocked," and the forgetting of what was just said or done.

WHAT ABOUT THE EFFECT OF DRIVING SKILLS FROM SMOKING POT?

Current studies indicate a prolongation of braking time in responding to a sudden stop signal while under the influence. In addition, recovery from glare was found to be prolonged under marihuana intoxication. Complex reaction time is impaired. These factors plus the visual and time distortion make driving a hazard.

WHAT IS "CONTACT HIGH"?

"Contact high" is the influence of those "stoned" upon experienced, non-indulging participants. Certain individuals exposed to those intoxicated by marihuana or other psychedelics feel euphoric. This is a reflection of the suggestibility of such persons.

WHAT IS THE EVIDENCE REGARDING BRAIN DAMAGE IN CHRONIC MARIHUANA USERS?

Most reports on this question have been either anecdotal or poorly controlled. A recent report from England using pneumoencephalography states that 8 of 10 young users showed evidence of cerebral atrophy.(1) The subjects were multiple drug users so that it is difficult to know what role marihuana played. No control group was studied. The authors presented the findings as preliminary, and the work is being repeated.

IS THERE A CUMULATIVE EFFECT FROM MARIHUANA?

Because of its lipid solubility, THC accumulates in fat-rich tissues. Its half life is between two and three days. Therefore tissue cumulation occurs. Whether this leads to detectable subjective effects is doubtful.

DOES MARIHUANA CAUSE CHROMOSOMAL STRUCTURE MALFORMATION OR BIRTH DEFECTS?

The *in vitro* animal and human examinations of chromosome morphology indicate that chromosomal anomalies do not occur. When multiple drugs are abused, the number of abnormal cells tend to be increased. Scattered reports of birth defects of children born of marihuana-smoking mothers are available. Whether the number of congenital anomalies exceeds the "normal" incidence (1 in 50 live births) is not known.

DOES MARIHUANA EXHIBIT CROSS TOLERANCE TO OTHER DRUGS?

There is increasing evidence that alcohol potentiates and produces cross tolerance to cannabis. Heavy marihuana users are prone to combine their smoking with drinking sweet wine. The combination of alcohol and THC produces an additive decrement on tests of performance and memory.

DOES TOLERANCE OR REVERSE TOLERANCE TO MARIHUANA DEVELOP?

Tolerance to marihuana preparations has been demonstrated in many species including man. Some effects of THC are diminished during chronic administration of the drug (sedation), but not others (conjunctival injection). The fact that consistent users may require less of the drug over time is apparently explained on the basis of behavioral tolerance. They have learned how to identify the effects more readily. There is some evidence that they can induce the state by responding to the non-specific cues, for example, they may feel "stoned" after smoking a placebo "joint."

HOW MUCH CRAVING TO CONTINUE THE USE OF MARIHUANA IS PRESENT?

Occasional users experience little compulsion to repeat the marihuana experience. Heavy users have a psychological dependency upon the drug and may feel tense or uneasy when it is unavailable, or when abstinence is necessary. Actual physical withdrawal symptoms are non-specific and should not be considered a withdrawal syndrome such as the DTs or the opiate withdrawal syndrome. People have been able to stop using after heavy involvement with only slight difficulty.

WHAT ARE THE LEGAL TRENDS?

The tendency is to reduce penalties for possession of small amounts of marihuana while retaining controls against traffickers and dealers. At present federal and many state laws provide misdemeanor penalties for users or simple possessors. Some states are considering a reduction in penalties so that the consumer will be charged with a minor violation. Legalization of marihuana, if and when it comes, would entail a legal manufacture and distribution system with penalties only for selling to a juvenile, being intoxicated and disorderly, or driving under the influence. In other words, a situation like that regulating alcohol would be one possibility.

The recommendation of the President's Commission on Marihuana to decriminalize private use and possession of small amounts of the drug is apparently a more rational approach than the severe penalties for this offense that now exist in several states. The recommendation is consistent with the new information about its relative harmfulness. This seems to be presented as an interim solution. A more definitive legal posture will be resolved as additional data are gathered regarding the risk-pleasure ratio of the substance.

The Commission's recommendation opens the possibility of legalizing and regulating cannabis use if it turns out to be a low risk item. Meanwhile, if future studies reveal definite evidence of substantial long term adverse effects, the option of excluding cannabis from social usage remains available.

IS POT JUST A FAD?

One argument in favor of keeping cannabis socially unacceptable is that it is just a fad. Marihuana does have certain qualities of a fad: its rapid acceptance by young people, its anti-establishment quality, the fact that drug popularity changes from year to year. Nevertheless, marihuana seems more durable than saddle shoes and hula hoops. It provides many with pleasurable feelings of relaxation, a sense of togetherness, and in large doses, a detachment from frustrating reality. In other cultures it has been accepted by large numbers of people for long periods of time. Although world events may change any prediction, it is likely that marihuana use will be continued by millions of people over the next decade.

WHAT WOULD HAPPEN IF POT WERE LEGALIZED?

A number of future developments are predictable if this country legalizes (regulates) marihuana.

1. The number of those who will try marihuana will increase markedly. Surveys have shown that about 10% of students do not use because of legal concerns. Larger numbers of people over 25 have desisted for similar reasons. These groups and others who have hesitated will at least experiment. On the other hand, a few people who smoke "pot" as a symbolic gesture of defiance might stop using.

2. Increased numbers of users will become daily indulgers. In every survey that showed an increased prevalence, the number of heavy users also increased. At present about a million people smoke pot daily in the United States.

3. The potency of the cannabis used will increase. At present the United States is one of the few Western countries that consume the plant material. The resin is preferred in Europe and most other countries. Hashish is being brought into this country in increasing quantities satisfying the demand for a more reliable, less bulky, stronger product. American soldiers in Europe can buy hashish for $1.00 a gram. Some of them use more than a 100 grams a month, which amounts to about 300 mg of THC daily compared with the estimated 15 mg a day for the heavy user in this country.

4. Children will become involved in marihuana smoking at an early

age. This trend is already discernible. With greater availability children will mimic the behavior of their older brothers and sisters sooner.

5. The consumption of alcoholic beverages will not decrease. Among many cannabis smokers a preference for wine and beer rather than distilled spirits is noted. Except in individual users there is no pattern of abstaining from alcohol.

6. Tobacco smoking will be relatively unaffected. Signs of a shift away from tobacco are not substantial.

7. Increased federal and state revenues would accrue. A rough estimate of a half billion in taxes and licensing fees might result from regulating marihuana.

8. An industry with sale over two billion dollars would be created. Ten thousand acres would be placed into cultivation of cannabis.

NOTES

1. Campbell, A.M.G., Evans, M., Thomson, J.L.G. and Williams, M.G., "Cerebral Atrophy in Young Cannabis Smokers." Lancet 2(7736): 1219-1224 (Dec. 4) 1970.
   "Cannabis Encephalopathy." Lancet 2(7736): 1240-1241 (Dec. 4) 1971.
2. Tennant, F.S., Preble, M., Pendergast, T.J. and Ventry, P., Medical Manifestations Associated with hashish." J.A.M.A. 216:1965-1969 (June 21) 1971.

REFERENCES

1. Spencer, D.J., "Cannabis—Induced Psychosis." Int. J. Addictions 66:141-150, 1971.
2. Marihuana and Health. Second Annual Report to Congress from the Secretary, HEW, 1972, U.S. Gov't. Printing Office, Washington, D.C. 20402.
3. Marihuana: An analysis of use, distribution and control. June, 1971, Bureau of Narcotics and Dangerous Drugs, U.S. Dept. of Justice, Washington, D.C. 29537.
4. Marihuana: A signal of misunderstanding. First report of the Na-

tional Commission on Marihuana and Drug Abuse, 1972, Supt. of Documents, U.S. Gov't. Printing Office; Washington, D.C. 20402.

4. Marihuana Issues

During the past few years, marihuana research has produced a considerable amount of new information. Of the many reports, a number deal with changes that would result in adverse effects in users over a period of time. These reports will be summarized here. The material in this summary is taken from Hearings held during May and June, 1974, by the Senate Subcommittee to Investigate the Administration of the Internal Security Act and other Internal Security Laws (Chairman: Senator Eastland). These Hearings were deliberately arranged to present the negative side of the marihuana story. As the Chairman stated in his summarizing remarks: "Part of the purpose of our recent Hearings was to correct this imbalance (the many reports of marihuana's harmlessness) and to present the "other side" of the story—to establish the fact that a large number of highly reputable scientists today regard marihuana as an exceedingly dangerous drug. We make no apology, therefore, for the one-sided nature of our Hearings —they were deliberately planned that way."

The conclusions mentioned by the Subcommittee will be stated in bold type. In the first paragraph following the conclusion a summary of the evidence will be given. In subsequent paragraphs additional information and opinions will be offered.

THC (THE ACTIVE COMPONENT OF MARIHUANA) ACCUMULATES IN THE BRAIN AND GONADS AND OTHER FATTY TISSUES IN THE SAME MANNER AS DDT

The statement was based on the testimony of Julius Axelrod of the NIH, Nobel Prize laureate for 1970. Dr. Axelrod presented the findings that THC is soluble in lipids and is only slowly excreted. In response to a question he stated that THC did accumulate in fatty tissues as DDT did because they were both lipid soluble.

Any further comparison between DDT and THC is inappropriate. Many necessary substances, for example, Vitamins A and D are also fat soluble. Further, in the tables presented by Dr. Axelrod, the brain shows the lowest concentration of THC of any organ examined.

MARIHUANA, EVEN WHEN USED IN MODERATE AMOUNTS, CAUSES MASSIVE DAMAGE TO THE ENTIRE CELLULAR PROCESS.

It Reduces DNA and RNA Synthesis which Reduces the Mitotic Index (the Rate at which New Cells are Produced).

Nahas testified that chronic marihuana users (defined as having smoked at least one cigarette a week for at least a year) have a diminished immune response as evaluated by their lymphocyte reaction *in vitro* to standard challenges. He ascribed the impairment to decreased DNA synthesis. The reduction of immune response was of the order of that found in patients with cancer. Zimmerman has reported that modest dosages of THC reduces and delays cell division and growth in a protozoan, *Tetrahymena*. These effects are ascribed to a reduction in the cell's ability to synthesize RNA, DNA, and other proteins. Leuchtenberger, using mouse and human lung cultures exposed to marihuana smoke for five days, found marked changes in cell structure, cell division, DNA content, and DNA synthesis.

Although these are test tube studies, they should be seriously considered for they may reflect changes in the body. A UCLA group (Silverstein and Lessin) recently reported no impairment of immune response on skin testing of moderate and heavy cannabis users.

It Results in Chromosomal Changes Including a Reduction in the Numbers of Chromosomes and Chromosomal Deformities.

Morishima stated that of lymphocytes from marihuana smokers 30.6 percent contained only 5 to 30 chromosomes whereas 7 percent of cells from the control group had a reduced number. Stenchever reported that when 49 users of marihuana were compared to 20 controls, the number of cells with chromosome breaks were 3.4 in the users compared with 1.2 cells with breaks per 100 in the control group.

A number of researchers have found no significant differences in chromosomes of users and non-users (Matsuyama, Legator, Dorrance, Gilmore, Rubin, etc.).

MARIHUANA CAUSES IRREVERSIBLE DAMAGE TO THE BRAIN INCLUDING BRAIN ATROPHY WHEN USED CHRONICALLY

Utilizing air encephalography in 10 patients with histories of consistent cannabis smoking over a period of three to 11 years, evidence of brain atrophy was demonstrated by Campbell. The subjects were males, average age 22, who had also used amphetamines and LSD in smaller amounts. Their cerebral ventricles were significantly larger than 13 controls of a similar age group. Heath, using his technique of depth electrodes in monkeys, demonstrated recording changes in the septal region and other areas following marihuana exposure. In one human with implanted electrodes, high amplitude, slow wave activity occurred in the septal region. The surface EEG was normal. When amphetamines, alcohol, and tobacco were used, septal changes did not occur.

Two CAT scan studies on heavy pot users have failed to confirm the presence of a brain atrophy.

ADVERSE EFFECTS UPON THE REPRODUCTIVE PROCESS INCLUDING DANGER OF GENETIC DAMAGE AND EVEN GENETIC MUTATION BY MARIHUANA.

Kolodny has shown that testosterone levels were temporarily reduced by 44 percent in young males who had used marihuana at least four days a week for at least six months. Sperm counts in 6 of 17 were reduced, falling to a level in the heavy smokers that would render them sterile. Kolodny has further observed that a small number of the subjects complained of impotence, which improved on discontinuing marihuana use. Leuchtenberger has some preliminary data that mice exposed to marihuana smoke for three months equivalent to 100 marihuana cigarettes have a disturbance of spermatogenesis. Miras found that female rats exposed to marihuana extract for several months manifested a diminished fertility and growth rate.

It appears that Kolodny's findings are valid. They have been replicated in animals, and, at UCLA, in man. It is the significance of the testosterone reduction from normal to low normal values that remain to be determined. Is this the reason some people seem to lose their drive and motivation after a long period on marihuana? What happens to the sexual differentiation of pubescent boys who smoke regularly?

HEAVY CANNABIS SMOKING CAN PRODUCE SINUSITIS, PHARNYNGITIS, EMPHYSEMA AND OTHER RESPIRATORY DIFFICULTIES IN A YEAR AS OPPOSED TO 10 TO 20 YEARS OF CIGARETTE TOBACCO SMOKING TO PRODUCE COMPARABLE COMPLICATIONS.

Tennant reported on hashish use among soldiers in West Germany where considerable amounts of this strong preparation have been used by some enlisted men. This group had frequent upper respiratory infections, and biopsies of the bronchi showed chronic inflammatory and metaplastic changes in the mucous membranes. Leuchtenberger believes that long term inhalation of marihuana can contribute to the development of lung cancer. This is based on the irregular growth patterns of human and animal cells under the exposure to cannabis, which resemble precancerous lesions. The older Indian literature contains reference to bronchitis, asthma, and other respiratory problems being caused by excessive hashish smoking.

The evidence that cannabis may cause lung cancer is minimal. Nevertheless, as pointed out in an earlier essay, the plant contains coal tars, and the possibility that it can be carcinogenic is present. As to bronchitis and pharyngitis, common experience indicates that heavy users are susceptible.

CHRONIC CANNABIS USE RESULTS IN DETERIORATION OF MENTAL FUNCTIONING, PATHOLOGICAL FORMS OF THINKING RESEMBLING PARANOIA, CHRONIC PASSIVITY, AND LACK OF MOTIVATION (THE SO-CALLED AMOTIVATIONAL SYNDROME).

A number of clinical reports are available that claim that psychological impairment can occur in connection with cannabis use. Only a few of these can be mentioned because of insufficient space. Kolansky has followed 38 young people and states that moderate or heavy marihuana usage produced serious neuropsychiatric sequellae. The impairment ranges from mild ego disturbances to psychosis. He believes that the adolescent is particularly vulnerable because he is in a period of critical psychic and somatic development. The disabilities included: poor social judgment, poor attention span, poor concentration, confusion, anxiety, depression, apathy, indifference, suspiciousness, and a slowed, slurred speech. Since the time of the first report Kolansky has seen hundreds of similar cases, including adults. Powelson has pointed out that the user has no insight into his gradual mental impairment. He believes that sometimes the changes are not reversible after the drug is discontinued. West was among the first to use the term "amotivational syndrome" in describing chronic users. He described the syndrome as follows:

> The experienced clinician observes in many of these individuals personality changes that seem to grow subtly over long periods: diminished drives, lessened ambition, decreased motivation, apathy, shortened attention span, distractibility, poor judgment, impaired communication skills, loss of effectiveness, introversion, magical thinking, derealization and depersonalization, diminished capacity to carry out complex plans and prepare realistically for the future, a peculiar fragmentation in the flow of thought, habit deterioration and progressive loss of insight.

Other recent publications along similar themes have come from Berjerot, Zeidenberg, Malcolm, Schwartz, Hardin Jones, Hall, and Soueif.

The question about the amotivational syndrome is: What is cause and what is effect? Does cannabis produce sedation, apathy, passivity, and reduction of active involvement in living? Or, do amotivated individuals find in cannabis a pharmacological reinforcement of their pattern of existence? Possibly both processes are at work. Many who smoke pot are also achievers. In Jamaica it is used by laborors to get ready for a day's work. They also have ganja breaks just as we have coffee breaks.

The literature on chronic marihuana use leading to psychosis is completely confusing. While it can be said with assurance that a few people, usually neophytes, who smoke potent materials can have an acute psychosis, the incidence and nature of long lasting psychotic reactions is strongly disputed. The older literature from Asian and African investigators tended to assert that cannabis was the reason for large numbers of their psychiatric patients. Most of them appear to have been schizophrenics who also smoked hashish. Cannabis psychosis is rarely diagnosed in this country, and the number of "potheads" requiring psychiatric hospitalization is not great according to mental hospital statistics.

SUMMARY

The transmission of accurate scientific data to the public in an emotionally charged issue like marihuana is very difficult. Some of the data are preliminary and some are contradictory. Nevertheless, the person intent on proving his particular notions can use the scientific literature to confirm his position. He can selectively cite studies, quote out of context, and overinterpret the data.

What attitude should the non-expert in the field adopt? We have gone through a period in the 1930s during which marihuana was accused of inevitably leading to "reefer madness," heroin addiction, and sexual depravity. Such propaganda may have frightened some youngsters away from the "killer weed," but as it became clear that these were gross overstatements and lies, a whole generation came to mistrust the information given them about marihuana and drugs in general. As a reaction against these excessive statements, the folklore of the past dozen years was that pot was harmless. This is as untrue as the opposite view of the early 1900s. The pothead is at real risk. Whether the occasional user is liable to develop some difficulty remains uncertain.

REFERENCES

1. *Marihuana-hashish epidemic and its impact on United States security. Hearings before the Subcommittee to investigate the administration of the internal security act and other internal security laws.* Senate Committee of the Judiciary, 1974, U.S. Gov't. Printing Office, Washington D.C. 20402.
2. *Marihuana and Health. Fourth Report to the U.S. Congress from the Secretary of HEW, 1974*, U.S. Gov't. Printing Office, Washington, D.C. 20402.
3. *Final Report of the Commission of Inquiry into the non-medical use of drugs.* Information Canada, Catalogue No. H21-5370/2, Ottawa, 1973.
4. *Drug Use in America: Problem in Perspective. Second report of the National Commission on Marihuana and Drug Abuse, March, 1973,* U.S. Gov't. Printing Office, Washington, D.C. 20402.

5. The Sex-Pot Controversy

A thousand years ago and longer the effects of marihuana upon sexuality were explored. This was the potion allegedly given to the Hashishim before turning them loose to assassinate (Hashishim—assassin?) the Crusaders and sundry other victims. While under its influence the new members would be transported to a ready-made paradise complete with luscious maidens.

Thereafter, it was easy to have them obey the bidding of the Old Man of the Mountain. A successful mission allegedly was rewarded by a return to the earthly paradise. An unsuccessful one merely meant that the real paradise was at hand.

This folk myth, brought back from the East by Marco Polo, is probably just another Arabian Night's Tale. But it serves to link cannabis with sex fantasies and activities, and it was actually used during the 1930s in this country as further evidence to classify marihuana as a narcotic drug.

One of the main reasons for the public's reluctance to lessen legal penalties for marihuana offenses is the residual belief that it promulgates promiscuity, licentiousness, and loss of controls over sexual acting out. Actually, the relationship between cannabis and sexuality is much more complicated, and some of the interactions are worth reviewing.

Almost every report, anecdotal or scientific, mentions the passivity that accompanies the use of marihuana. In fact, it is the loss of drive and motivation that concerns even more citizens than its potential for dissolving sexual controls. It is odd that the same drug should be accused simultaneously of promoting behavioral passivity and sexual aggressiveness.

The question of pot and sex was first thoughtfully dealt with by the Indian Hemp Drugs Commission in 1894. After years of interviewing and studying data, the commission concluded that cannabis had "no aphrodisiac power whatever." It continued: "As a matter of fact, it is used by ascetics in this country (India) with the ostensible object of destroying sexual appetite."

In our own research with LSD, we encountered a similar phenomenon. Over the years we gave more than a thousand people LSD in a hospital setting. Not one instance of erotic activity was observed, and sexual fantasies were most infrequent. When direct inquiry was made, subjects said their experience was "beyond sex." Meanwhile, LSD was being extolled on the street as a most effective enhancer of sex.

RECENT STUDIES

Kolansky and Moore's report on adverse reactions to marihuana included 13 females who had an "unusual degree of sexual promiscuity, which ranged from sexual relations with several individuals of the opposite sex to relations with individuals of the same sex, individuals of both sexes, and sometimes, individuals of both sexes on the same evening.

"In the histories of all these individuals, we were struck by the loss of sexual inhibition after short periods of marihuana smoking. Seven patients of this group became pregnant (one on several occasions), and four developed venereal disease. In no instance was there sexual promiscuity prior to the beginning of marihuana smoking.

"We take these results to indicate marihuana's effect on loosening the superego controls and altering superego ideals."

Practically every survey published has confirmed that sexual activity correlates directly with the degree and duration of marihuana use. For example, the Brill and Christie data indicate that claims of virginity decrease with continuing marihuana use, as does the mean age of first intercourse. The mean frequency of intercourse increases as use increases.

They also found that heavy users gave "increased sexual pleasure" as the second most common response (83 percent) to question about marihuana effects. Half of the moderate users reported this effect, and it was eighth in their list of effects.

In a survey conducted at the Haight-Ashbury Clinic the great majority of respondents (80 percent) said the enjoyment of sex was enhanced with marihuana. Enhanced sensory awareness, the relaxation of inhibitions, and a greater empathy with others were cited as reasons for the increased enjoyment.

Goode has compiled eight reasons for sexual enhancement from marihuana. These were given to him in his anonymous survey of college students in his class. They include: an increased sense of touch, a feeling of skin warmth, intensification of emotions, feeling of affection for one's partner, subjective prolongation of time, feeling of relaxation, ability to focus only upon the sex act itself, and the greater intensity of orgasm. He hastens to point out that many of these effects are not due to the action of the drug. Rather, they may be a reflection of marihuana's positive evaluation by the counter culture since it is a symbol of disaffiliation, and therefore, it is overvalued.

What seems to happen is that a selective recruitment process takes place. Sexual permissiveness and marihuana use are not necessarily cause and effect, rather both characteristics are indicators of the young person's involvement in a subculture that is tolerant of a wide range of non-traditional values and activities. A high correlation also exists between marihuana use and other attitudes and behaviors. In fact, in Goode's sample, 97 percent of the non-religious, liberal, cigarette-smoking men had tried marihuana, and 62 percent smoked it weekly or more. But only 4 percent of the religious, politically conservative, non-smoking women had ever tried marihuana, and none was a weekly smoker.

Just as we would not say that marihuana use causes the person to become a political liberal, we should not draw hasty cause and effect relations between marihuana and sexual permissiveness. Rather, a powerful selective recruitment process might account for the high clustering of such behaviors. It is a life style that includes sexual hyperactivity, liberal political beliefs, tobacco and marihuana smoking, a certain uniformity of hair styling and wearing apparel, a hang loose ethic, etc.

Marihuana is a drug that heightens suggestibility. If it is believed by large numbers of its users that it is an aphrodisiac, then, by suggestion, it will be. It is a self-fulfilling prophecy—a magnificent placebo effect. If that effect is anticipated, it will happen. Theoretically, then legalization of the drug would cause numbers of marihuana users to lose its sex-enhancing quality.

The National Comission on Marihuana and Drugs conducted an opinion survey that inquired of a sample of youth and adults whether sexual pleasure was enhanced by marihuana. About a quarter believed that it was, half were uncertain, the remainder either did not respond or said it was not.

The commission also reviewed the literature to determine whether sexual behavior on the part of the user would lead to "sexual aggression, profligacy, promiscuity and other aberrant activities." The commission concluded the degree of psychosexual stimulation induced by marihuana depended on the personality of the user and the extent that he came to anticipate such an effect.

Women were more likely to report heightened sexual desire than men, young people more arousal than older users, and the frequent users more interest than infrequent ones. The commission could determine nothing inherent in the drug itself that produced heightened sexual interest, desire or arousal, nor any evidence that marihuana has a specific action on the sex centers in the brain or an effect upon the sexual organs.

As in other studies, the commission concluded that marihuana influences sexual responses by acting on higher brain centers to relax inhibitions and loosen the usual restraints on social behavior. Much of the response is modified by the individual's own expectations and by the set and setting in which marihuana use takes place. They also noted the intensification of sensory input under the drug.

The commission conclusion was that a study of the available evidence lent little support to the belief that marihuana is a significant factor in sexual aggression or in the carrying out of sexual offenses. Although sexual activity may be increased, it does not appreciably alter established patterns of such behavior. The commission found that arrests for sex offenses were rare in the United States, and that marihuana was not a significant contributor to the commission of criminal sexual acts.

Scher has stated that 10 to 20 percent of marihuana users become troubled enough to require psychiatric attention. This, too, may be a self-selection factor since emotionally labile people may seek out a drug like marihuana in an effort to treat their anxiety or depression. He also has observed that his heavy marihuana-using patients tend to lose interest in sex over a period of time. The loss of sexual interest in chronic "potheads" also has been remarked upon in the older Indian literature among hashish-dependent people. One wonders whether it could be a reflection of the lowered male sex hormone levels noted in animals and man during the past year.

ENDOCRINE STUDIES

The recent finding that moderate or heavy marihuana use has definite effects upon sex hormone levels in men now has been confirmed in four studies and not been found to be the case in one. Kolodny reported that the plasma testosterone level of 20 pot users was 44 percent lower than a similar group of non-using males. In addition, a third of them had sperm counts below normal, and in a few cases they were so low that the men could be considered functionally sterile. Two of the 20 reported impotence. In one person who elected to quit smoking potency was regained.

These studies have been continued on your author's group of subjects on the Marihuana Research Suite at UCLA. Since these subjects are hospitalized with research assistants in attendance day and night, it is highly unlikely that they are taking drugs other than marihuana. An acute drop in plasma testosterone levels occurred within an hour after smoking a "joint" containing 19 mg of THC. The decrease continued over the next five hours. It is believed that the finding of a reduction in plasma testosterone is a valid one, but its exact significance remains to be determined.

Kolodny suggests that if a woman is carrying a male fetus, its sexual differentiation may be inhibited by regular marihuana smoking during the first trimester. He also suggests that the pubescent boy who smokes consistently may have problems in the development of his secondary sexual characteristics.

Whether the dozen or so cases of gynecomastia reported in heavy marihuana smokers can be attributed to the hormonal change remains unknown. Testosterone is involved in the development of secondary sexual characteristics (hair growth, voice, baldness, etc.). It has some influence on male and female sex drive, and large quantities are injected for that purpose. Testosterone also has some influence upon non-sexual drive states, perhaps because of its anabolic effect.

Could a reduction in testosterone level over long periods be the biochemical substrate of the amotivational syndrome?

SUMMARY

At our present level of ignorance about sexuality and about cannabis, what rational position can be adopted?

First, we must recognize that even without cannabis, our involvement in sex-related activities may well have been called "promiscuous" by our grandfathers. The general loosening of morality, the erosion of family, church and other authoritarian controls, the Pill, antibiotics, and other recent developments have produced the current casual attitudes. Although we may not perceive it, countercultural beliefs have had their impact upon the dominant culture.

Marihuana has some enhancing effect upon sexual proceedings for some. It may be sexually provocative for some. Nonspecific factors play an important role in this matter. Opposite effects also occur, and an endocrinologic basis for actual diminition of drives and potency may exist.

It may be well to close with a quote from Hollister: "If marihuana is a sexual stimulant, it should be limited to people over 40. It is a great paradox that sexual stimulants are sought by those who have the least need for them."

REFERENCES

1. Koff, W. C. *Marihuana and sexual activity*. J. Sex Research. 10: 194–204 (Aug) 1974.
2. Gay, G. R. and Sheppard, C. W. *Sex in the drug culture. Medical Aspects of Human Sexuality*, pp. 28–50, (Oct) 1972.
3. Goode, E., *Sex and Marihuana*. Sexual Behavior. 2:45–51 (May) 1972.
4. Goode, E. *Drug use and sexual activity on a college campus*. Am. J. Psychiat. 128:92–96 (Apr.) 1972.
5. Kolodny, R. C., et al., *Depression of plasma testosterone levels after chronic intensive marihuana use*. N.E.J. Med. 290:872–874 (Apr. 18) 1974.
6. Marihuana and Sexual behavior. In: *Marihuana: A Signal of Misunderstanding*. First report of the National Commission on Marihuana and Drugs. Appendix, VOL. I, Washington, D.C., U.S. Gov't Printing Office, March, 1972, pp. 434–439.

6. Science, the Press, and Marihuana

Since the scientific revolution began during the eighteenth century, scientists have assumed the role of arbiters and even oracles over the vast territory called scientific—and over the terrain beyond. As health care scientists, doctors generally have made the final pronouncements about health, illness, and related matters. This is probably as it should be. After all, what other group is better qualified to offer opinions about public health?

Unfortunately, despite a flood of medical news in the media, the public is often confused. What people hear are authoritative pronouncements that are contradictory and quite irreconcilable.

"Is there anything that is not cancer-producing?" was the plaintive question posed in a recent letter to a newspaper editor. To read of the conflicting scientific assertions about cholesterol, various reducing diets, certain operations, and many drugs must be puzzling to the lay person who would like to be well informed.

Perhaps a part of the dilemma is a misunderstanding about the nature of the scientific process. When some of the problems of research and its reporting are understood, the controversies may become more comprehensible. Conflicting medical press releases must be understood for what they are: incomplete evidence, sometimes misinterpretation of data, excessive drawing of conclusions, or the biases that scientists—and everyone else—possess.

This essay will deal with some of the problems of scientific reporting and it will use the current marihuana controversy to illustrate them. The harm or harmlessness of marihuana is a heatedly debated item these days. Dozens of court cases have sprung up across the land. And the experts, pro and con, are doing verbal battle with each other before a puzzled judge and sometimes a bemused jury. If science is a precise discipline, why should this be so? Why shouldn't there be one simple truth about questions that can be answered by research?

It is not sufficiently recognized that scientific investigation is not as precise or absolute as we might expect, and scientific reporting in the media is even less so. The following are some of the perennial problems in obtaining data, drawing the proper conclusions, and reporting the conclusions to the public.

THE PROBLEM OF EXTRAPOLATING FROM ANIMAL OR TEST TUBE STUDIES TO HUMAN EFFECTS

That something happens in a test tube or in an animal does not necessarily mean that it has direct applicability to the human situation. At best it should be considered an indicator, and further observations must be made in man.

Often the dose used in obtaining positive results is so out of line with maximum human dose ranges that conclusions beyond the animal species and dose used should never be drawn. On the other hand, in the rat that metabolizes THC very efficiently, very large amounts must be given to achieve any effect at all. An example of the variability of species response to marihuana is reflected in the heart rate. In the dog, marihuana evokes a bradycardia; in people, a tachycardia. So while basic animal or *in vitro* work is necessary and important, its unqualified translation to the human situation is unjustified.

THE PROBLEM OF EXTRAPOLATING INFORMATION OBTAINED FROM ONE CULTURE TO ANOTHER

Although humans resemble each other more than they differ, transposing information gathered in one cultural setting to another can be precarious. Not only may there be certain genetic differences but there also are intervening dietary, economic, and life-style differences that may alter the response as much as the pharmacologic effects of a drug. For example, extrapolating the results of the Jamaican marihuana study without considering that the subjects were rural, unskilled laborers using "ganja" to a completely different setting and set—namely the middle class, urban smoker in the United States who also operates a car and other complex machinery—may not be justified.

THE PROBLEM OF UNCONTROLLED VARIABLES

The spectacle of competent scientists obtaining diametrically opposed findings must be puzzling to the public. After all, the basic tenet of the scientific method is that an experiment can be repeated anywhere with identical results.

The problems arise when exactly the same conditions, the same animal strain, the same dosages in the same concentrations are not used. Ideally, every variable should be controlled, but this is not possible when dealing with living systems, especially humans. Therefore, the results will vary from laboratory to laboratory, or even with the same investigator doing the same study at different times. This does not mean that the scientific method is useless. It means that it must be rigorously practiced and differing results studied to determine why they differ.

In marihuana research contradictory findings have been reported for a series of important issues: plasma testosterone levels, chromosome breaks, immune responsivity, brain atrophy, and others. The divergent results were usually due to uncontrolled variables or differences in the design of the studies.

Marihuana research has a built-in variability that makes its study even more difficult than other drug investigations. It is a mishmash of more than a dozen cannabinoids, about 30 terpenes, assorted sterols, and variable amounts of other compounds. Each sample tends to be different from the others. This variance may account for some of the divergent results.

THE PROBLEM OF RARE COMPLICATIONS

It would be nice to know what sort of adverse affects we might expect from a drug before it is approved and accepted into the culture, including the rare but serious complications. These might only be determined by following large populations of users for long periods of time. One might reflect on the fact that it took more than 200 years to establish a link between tobacco and bronchogenic carcinoma, and that disorder is not a rare event.

The question of the human carcinogenicity of cannabis has not been answered, nor will it be in the foreseeable future. Nor will animal models do more than make a contribution to that answer.

Someone might ask: "How many pot smokers with lung cancer have you seen?" A reasonable answer might be: "As many cigarette smokers with lung cancer as were seen before World War II." If an observer is not alert to such a relationship he might never see it.

THE PROBLEM OF REPORTING PRELIMINARY RESULTS

Another problem arises when a preliminary report is presented at some scientific meeting and it is written up as a definitive study in the press, or it is presented on radio or television as conclusive. Part of the problem lies with the investigator who does not object to the publicity and part is in the nature of the communications system which cannot distinguish between a tentative research report with a few subjects and a final, completed piece of work.

Press releases and news items have been seen by the public asserting that marihuana acts like DDT in the brain, that even in moderate doses it causes massive damage to the entire cellular process, that it causes actual brain atrophy and that cannabis smoke is more carcinogenic than tobacco smoke, etc. From the other side of the aisle we hear: marihuana can cure alcoholism, marihuana is safe, marihuana is not a drug. To be generous, all of these statements are extremely preliminary. Some of them are distortions of the data, and others are expressions of feelings, not fact.

THE PROBLEM OF INTERPRETING RESULTS

Scientists are prone not only to report their results but also to suggest their possible significance. It is rare for a researcher to underestimate the importance of his investigation. The tendency is to go beyond the data in interpreting it. Therefore, the data may be accurate but its meaning is exaggerated or even incorrect.

It is hardly possible to say from some *in vitro* or animal experiment what will happen in man, yet we can read such statements every day. Even human studies cannot be extrapolated to the entire population. They may have had a small number of subjects, the selection of subjects may have been skewed, they may not have been well controlled, and so on.

For example, cellular immunity was found to be greatly impaired in marihuana smokers in an *in vitro* experiment. The loss of immune responsivity was as great as that of cancer patients or patients with kidney transplants on immunosuppressive therapy. Even if the test tube findings were correct, the interpretation that moderate marihuana users have a drastically reduced immunity to cancer and viral or other infections is excessive. At the very least, before such a statement can be made, a controlled epidemiologic study of the health of marihuana smokers versus nonsmokers should have been done to demonstrate that they were actually more susceptible to infections. Even if it is found that they are, their lifestyle and personal hygiene would have to be ruled out as possible factors.

THE PROBLEM OF POOR RESEARCH

Like all other human endeavors, research can be faulty and give rise to erroneous information. This may be due to defects in the design of the study, in its execution, in the way the data are analyzed, or in the manner the project is written up. Poor research is worse than no research because once it enters the scientific literature it takes a series of subsequent investigations to refute the original incorrect conclusions.

The earlier studies of cannabis were impressionistic, rarely controlled, and not rigorously conducted. During the last 10 years a more orderly research effort has developed a solid body of information about marihuana. A number of important questions remain unanswered or only partially answered, but this is true of every sector of scientific scrutiny—of tobacco and alcohol research, for example.

THE PROBLEM OF THE NEWS MEDIA

News is what is new and different, and it is even better news if it is sensational. Deliberate distortions of scientific information by reporters are infrequent these days, but highlighting, overemphasis, or slanting of the facts can distort the data. Even simplifying or abbreviating a research report might result in serious inaccuracies.

Many scientific communications are so technical and complex that they need translation into popular English, but there is still the risk that meanings might be changed in the process. Every investigator has had the embarrassing experience of having a sentence pulled out of context, or a carefully hedged statement printed without any disclaimers whatsoever.

In the emotionally charged area of what to do about marihuana, reporters' or publishers' prejudices may also intervene. We all tend to extract from a body of information those elements that confirm our beliefs. This is true for science writers—and for scientists.

SUMMARY

What Is To Be Done When an Opinion Must Be Formed or a Decision Made on the Basis of Incomplete or Questionably Accurate Information?

The reasonable response would be to make a best guess. The important point is that the opinion should be recognized as a guess and that we should be ready and willing to alter it as we encounter additional information.

What Is To Be Done by the Scientific Community about Incorrect or Inept News Items?

It would be helpful to have consultant scientists in each subspecialty review items within their area of expertise, but this seems like a ponderous and time-consuming solution. It would be preferable if each investigator would take full responsibility for his reports, if possible, including the actual material printed in the press or heard on radio or television.

What Should our Posture Be Toward the Marihuana Issue?

We ought to recognize that the facts are not all in—and may never be. Extreme positions on either side are not justified by the available experimental work or by clinical experience. Decriminalization, such as the California legislation affords, appears justified at our current level or ignorance since the legislation does not seem to increase morbidity and it does decrease the numbers of arrests on criminal charges for possession of small amounts. We have not approved the use of the drug and we have managed to reduce the damage done to the young adult who would have the stigma of an arrest record under the previous legislation.

What Should the Public Attitude Be toward Medical News in the Media?

Health information is said to be among the most widely read or listened to material in the media. A well informed public can prevent many illnesses and so magazine and newspaper articles and radio and television features are valuable to the public health. When new discoveries and breakthroughs are reported, however, they should not be uncritically accepted. It would be well to read the item carefully or wait for further confirmation. When such information has direct relevance to one's own, or one's family's health, then a physician or other health professional should be consulted.

It is not to be expected, however, that physicians will be able to answer all questions on recent research information.

7. Marihuana: A New Ball Game?

In earlier comments on cannabis an attempt was made to present timely research and clinical findings in an evenhanded manner. Naturally, not everyone was pleased with the information.

Some members of NORML (National Organization for the Reform of Marihuana Laws) objected to the recital of possible adverse consequences of consistent use. On the other hand, those who were convinced that cannabis is an evil weed did not appreciate my cautionary comments about drawing final conclusions about marihuana complications from test tube and animal data, accepting unreplicated reports, and maintaining a reserved attitude toward sensationalized news media condemnation of the drug.

A number of reports have come forth recently that have produced an increased concern about the marihuana situation. Some of the reports are not yet general knowledge, and a review of these findings seems appropriate.

WHO SHALL SAY WHEN SCIENTISTS DISAGREE

Because of the nature of the scientific process, we never will have all the facts concerning the safety or toxicity of marihuana. The observation that contradictory reports emanate from well-run laboratories is not surprising to those who understand the subtleties of the scientific method. The multitude of variables when the subjects are humans, makes occasional contradictory results quite probable.

It is now possible to selectively cite the scientific literature and prove that: (1) cannabis is an extremely hazardous material, or (2) that it is completely safe. A preferred alternative to understand the situation would be to carefully evaluate all the data and construct a best estimate of the actual problems involved.

PREVALENCE

The use of marihuana continues to increase each year with the 12 to 25-year-old age group showing the highest prevalence. What is important is that the number of daily users also has increased so that about 10 percent of all high school seniors in one survey smoked at least once a day. In another age group the frequency and prevalence of use also has increased markedly. These are the pre-teenagers, the 8 to 11-year-olds. Daily juvenile marihuana smoking is a vastly different matter than occasional adult indulgence. If some of the physical problems to be discussed are clinically significant, it is the prolonged patterns of heavy use by children that will bring them out.(1)

Even more important than physical problems, youth is a time of learning to deal with life's difficulties. If coping techniques are not acquired, if methods of managing stress are not developed, then a sort of maturation arrest occurs. Thus, long periods of intoxication with marihuana or any other drug produces a psychological deficit that may never be made up. Therefore, heavy involvement with a drug that distances the user from life problems during pre-adolescence and adolescence is very different from a similar situation in an adult who hopefully already has learned to surmount frustrations and ambiguity.

THE STREET SCENE

It is clear that the marihuana business is now one of our largest growth industries. When seizures of 100 tons of high grade marihuana are made from a single shipment, the quantity that reaches the street must be enormous. Furthermore, the quality has improved so that the weak United States grown and the medium grade Mexican varieties have given way to Colombian, Thai, and other high quality merchandise that is two to 10 times stronger than it was only a few years ago. Hash oit, a distillate of cannabis leaves now can be produced with a 10 to 40 percent content of THC. This is in contrast to the 1 percent or less found in street samples in the past.

HORMONAL EFFECTS

The testosterone and leutinizing hormone reduction by cannabis in male humans and animals has been fairly well established, although other studies have not replicated this finding. The divergent results seem to depend upon when the tests are done. It is also unknown just what the significance of a decrease to a low normal plasma testosterone level is. It is speculated that during developmental periods (pregnancy with a male fetus, male adolescence) such decrements may be meaningful. Instances of gynecomastia (enlargement of the male breast), male impotence that improves after stopping cannabis, and diminished sperm counts with abnormal forms are being reported.

In a meeting in Reims, France, during the summer of 1978, reports of the lowering of leutinizing and follicile-stimulating hormones in female monkeys were presented.(2) Absence of ovulation was found in those monkeys receiving THC, but not in the control group. In a group of mice with newborn offspring, lactation was abolished by injected THC. Reports of an embryocidal effect of cannabis on pregnant rats and primates were presented. Equivalent studies in humans are unavailable since research on females has not been permitted by the FDA until recently. It is important to be aware that the animal investigations mentioned employed doses that were deliberately kept within the range used by smokers in this country.

PULMONARY EFFECTS

Chronic bronchitis from heavy cannabis use is an ancient story well described in the scientific literature of India, Egypt, and other lands where cannabis smoking is traditional and widespread. That some young North Americans will smoke similar larger quantities of cannabis was demonstrated by studies of American soldiers stationed in West Germany. They developed inflammatory changes of the upper airway.(3) Bronchial biopsies showed metaplastic changes of the bronchial epithelium. Chronic heavy smoking of marihuana has resulted in changes similar to heavy tobacco smoking and suggests a potential for pulmonary emphysema and fibrosis in both conditions.(4) It is possible that marihuana smoke produces narrowing of the larger airways more than tobacco smoke.(5) Whether this is due to the difference of quality of the coal tars in the two plants, or whether it is a reflection of the difference in marihuana smoking techniques is undetermined. Hoffman, *et al*, suggests that due to its poorer combustibility, marihuana smoke contains about 50 percent more of the carcinogenic hydrocarbons.(6) This group's results from painting marihuana and tobacco tars on mouse skin indicated that both had tumor-promoting properties with tobacco tar producing more tumors. Using marihuana smoke condensates, Cottrell, *et al*, painted mouse skin and obtained metaplasia of the sebaceous glands, a finding that apparently correlates with carcinogenicity.(7)

MIND-BRAIN ISSUES

Acute

The acute affects of cannabis intoxication are well known and little new knowledge is available. The infrequent episodes of anxiety, panic and paranoid reactions require no further elaboration since they also are well known. It is now evident that complex tasks such as driving a car or flying an airplane are done much more poorly under the influence of marihuana. Immediate recall suffers, resulting in halting or blocked speech and difficulty in remembering actions just taken. The impairment of immediate memory appears to be caused by a disturbance in the transfer of information from short-term to long-term memory.(8) These immediate effects are not as much a matter of concern as the longer term, high dose consequences.

Chronic

One subject of debate is the amotivational syndrome: the loss of drive, the increase in passivity, and the sluggish mentation of certain, not all, chronic users. What must be remembered is that large amounts of cannabis have a depressant effect upon the central nervous system, and equivalent amounts of alcohol or sedatives also would produce a decreased desire to work, poor performance, and a blunted emotional response. One difference is that THC is retained in the brain lipid phase for long periods because of its aqueous insolubility.

Some young people do become sedated from considerable cannabis consumption. Others may become amotivated from discouragement about their situation, and marihuana ingestion simply reinforces their dropout from active participation in life. In our study of highly motivated young men and in the Jamaica study, a loss of motivation was not perceptible. Evidently, sufficient drive will overcome marihuana sedation; low drive levels will be overwhelmed by the drug.

The controversy about heavy cannabis use causing brain atrophy has been resolved. In two experiments, much better designed and controlled than the original report, no evidence of cerebral atrophy could be found. What is not so easily reconciled is Heath's work in which implanted electrodes in the limbic system of monkeys demonstrated persisting and specific abnormal EEGs.(9) Postmortem examination of these areas indicated rather serious microscopic neuronal alterations.

OTHER AREAS OF DISCUSSION

If the consequences mentioned of protracted and considerable marihuana use compels us to assume a more guarded attitude toward the weed, the following problem areas remain undecided at present. They should be kept in mind, but held in abeyance until additional and more definitive work is done.

1. The reports of chromosome damage are difficult to evaluate because of the many intervening variables and because universal standards for measuring chromosomal alterations are lacking. Therefore each laboratory has its own standards and intralaboratory comparisons are difficult to make.

2. A few studies of markedly impaired immune responsivity are puzzling to explain. If the results were to be extrapolated to the real life situation, chronic marihuana smokers would be laid low in substantial numbers from infections or cancers.

3. Interference by THC with the synthesis of DNA and other proteins causing impairment in cellular metabolism has been reported by at least three groups. This would have such serious consequences in humans that it does not appear to be compatible with continued survival. It is therefore difficult to reconcile with common observations.

SUMMARY

The combination of the increasing youthfulness of current cannabis users, the greater frequency of use, and the greater potency of the smoked material make for a completely changed situation than existed only a few years ago. Therefore what was said then may no longer apply now.

A new educational effort is needed to bring potential or actual users up to date. Just as the scare campaign of the Anslinger era was not based on evidence, so also the benign reputation of cannabis during the past decade also lacks a factual base. There are real areas of concern, some serious, that health professionals and the public should know about.

Most thoughtful members on all sides of the marihuana controversy would agree with the following statements.

1. Pregnant women should not use the drug.

2. Adolescents should be discouraged from use, especially heavy use.

3. People with heart problems may be further impaired by the heart-accelerating property of cannabis.

4. People with lung disease should not use the drug because of its irritant effects.

5. The infrequent use of marihuana (less than once a week) probably will not result in ill effects except when one of the infrequent acute reactions mentioned happens to occur.

6. Continued work on the therapeutic potential of cannabis should proceed, especially in the control of nausea and vomiting and in open angle glaucoma.

It is in the adult use in considerable quantities that much of the strong differences of opinion reside and will continue to reside. Even if marihuana casualties begin to accumulate as smokers in this country consume more over time, the differences will remain. We have learned that persuasive statistics about morbidity and mortality from recreational drugs do little to change the usage pattern of those with ingrained habits.

CONCLUSION

It appears that cannabis use in this country is evolving in new directions that will increase its morbidity. To prevent the mental and physical consequences, high priority should be given to deterring children from becoming involved and overinvolved. Legalization of the drug is not indicated in view of the recent research findings. Decriminalization of the possession of small amounts remains a tenable position. The harmfulness of making users of marihuana criminals is as serious as their occasional use. The unsatisfactory attempts to arrest and prosecute the large number of marihuana smokers also supports the decriminalization statute.

NOTES

1. Abelson, H. I., Fishburne, P.M. and Cisin, I. *Nationwide survey on drug abuse: 1977*, Vol. I. Superintendent of Documents. U.S. Government Printing Office, Washington, D.C. 20402. Stock No. 017-024-00707-2.
2. International symposium on cannabis. July, 1978. To be published.
3. Tennant, F. S., Preble, M., Pendergast, T. H. and Ventry, P. Medical manifestations associated with hashish. JAMA 216:1965–69, 1971.
4. Henderson, R. L., Tennant, F. S. and Guerney, R. Respiratory manifestations of hashish smoking. Arch: Otolaryngol. 85:248–251, 1972.
5. Tashkin, D. P. Respiratory status of 74 chronic marihuana smokers: Comparison with matched controls. To be published.
6. Hoffman, D., *et al.* On the carcinogenicity of marihuana smoke. In: *Recent Advances in Phytochemistry*, Vol. 9, Ed.: V. C. Runeckles, Plenum, New York, 1975.
7. Cottrell, J. C., *et al.* Toxic effects of marihuana tar on mouse skin. Arch. Environ. Health 26:277, 1973.
8. Melges, F. T., Tinklenberg, J. R., Hollister, L. E. and Gillespie, H. K. Marihuana and temporal disintegration. Science 168:1118–1120, 1970.
9. Heath, R. G. International symposium on cannabis. July, 1978. To be published.

8. Solvent and Aerosol Intoxication

INTRODUCTION

The use of industrial solvents and aerosol sprays to achieve an intoxicated state would seem like an undesirable way to arrive at an alteration of consciousness. Nevertheless, a number of juveniles experiment with or habitually use these substances by sniffing or inhalation. In some urban centers endemic abuse of model airplane glue, paint thinner, gasoline, or some other commercial solvent or propellant is well known.

The volatile substances are generally aromatic or aliphatic hydrocarbons, sometimes chlorinated or fluorinated. They are liquid at room temperature, but evaporate readily. Inhalation provides rapid access to the brain via the lungs, assuring immediate onset of action and relatively short duration of effects.

CLASSIFICATION

The classification of the solvents is difficult because household and commercial products may have unknown formulations, which need not be chemically pure. In addition, they may contain ingredients that are more toxic than the solvent itself. For example, chronic gasoline sniffing has resulted in lead poisoning. The aerosols are used to propel a spray of insecticide, furniture polish or other noxious material. The toxicity of the active ingredient may be much greater than the solvent.

The table provides a listing of the common solvents and some of their commercial uses (see page 42).

The number of household products being packaged in spray cans increases daily. A partial list includes window cleaners, glass chillers, air sanitizers, furniture polishes, insecticides, disinfectants, various medications, deodorants, hair sprays and anti-perspirants.

The volatile solvents are properly classified as anesthetics along with ether and alcohol. Like the latter, they may produce a temporary period of stimulation before depression of the central nervous system occurs.

SYMPTOMS AND SIGNS

The clinical picture is that of a delirium. Mental confusion, psychomotor clumsiness, emotional lability, and impairment of thinking are routinely seen. Early symptoms consist of dizziness, slurred speech, unsteady gait, and drowsiness. Sometimes impulsiveness, excitement, and irritability develop, and injuries can take place during periods of overactivity. As the state deepens illusions, hallucinations, and delusions may be identified. Ordinarily an euphoric, dreamy "high" is described with sleep a frequent end point. The periods of intoxication last from minutes to an hour or two.

Respirations may be depressed, the pupils somewhat dilated, and the heart rate accelerated. Chronic users may have a persistent cough. A glue sniffer's rash around the nose and mouth has been described.

A partial tolerance to these fumes develops with daily use. They are potentiated by other CNS depressants, alcohol being occasionally imbibed

Table I-3: The Major Volatile Solvents

Chemical	Commercial Products
Toluene	Plastic cement Airplane glue Lacquer thinner
Xylene	
Acetone	Fingernail polish remover Model cement
Gasoline	Motor fuel
Benzene	Rubber cement Cleaning fluid Tube repair kits
Naphtha	Lighter fluid
Hexane	Plastic cement
Chlorinated hydrocarbons: Carbon tetrachloride	Spot remover Dry cleaner
Trichlorethylene	Degreaser Dry cleaner Refrigerant
Freons: Trichlormonofluoromethane	Aerosols, refrigerant
Dichlordifluoremethane	Aerosols, refrigerant

for this purpose. A withdrawal syndrome has not been described. Psychological dependence is well known.

THE ABUSERS

Those who abuse the volatile solvents tend to be a more homogenous group than abusers of other drugs. They are underprivileged, young (age range 7-17), with males outnumbering females. Solvent sniffing by adults is quite unusual. It is found almost exclusively among prisoners and employees in factories where the substances are used. Gasoline sniffing is more common in remote rural areas than in cities.

Most youngsters who try these intoxicants will sniff the currently popular solvent once or a few times and then desist. A smaller number will become heavy users, using daily for years. By their late teens solvent sniffing is abandoned. "Maturing out" of the solvent habit is a well established observation. Unfortunately, many chronic sniffers will become chronic alchoholics or barbiturate addicts.

Inquiry into the reasons for using generally elicits comments like "wanting to get away from it all" or "liking the high." Many sniffers appear to suffer with excessive feelings of shyness, insecurity or inferiority, and they may use these intoxicants in an effort at self treatment. Juvenile courts see chronic solvent users frequently. It is not clear whether solvent abuse causes delinquent behavior or is a further manifestation of it. It is not known whether the practice makes these young people more inept at their criminal activities, and therefore more likely to be apprehended.

Almost all reports indicate that solvent abuse is caused by a disorganized existence. The disorganization may originate within the individual; he may be schizophrenic or have a character disorder. His home life may be chaotic with unloving, hostile, or absent parents. The social situation may be demoralizing and hopeless. Another variable of considerable weight is the current substance the peer group is using.

MODE OF USE

The commercial solvents are poured onto a rag, balloon, or plastic bag and sniffed. Even more frequently they are inhaled through the mouth. The aerosol spray may be inhaled directly from the can or first sprayed into some container. Solvent sniffing may be a private or a group activity. As the action of the drug develops, even group "glue" parties are marked by withdrawal and low levels of communication.

COMPLICATIONS

Toluene, naphtha, and acetone are supposed to be less toxic than xylene, benzene, gasoline, trichloroethylene, and carbon tetrachloride. Just how lethal the practice of solvent inhalation is, is not precisely known. The acute hazards are unquestionably real. During 1968 in Japan, 104 persons died of acute solvent poisoning. One investigator had no difficulty finding 110 cases of recent, sudden sniffing deaths in the American literature that was not caused by plastic bag suffocation. The majority of these were due to aerosol abuse.

Many of the hazards associated with solvent abuse are due to impaired judgement and irrational, reckless behavior. These people are accident prone and can also injure those in their vicinity.

A number of reports attest to injury to various organ systems. Brain, liver, kidney, and bone marrow damage to individual users is claimed. When it occurs it probably represents either a hypersensitivity to the solvents or a continuing, heavy exposure to these agents.

Death was earlier thought to be caused by respiratory arrest. Some sudden deaths are now known to be due to a cardiac arrhythmia especially when, concurrently, oxygen intake is impaired or physical exertion occurs. Carbon tetrachloride can produce a hepatorenal syndrome. The aerosols may occlude the airway by freezing the larynx. The aerosols are not considered toxic chemicals, but it is believed that they exert their adverse effects by preventing the transfer of oxygen in the lungs by occluding the alveolar surface. A number of spray-can deaths involve the use of plastic garment bags positioned over the head or by retiring to sealed closets in order to achieve a higher concentration of the volatile material. Another accidental form of death occurs when the sniffer passes out onto the rag or plastic bag containing the solvent and suffocates.

CONTROL

Legislation in many communities and states makes the sale of model airplane cements to juveniles without parental permission a misdemeanor. Other solvents may be included in such statutes.

A major model airplane cement manufacturer has added a small amount of synthetic oil of mustard to his preparation. This is apparently insufficient to produce nausea under normal usage, but is unpleasant when the contents are used for sniffing. Another producer claims to have developed an airplane glue that is non-intoxicating when inhaled. Although these are encouraging developments, the variety and availability of the inhalants in every kitchen, laundry, and bathroom make other measures necessary. These include the generation of internal controls in a child so that the use of dangerous substances is excluded as one of the options for problem-solving purposes.

TREATMENT

The management of the acutely intoxicated sniffer requires no special procedures. He should be observed and prevented from hurting himself. Bedrest is indicated, and he should be quieted by reassurance rather than drugs or physical restraints. If carbon tetrachloride was used, urinary output should be monitored. There are no specific tests for the detection of these substances, but their odor generally is detectable for a few hours.

The treatment of the solvent-dependent youngster is difficult, and relapse is frequent despite knowlege of the physical dangers and the possibility of punitive action. The child, the family, the school, and the "gang" may have to be dealt with if any definitive gains are to be made. The patient's self image must be changed from that of a "loser" and a "loner" to that of a person who is respected and loved. Every effort should be made to reduce the youngster's demoralization. As confidence and self-respect increase, his ability to cope with the problems of everyday life begins to improve.

REFERENCES

1. Bass, M. Cardiac toxicity of aerosol propellants. J.A.M.A. 215: 1501, 1971.
2. Bass, M. Sudden sniffing death. J.A.M.A. 212: 2075, 1970.
3. Chapel, J.L. and Thomas, G. Aerosol inhalation for kicks. Missouri Med. 67: 378, 1970.
4. Crooke, S.T. Solvent inhalation. Tex. Med. 68: 67, 1972.
5. Flowers, N.C. et al. Nonanoxic aerosol arrhythmias, J.A.M.A. 219: 33, 1972.
6. Law, W.R. and Nelson, E.R. Gasoline sniffing in an adult. Report of a case with the unusual complication of lead encephalopathy. J.A.M.A. 204: 1002, 1968.
7. O'Brien, E.T., Yoman, W.B. and Hobly, J.A.E. Hepatorenal damage from toluene in a "glue sniffer". Brit. Med. J. 5725: 29, 1971.
8. Press, E. and Done, A.K. Physiologic effects and community control measures for intoxication from intentional inhalation of organic solvents. I. Pediatrics, 39: 451, 1967.
9. Press, E. and Done, A.K. Physiologic effects and community control measures for intoxication from the intentional inhalation of organic solvents. II. Pediatrics 39: 611, 1967.
10. Rubin, T. Glue sniffing: A rehabilitation approach. In: Resource Book for Drug Abuse Information, National Clearinghouse for Mental Health Information, Rockville, Md., 1969.
11. Taylor, G.J. and Harris, W.S. Cardiac toxicity of aerosol propellants. J.A.M.A. 214: 81, 1970.

9. Inhalant Abuse

The deliberate use of industrial solvents for purposes of intoxication is a rather surprising leisure time activity of the past quarter century. The practice points up the willingness of some individuals to accept the dangers of exposing themselves to chemicals of unknown or incompletely known toxicity in order to achieve periodic inebriation.

The problem of toxicity is quite unlike that encountered in industrial plants. In industry the exposure is in low concentrations over a long period. As employed by juveniles the impact is brief, intermittent, but of an extremely high concentration of the hydrocarbons—hundreds of times the permitted maximum limits.

THE ATTRACTIVENESS OF SOLVENTS

Adolescents may prefer inhalants for reasons not completely obvious to adults. The following are some reasons given by adolescent solvent users.

They Are the Most Readily Available "High" Producers

Aerosols and cans of paint, gasoline, lacquer thinner, etc., are found in homes, schools, garages, and in a variety of stores. In poor households a stockpile of alcohol may not exist but almost every home has one or more solvents.

They Are Inexpensive or, Alternatively, Easy to Steal

Solvents have been called the "poor man's pot" by some users. They may perfer marihuana but the inhalants are more cost effective. For less than a dollar a pint, varnish remover will provide dozens of intoxications.

They Are Legal

Although some communities have laws about selling model airplane glue to unaccompanied minors, anyone can buy a can of spray paint. Airplane cement is not used very much at the present time. The aerosols and paint solvents are preferred.

The Packaging Is Compact

A tube or jar of plastic cement, lighter fluid, spot remover, or fingernail polish fits into a pocket and can intoxicate as readily as a quart of whiskey.

They Work Quickly

A few deep inhalations bring on the "stoned" state. Drugs that are absorbed by the lungs reach the brain in seconds, almost as rapidly as the intravenous route.

They Don't Last Too Long
Depending on the dose, the inebriation is over in minutes, or one can sniff all day long and stay stoned.

The Hangover Is Not as Bad as Alcohol
Headache seems to be the most common post-intoxication complaint.

TECHNIQUE OF USAGE

In addition to the usual procedure of inhaling the fumes from a cloth or plastic bag, some other techniques have been described.(1) One is to place a soaked rag into the mouth and inhale. This is a particularly hazardous technique because even after the user becomes unconscious, he still continues to inhale the vapor and may overdose.

A second method that has been observed is to take the cap off a gasoline tank and inhale the fumes directly. Most gasoline contains lead, and cases of encephalopathy and neuropathy have been recorded. A third method is to spray the aerosol directly into the nose and mouth. In addition to the dangers inherent in the contents, the possibility of freezing the oral and pharyngeal tissues arises.

THE PROBLEM OF MIXTURES

Industrial solvents are never pure chemicals. At times, the trace amounts they contain may be more dangerous to health than the primary component. Also, the commercial products—whether they be paint thinners, liquid cements, or other items—are combinations of substances whose formulations are rarely found on the label. Furthermore, the formulation is changed from time to time so that what may have been relatively non-toxic last year can be poisonous this year. The mixtures have another hazard. A chemical may become lethal in the presence of a second substance although neither one alone is deadly.

THE JUNIOR "HIT" PARADE

A survey of San Francisco school children was taken by Linder.(2) In response to a query about use of drugs during the past year, elementary school children indicated that solvents were second only to alcohol and ahead of six other drug groups. Among the junior high school students solvents dropped to sixth place. Senior high school and college students used them seventh in frequency—ahead of heroin which ranked last. This report emphasizes the youthfulness of solvent abusers and the fact that with the passage of time, they tend to move on to other drugs, particularly sedatives and alcohol.

"HUFFERS" NEUROPATHY

Peripheral neuritis due to triorthocresyl phosphate, leaded gasoline, acrylamide, methylbutylketone, and hexane have been recorded in the past. Prockop and his associates at Tampa General Hospital reported a strange story recently that illustrates some of the problems in the diagnosis of solvent abuse pathology.(3)

Seven young men in the Tampa area had been "huffing" (inhaling) a popular lacquer thinner. After the oil embargo, and because of a subsequent increase in prices, the formulation was changed because some items had become too expensive. Soon after, the seven developed severe weakness and numbness in the extremities that ascended centrally. They sought help in a number of Tampa hospitals where a variety of diagnoses were made. Eventually, the common use of the solvent was discovered. One person died after two weeks of artificial respiration. Two have bulbar paralysis and require respirator care. Four are in wheelchairs with muscle wasting, motor loss, and some sensory impairment.

The company was notified and they quickly changed the formula. People who "huff" the new material do not seem to become afflicted with the peripheral neuropathy. The offending agent may be methylamylketone, which was not in the original formula or in the present one, but was included in the suspected formula. This is uncertain because 10 other chemicals were also present.

GOLD AND BRONZE SPRAY PAINT INHALATION

During the past few years an increasing misuse of metallic paint aerosols has been identified, beginning in the southwestern United States and now spreading to other areas.

Gold and bronze paints are preferred. They are sprayed onto a rag or a plastic bag and deeply inhaled orally. These aerosols contain metallic copper and zinc with other heavy metals present as impurities. In a small number of cases studied in Fresno, California, by Wilde, high levels of copper were found in the urine.(4) This may indicate systemic copper absorption from the lungs along with the solvent. If so, prolonged exposure to copper containing sprays might lead to hepatolenticular degeneration (Wilson's disease). If any of the paints contain appreciable amounts of cadmium, this metal is also very toxic.

SOLVENTS AND VIOLENCE

Vargas emphasizes the violent behavior of some huffers.(1) In the past it was believed that since the period of intoxication was brief, and the state often terminated in sleep, violent behavior was uncommon. Early in the intoxication, however, impulsive and aggressive behavior is quite possible. He quotes Done who says: "Among the various forms of abuse, inhalant use is the most likely to cause violent, antisocial behavior during intoxication."

The solvents belong to the same pharmacologic class as alcohol, a substance well known for its ability to unleash destructive behavior.(5) Why these anesthetics are producers of aggression is complicated, but there also is a simple answer. These drugs extinguish control over behavior before they extinguish control over motor activity. Thus the intoxicated person has lost his inhibitions about acting out while he still remains capable of acting.

DEATHS ASSOCIATED WITH SOLVENT ABUSE

More than 100 deaths a year in this country are estimated to result from intentional inhalation of volatile hydrocarbons. The mechanisms vary. The major causes are as follows.

Death Due to Chronic Damage to a Vital Organ

The chlorinated hydrocarbons (carbon tetrachloride), the five and six carbon ketones (methylbutylketone), and certain aromatic compounds (benzol) are cytotoxic. Death can occur from liver, kidney, bone marrow or other organ failure.

Acute Sniffing Death

Venticular fibrillation can be induced by central respiratory depression. The combination of physical exertion, low blood oxygen levels due to depression of the breathing center and certain solvents predisposes to an abnormal heart rhythm. Other acute deaths appear to be pulmonary with congestion and edema found at autopsy. Any solvent, including large amounts of toluene and gasoline, can cause paralysis of the breathing center.

Asphyxiation

The practice of inhaling a solvent in a closed space or with one's head in a plastic bag can cause death by oxygen deprivation.

Accidental Death

Poor judgment and impulsive behavior while intoxicated have resulted in fatal falls and other accidents.

COMMENTS

Although solvent toxicity is more serious than many other drugs of abuse, little has been done to study in depth the nature and extent of the problem. Since the very youngest age group is involved it seems imperative to know whether the growing human organism is particularly susceptible to the cerebral, neuromuscular, hematopoetic, and hepatorenal impairment that has occasionally been reported.

The National Institute on Drug Abuse has at last manifested an interest in the intentional inhalation of solvents and recently held a workshop on inhalant abuse. A small number of contracts and grants have been let in this area. Animal models that will reproduce the human abuse situation are being developed. Individual solvents and combinations will be tested for toxicity. From the information acquired, strategies for finding preventive and rehabilitation programs can be developed.

Solvent sniffing is a low status avocation. No one, except the sniffers, has a good word for it. Perhaps the experimental use of a volatile substance can be understood as the exploratory behavior of adolescents who are willing to try anything once. But their chronic use, solventism, is difficult to justify in people who have any respect whatsoever for their bodies and minds.

NOTES

1. Vargas, P. *The hidden dangers of aerosols.* Unpublished manuscript, The Drug Abuse Council, Washington, D.C.
2. Linder, R. L., *et al. Solvent sniffing: A continuing problem among youth.* Proc. West. Pharmacol. Soc. 18:371, 1975.
3. Prockop, L., *et al., "Huffers neuropathy."* JAMA 229:1083, 1974.
4. Wilde, C., *Aerosol metallic paints: Deliberate inhalation. A study of inhalation and/or ingestion of copper and zinc particles.* Int. J. Addictions. 10:127, 1975.
5. Cohen, S. *The volatile solvents.* Pub. Health Rev. 2:185, 1973.

10. Amyl Nitrite Rediscovered

An upsurge of amyl nitrite sniffing during the past few years has been amply documented in the news media but not in scientific journals. A review of this volatile solvent is therefore indicated from both a medical and a sociologic standpoint.

PHARMACOLOGY

Amyl nitrite (more properly isoamyl nitrite or insopentyl nitrite) is a yellowish, volatile, inflammable liquid with a fruity odor. It is unstable and decomposes in the presence of air and light. The chemical was introduced into medicine over a century ago when it was found to relieve angina pectoris by dilating coronary arteries and temporarily improving the perfusion and oxygenation of heart muscle. The severe chest pain of coronary insufficiency following exertion could be relieved within 30 seconds and its effects would last five minutes or more. It accomplished the relief of coronary spasm by relaxing smooth muscles in the arterial walls.

Amyl nitrite was marketed under the trade names of Vaporole and Aspirole in fragile glass pearls containing 0.3 ml of the substance, the glass being covered with a woven absorbent material. The pearls could be safely crushed in the hand and the liquid inhaled. Currently, other vasodilators —sublingual nitroglycerin, for example—are preferred and amyl nitrite is less frequently used for angina pectoris.

Smooth muscle fibres in other parts of the body are relaxed by amyl nitrite as well. Of importance to this discussion is the dilation of the meningeal arteries over the surface of the brain. These arteries expand and produce feelings of suffusion and fullness in the head. At the same time oxygen supplied to deep areas of the brain may be diminished because these arteries contain few muscle fibres and do not dilate as much as arteries in other organs. Because of the vasodilation, the return of blood to the heart is reduced, lowering the blood pressure and further reducing perfusion of the cerebral arteries. This would explain the occasional complaints of giddiness, dizziness, and faintness, with occasional syncope.

The subjective experience of time is slowed down. It is this slowing of the perception of time that started a modest amount of non-medical use of the drug that extends back to the 1930s and continues with increasing frequency. Just prior to climax a pearl would be crushed and inhaled, extending the sensation of orgasm. The effects were alleged to be satisfactory. In addition to the cerebral vasodilatory effects, some direct mental changes have been described. Mild sensory intensification, a diminution of ego controls, and some increase in aggressiveness have been mentioned.

These "snappers" or "poppers," so called from the sound made when they were broken, also have other actions. The smooth muscles in the bronchial tree and the bile duct dilate. It is hardly ever used to provide relief from asthma or spasm of the common bile duct, probably because its effects are too transient. The smooth muscles in arteries and other organs also dilated but not as markedly as the coronaries, the meningeal vessels, the bronchi, and the bilary system. Until better treatments came along, amyl nitrite was used in the treatment of cyanide and hydrogen sulfide poisoning and as a diagnostic tool in the identification of cardiac septal defects.

When the nitrites, including the volatile nitrites, are used, frequently tolerance will develop within two or three weeks. Larger doses will then be required to achieve the initial effects. The mechanism of tolerance acquisition in unknown. Withdrawal symptoms have not yet been described. Cessation of the administration of nitrites will reestablish the original level of sensitivity in a few days.

Interestingly, the tolerance to nitrites was first discovered in munitions factories where the new workers would suffer from headaches upon exposure to nitroglycerin. These nitrite headaches would subside within a few weeks, however, after their vacation and would reoccur upon resumption of work. Some workers lost their tolerance during a weekend away from the job and had the "Monday disease" on reporting back. Many of them learned to maintain their tolerance while on weekends or vacations by rubbing a little nitroglycerin on their skin.

CURRENT STATUS

Recently, amyl nitrite has become more and more popular as an orgasm expander. This has been particularly true among male homosexuals, but heterosexual men and women also indulge. Occasional reports of increased sexual aggressiveness have been received. Since the pearls of amyl nitrite were usually prescription items and therefore somewhat difficult to obtain, new products appeared and were sold through adult bookshop outlets.

These included such exotic trade names as Locker Room, Rush, Jac Aroma, Aroma of Men, Kick, Bullet, and Toilet Water. They were alleged to be used as room odorizers. The Food and Drug Administration is studying the problem, but it has not yet taken any action on it.

The Consumer Products Safety Commission will soon file a brief against the various manufacturers stating that they have mislabeled their product. The porno shops sell small bottles of either amyl or isobutyl nitrite at an excellent profit. Isobutyl nitrite is presumed to act similarly to the amyl analogue but its pharmacology remains essentially uninvestigated.

A more recent development has been the sniffing of the aliphatic nitrites for whatever intrinsic mental effects they have rather than as modifiers of the sexual response. Increasing numbers of people are inhaling them throughout the day. Since the effects last only a minute or two, they may be sniffed a dozen or more times an hour.

It would be nice to know exactly which psychic effects are so attractive and desirable. Is it the mild disinhibitory action, the feeling of fullness in the head, or perhaps, the giddiness and light headedness mentioned earlier? It certainly is no profound alteration of consciousness, rather it is more like the effect noted by children who spin around until dizzy. The increased interest in the volatile nitrites is reminiscent of the methaqualone fad of a few years ago when this very ordinary sedative was touted as "heroin for lovers."

It is strange that among the people who are prescribed amyl nitrite for heart pain, pleasurable effects are never described. Instead, they complain of the odor, the pounding headache, or the feeling of fullness in the eyes. The pulsing headache is a typical nitrite headache due to stretching of the meninges by the distended arteries. An instance of psychological dependence on amyl nitrite by cardiac patients could not be found in the literature. Many years ago I knew of one patient who compulsively inhaled amyl nitrite, but this practice was secondary to his apprehension and ruminations about the recurrent anginal attacks. It was not a search for kicks.

If is of interest that a Haight-Ashbury Clinic patient group, when asked about their drug-taking practices in connection with sex, gave amyl nitrite low ratings in comparison with a number of other drugs. Marihuana, hallucinogens, amphetamines, cocaine, and even opiates were ranked higher.

TOXICOLOGY

Only limited toxicological data are available. Amyl nitrite is rapidly absorbed through the lungs. Gastric secretions decompose it, and it is ineffective when swallowed. Animals given increasing doses become ataxic, vomit, and develop convulsions that can terminate in death. A small number of dogs was subjected to repeated inhalations of amyl nitrite at 20 to 90 second intervals for up to seven minutes. Gagging, involuntary urination and defecation, and twitching muscular movements were noted.

In humans complaints of nausea, dizziness, and weakness have been described. These symptoms are due to the drop in blood pressure and increase in heart rate. Fainting, especially from the erect position, can occur. The combined use of alcohol and amyl nitrite apparently can produce syncope. The pulsating headache is frequently mentioned by heart patients and by recreational inhalers. A deep flush over the head and neck is another complaint.

Nitrites are known to cause methemoglobinemia. If the volatile nitrites are inhaled in substantial amounts consistently, it is possible that the conversion of hemoglobin to methemoglobin will take place. In a patient with a history of chronic abuse, the possibility of methemoglobinemia should be kept in mind.

The use of amyl nitrite could be dangerous in people with cerebral hemorrhage, recent head injury, hypotension, or glaucoma. Those with heart disease other than coronary spasm will not be benefited and may be harmed by the hypotension and tachycardia.

SUMMARY

The rationale of using amyl nitrite to prolong the sensation of orgasm may be based on some psychophysiologic mechanism. Its use to induce a desirable altered state of consciousness is more difficult to understand.

We know so little of its side effects, particularly in the manner it is currently being used, that it is difficult to say whether it is accompanied by harmful sequellae. The all–day–long inhalation of amyl nitrite is another example of people doing to themselves what research pharmacologists would not be permitted to do under carefully supervised conditions by a university committee established to safeguard human rights.

The preoccupation of certain groups of people with isoamyl and isobutyl nitrite as a means of changing their consciousness is a reflection of their willingness to use chemicals for this purpose without appreciable safety data. The long-term effects of all–day sniffing are completely unknown. They will remain unknown for many years because the studies to determine any adverse consequences have not even begun.

ADDITIONAL READING

1. Bruckner, J. V. and Peterson, R. G. Review of the aliphatic and aromatic hydrocarbons. In: *Review of Inhalants: From Euphoria to Dysfunction*. Eds.: C. W. Sharp and M. L. Brehm, NIDA Research Monograph, Rockville, Maryland 20857, 1978.
2. Everett, G. Effects of amyl nitrite ("poppers") as an aphrodisiac. In: *Sexual Behavior. Pharmacology and Biochemistry*. Eds.: M. Sandler and G. Gessa, Raven, New York, 1975.

3. Gay, G. et al. Drug-sex practice in Haight-Ashbury, or the sensuous hippie. In: *Sexual Behavior: Pharmacology and Biochemistry,* Eds.: M. Sandler and G. Gessa, Raven, New York, 1975.
4. Hollister, L. Drugs and sexual behavior in man. Life Sciences 17:661, 1975.
5. Dewey, W. L. et al. Some behavioral and toxicological effects of amyl nitrite. Res. Comm. Chem. Path. Pharm. 5:889, 1973.
6. Knoepfler, P. Pleasure enhancing sex devices. Med. Aspects Human Sexual. 11:17, 1977.
7. Louria, D. Sexual use of amyl nitrite. Med. Aspects Human Sexual. 4:89, 1970.
8. Pearlman, J. and Adams, G. Amyl nitrite inhalation fad. JAMA 212:160, 1970.

11. Household Hallucinogens

Substances that produce hallucinations and delusions are commonly thought of as exotic, out-of-the-way, tropical mushrooms, vines or cacti. Alternatively, they are imagined as the esoteric brew of some odd psychedelic chemist. In fact, a fair number of common items found in the home can disrupt mental functioning. Both accidental or intentional intoxications have occurred from household products. A review of these substances may be worthwhile if only to understand some delirious reactions whose cause is obscure until a detailed history of exogenous substance intake is taken.

IN THE KITCHEN CABINET

Nutmeg

Nutmeg is the dried seed of *Myristica fragrans*, which appears on the kitchen shelf as a coarsely ground powder or as the whole seed. When taken in sufficient quantities a confusional state with variable autonomic symptoms can develop. Prisoners have been known to steal or buy nutmeg when better hallucinogens were unavailable to them. Some college students have shown a recent increased interest in nutmeg swallowing or sniffing. The amount ingested in any number of eggnogs is insufficient to contribute to the effects of this concoction. During the past century a few deaths were recorded in women who took very large amounts of nutmeg in an effort to abort.

Mace

Mace is the orange colored, dried, lacy covering of the shell of the nutmeg. Both mace and nutmeg contain myristicin, a terpene, which is supposed to be the hallucinogenic agent. Ground or whole mace is also found in the kitchen, but it is less commonly used in cooking than nutmeg. An occasional student mace party has been described, but its misuse is very infrequent.

IN THE GARAGE, LAUNDRY, ETC.

The volatile substances are a heterogenous group of commercial solvents, aerosols, and anesthetics. They have in common that they are all inhaled, and their ability to produce an intoxicated state marked by confusion, slurred speech, incoordination, delirium, stupor, or coma.

Commercial Solvents

Many items found in or around a home contain toluene, benzene, xylene, hexane, naphtha, acetone, carbon tetrachloride, or trichlorethylene. Such common products as model airplane glue, varnish removers, lacquer and paint thinners, moth preventatives, furniture and clothing cleaning fluids, nail polish remover, and cigarette lighter fluid may have one or more of the above intoxicating substances. The liquid is ordinarily poured on a rag or into a plastic bag, and the fumes are inhaled. The drunken state lasts about a half hour.

Airplane glue was the most commonly abused substance. Gasoline is usually sniffed in remote, rural areas where other intoxicants are difficult to find. Small epidemics of paint thinner misuse have been reported. It is believed that the inhalation of volatile solvents is not increasing, rather it may be actually decreasing.

Aerosols

These are substances (e.g., furniture polishes, deodorants, insecticides, window cleaners, etc.) in a spray can. The propellant is usually a Freon, a fluorinated or chlorinated hydrocarbon. Freons intoxicate by obstructing the transfer of oxygen into the blood stream, thus producing cerebral anoxia.

Instances of death due to laryngospasm secondary to refrigeration of the larynx and by cardiac arrest have been described. The poisonous qualities of the basic substance contained in the spray is another factor in understanding the toxicity of this group.

Anesthetics

Nitrous oxide (laughing gas) is available in certain industrial operations, for example, as a tracer gas to detect pipe leaks and to reduce pre-ignition in racing cars. It may be found in homes as a whipped cream propellant. Nitrous oxide inhaling is occasionally encountered. Ether may occasionally find its way into the home as an adhesive tape remover or spot eradicator. Ether had considerable popularity over a century ago as an euphoriant by sniffing or drinking. Although not considered an anesthetic, 30 percent carbon dioxide gas produces transient states of unconsciousness, which are relished by a few people. The compressed gas is used in a number of commercial activities.

IN THE MEDICINE CHEST

In addition to the numerous prescription items that can be abused, the following are some mind altering substances that are encountered in the family medicine cabinet.

Cough Syrups

Cough syrups usually contain codeine, dextromethorphan, or some similar cough suppressant. Codeine has a low addiction potential, but it has been used by young people for its narcotic effects. It is also employed by addicts when they are unable to obtain heroin. It will partially suppress the heroin withdrawal symptoms. Dextromethorphan is still less addicting, but it, too, has been abused by a few people.

The cough syrups are exempt narcotics. They can be purchased without a prescription, and large amounts are consumed by habitual users. The alcohol content also contributes to the intoxicating effect of these preparations.

Nasal Inhalers and Sprays

Nasal inhalers originally contained benzedrine, but the contents were sometimes removed and swallowed for the stimulating effect. Currently, they are formulated with propylhexadrine, desoxyephedrine, or similar compounds that have the vasodilator effect of the amphetamines without the stimulant action. The consumption of nasal inhaler material is not a problem at this time. Nasal decongestant sprays ordinarily contain ephedrine or a related chemical. When used in large amounts, ephedrine is capable of inducing amphetamine-like effects.

Antihistamines

Certain antihistamines have a sedative quality, which is intoxicating in large amounts. Patent medicines that are sold for insomnia or as cold remedies contain antihistamines. Occasionally, prolonged release cold capsules are opened by youngsters and the colored pellets sorted out so that full doses of the contained antihistamine or the ephedrine-like material can be consumed.

Anticholinergic Drugs

Compounds containing belladonna or strammonium occasionally appear in the medicine cabinets of people who have ulcers or asthma. Scopolamine in over-the-counter sleeping medicines also belongs to the group of anticholinergic drugs. Accidental or purposeful overdosage results in a toxic-confusional psychosis. The patent medicine Asthmador, which could be purchased without a prescription, is now under more stringent control in most states. Until recently Asthmador "trips" were taken by adventurous experimenters.

FROM THE GARDEN

A half dozen seed varieties of the American morning glory (*Ipomoea purpurea*) if sufficiently chewed or ground, provide a drowsy, LSD-like experience. Underdoses and overdoses occur because of the variability of the alkaloid content. Morning glory seeds are attractive to those who prefer "natural" or "organic" substances to laboratory psychedelics.

The seeds of the baby Hawaiian wood rose contain a lysergic acid derivative (as do certain morning glory seeds). The experience tends to be more unpleasant than the LSD state, with nausea and vomiting troublesome for certain people.

The inside of the banana peel and the Scotch broom plant are placebos. Rumors to the contrary are incorrect.

ALCOHOL-CONTAINING HOUSEHOLD ITEMS

Alcoholic beverages are so ubiquitous that the search for alcoholic household preparations seems redundant. However, in some homes alcohol is forbidden, and substitutes may be sought out. In jail kitchens the inmates seek something that can inebriate, or they brew their own beverages from starch or sugar plus yeast. Aside from the cooking wines, the favorite potions apt to be used for purposes of intoxication are vanilla, almond, and similar extracts (35 percent alcohol). Eau de colognes and shaving lotions have a high ethanol content and have been swallowed when nothing more potable was available. Even Listerine (25 percent alcohol) has been imbibed by a few who could not tolerate temporary abstinence. During the Prohibition years poisonous items such as Sterno, rubbing alcohol, and Fluidextract of Jamaica Ginger were consumed by thirsty, desperate drinkers.

Another reason for being aware of the alcoholic content of substances not ordinarily considered to contain ethanol is the occasional person on

Antabuse who may be very sensitive to alcohol-Antabuse effects. One such person complained that the liberal application of his shaving lotion regularly resulted in nausea. The possibility that a conditioned reflex might explain the nausea was not excluded.

This array of home based intoxicants is presented to make a point. It demonstrates that cutting off supplies of one dangerous drug does not accomplish much more than shifting the seriously drug-dependent person to some other. We shall never be able to abolish all mind altering substances from our environment. Some are more harmful than others, and they require the wisest controls that can be devised. The analogy with disease producing microorganisms is obvious. We survive in the presence of pathogenic bacteria because we have developed an immunity to them, or because we have devised effective preventative measures to control them. With drugs of abuse a similar personal and social resistance to their use will be the definitive solution. It is obviously a long term project and has implications far beyond the area of drug abuse.

SELECTED REFERENCES

General
1. Gershon, S. and Angrist, B. Drug induced psychoses I. Hospital Practise. 35 (June) 1967.
2. Gershon, S. and Angrist, B. Drug induced psychoses II. Hospital Practise. 50 (July) 1967.

Nitrous Oxide
3. Brilliant, L. Nitrous oxide as a psychedelic drug. New Eng. J. Med. 283:1522, 1970.
4. Dillon, J.B. Nitrous oxide inhalation as a fad. Calif. Med. 106:444 (June) 1967.
5. Brown, R. Nitrous oxide theft control. Can. Anesthetics Soc. J. 17:661, 1970.

Morning Glory Seeds
6. Isbell, H. and Gorodetzky, C.W. Effect of alkaloids of ololuqui in man. Psychopharmacologia 8:331, 1966.
7. Cohen, S. Suicide following morning glory seed ingestion. Am. J. Psychiat. 120:1024, 1964.

Nutmeg
8. Myristica fragrans (Nutmeg) In "Ethnopharmacologic search for psychoactive drugs." Public Health Service Publication No. 1645,

Supt. of Documents, U.S. Govt. Printing Office, Washington, D.C. 20402, 1967.

Volatile Solvents

9. Kupperstein, L.R. and Susman, R.M. A bibliography on the inhalation of glue fumes and other toxic vapors. Int. J. Addictions 3:177, 1968.
10. Samples, V. L. Sniffing at McNeil Island. Am. J. Correction 30:11, 1968.
11. Preble, E. and Laury, G.V. Plastic cement: The ten cent hallucinogen. Int. J. Addictions. 2:271, 1967.
12. Press, E. and Done, A.K. Solvent sniffing. Pediatrics 39:611, 1967, and Pediatrics 39:451, 1967.
13. Durden, D.W. and Chipman, D.W. Gasoline sniffing complicated by acute carbon monoxide poisoning. Arch. Int. Med. 119:371, 1967.
14. Law, W.R. and Nelson, E.R. Gasoline sniffing by an adult. JAMA 204:1002, 1968.
15. Ackerly, W.C. and Gibson, G. Lighter fluid sniffing. Am. J. Psychiatry 120:1056, 1964.
16. Massengale, O.N. et al. Physical and psychological factors in glue sniffing. New Eng. J. Med. 269:1340, 1963.
17. Malcolm, A. On solvent sniffing. Addiction Research, Foundation of Ontario, 1969.
18. Musclow, C.E. and Owen, C.F. Glue sniffing: Report of a fatal case. Can. Med. Assn. J. 104:315, 1971.

12. Angel Dust: The Pervasive Psychedelic

Table I-4: Angel Dust

Generic Name:	Phenycyclidine
Trade Name:	Sernylan (Parke-Davis)
Chemical Name:	1-(1-phenycyclohexyl) piperidine
	CHI
Street Names:	Angel Dust, PCP (from chemical name or PeaCePill), Hog, LBJ, and some 20 other names. In addition, most material alleged to be THC, psilocybin, and mescaline is PCP. Some LSD and cocaine samples contain PCP.

BACKGROUND

Phencylidine was investigated during the 1950s as an anesthetic agent. Although it was found to be effective for analgesia and anesthesia, certain side effects, especially postoperative agitation and delirium lasting for hours, precluded its final acceptance.

Later, it was found to be a satisfactory anesthetic agent for certain animals, and it was marketed for that purpose until recently. A chemically related compound, ketamine, (Ketalar, Parke-Davis) is employed as a human anesthetic. Small quantities of ketamine and TCP, the thiophene analogue of PCP, have been found in analyses of illicit drug supplies.

Angel dust appears in multiple forms: as a crystalline powder, as tablets and capsules in a variety of colors, shapes and sizes. It is readily manufactured by kitchen chemists from available precursors. The procedure is not complicated and supplies are plentiful. This explains why it is the common substitute for less available psychedelics like mescaline. An occasional batch of PCP contains 1-piperidinocyclohexane-carbonitrile, a by-product of the synthetic process. Epidemics of abdominal cramps, bloody vomiting, diarrhea, and coma have been attributed to this contaminant.

PHARMACOLOGIC EFFECTS

Angel dust can be inhaled, smoked when sprinkled on parsley or marihuana, swallowed, or injected. Evidence of tolerance development or of a withdrawal syndrome is incomplete. Sympathomimetic effects such as tachycardia, hypertension, and increased deep reflexes are prominent. In addition, cholinergic activity, sweating, flushing, drooling, and pupillary constriction can be observed. Cerebellar signs include dizziness, ataxia, dysarthria, and nystagmus.

The rather remarkable psychological effects have been attributed to a defect in the integration of incoming sensory stimuli. They have been compared to prolonged sensory deprivation. An inability to process sensory information would give rise to secondary deficits including a loss of reality testing ability, dissolution of ego boundaries, and intellectual and emotional disorganization.

With large doses, coma occurs and major convulsions are a possibility. Causes of death may be from status epilepticus, cardiac or respiratory arrest, or a hypertensive crisis from rupture of a cerebral blood vessel. One author has reported 19 phencyclidine-related deaths.

CLINICAL PROBLEMS: ACUTE EFFECTS

A number of clinical problems arise in connection with PCP intake. These never have been adequately classified. The following is an attempt to organize the various conditions that have been seen.

Disinhibition
Low doses of phencyclidine (1-5 mg) may consist of the usual releasing effects of many psychoactive drugs upon cerebral functions. A floaty euphoria is described, sometimes associated with a feeling of numbness. Speech remains relatively intact. In fact, some people will take small amounts in order to make conversation more intense and meaningful. Behavior may be looser than when sober. Emotional lability is regularly seen. Ordinarily, problems do not arise during this phase.

Toxic psychosis
An excited, confused intoxication can develop with increasing doses (5-15 mg). Body distortions may be noted, possibly on the basis of impaired proprioceptive messages arriving from the body surface. Pain and touch perception is much reduced. Communication is definitely impaired. At times the person can hardly speak because of his internal turmoil. Psychological tests either cannot be performed or low scores are obtained. Disorientation for time, place, and even person may be elicited. The individual either moves about restlessly or is quiet and withdrawn.

Schizopheniform Psychosis
A number of clinical pictures can emerge after moderate or higher doses (10 mg and more) that resemble various acute schizophrenic syn-

dromes—and they can last for day or months. Sometimes they mimic the functional psychotic reactions so closely that the diagnosis of schizophrenia is made on admission to a hospital. The resemblance to schizophrenia is also of interest to those studying that disorder. Phencyclidine is considered a possible model of certain schizophrenic reactions. Furthermore, when the drug is given to chronic schizophrenic patients it reactivates their psychosis.

Stuporous catatonia. Mutism, grimacing, repetitive movements of the extremities or body, posturing, even waxy flexibility have been described in some who have adverse reactions to phencyclidine. The apparent mechanism for functional catatonic stupor and for the phencyclidine psychosis may be a similar difficulty with the integration of external and internal sensation resulting in accelerated and chaotic mental activity. The only way to cope is to "clam up" and withdraw completely.

Excited catatonia. Psychomotor agitation, incoherent, profuse speech and unpredictable destructiveness may be another cluster of behaviors following phencyclidine usage. The internal mental events are so disturbing and without meaning that certain people will respond by aimless running, by bizarre actions, and by striking bystanders. Catatonic excitement can be dangerous, not only because of the aggressive activity against one's self and others but because exhaustion can develop over a short period of time.

Paranoid schizophrenia. Some post-phencyclidine psychoses mimic paranoid states. Auditory hallucinations, ideas of reference with suspicious or grandiose content, and feelings of unreality and strangeness are experienced. Depersonalization may be so complete that "Me" cannot be separated from "Not-Me." In other instances impairment of ego functioning precludes the ability to differentiate between reality and fantasy.

Coma

Doses of as much as 1000 mg of PCP are said to have been taken, resulting in prolonged comatose states or death. Far lesser amounts can induce a complete unresponsiveness to painful stimuli and a decerebrate rigidity or opistotonus. If recovery occurs, amnesia for the entire episode will be evident. Marked slowing of the EEG is seen on tracings.

Other States

A variety of other conditions has been reported. Anxiety and panic can understandably result from the loss of ability to sort out sensory experience. Depressions with suicidal ideation have occurred. Some users have mentioned living through "sheer nothingness" for many hours. Others have spoken of an "endless isolation" apparently referring to the intense sensory blockade.

CLINICAL PROBLEMS: CHRONIC EFFECTS

After many exposures to PCP some of the acute states may become chronic. Recurrent psychotic reactions have been seen in people who decompensated, yet were unwilling to stop using the drug. Chronic depressive, anxiety, and confusional states also can be identified. In addition to these, two chronic conditions require further mention.

Organic Brain Dysfunction

Instances have been encountered in which taking PCP repetitively appears to result in a chronic impairment of mental functioning, apparently on an organic basis. During sober intervals the person demonstrates memory gaps, some disorientation, perhaps visual disturbances, and, commonly, difficulty with speech. The latter may be a blocking or an inability to retrieve the proper words. The condition may improve with time if phencyclidine exposure does not recur.

Behavioral Toxicity

Even in the interval between PCP trips, impulses controls might be loosened. This may be manifested by outbursts in school or at home, tantrums, easily aroused assaultiveness, and uncontrolled belligerence. Unusual car accidents or criminal acts may occur. A second type of behavioral deviancy is an extreme withdrawal from all people and activities.

DIAGNOSIS

Phencyclidine can be detected in urine qualitatively and quantitatively by commercial or hospital laboratories. High dose intake is associated with a leukocytosis and an elevated CPK. The presence of hypertension and tachycardia along with some of the aforementioned psychiatric disturbances is suspicious of phencyclidine ingestion. Similar symptoms, however, may also occur with amphetamines and cocaine poisoning. Normally, the history of PCP intake will be readily provided by the patient or accompanying person. However, they may speak of THC or provide a slang name for PCP that is locally popular.

TREATMENT

Because of the unusual clinical pictures it might be well to withhold drug therapy if the patient is not hyperactive. A quiet, non-stimulating environment may be all that is needed. Diazepam, 10 mg intramuscularly, and repeated, will help control muscle spasms and restlessness. Vital signs require frequent recording in case cardiorespiratory intervention becomes necessary. Dilantin may be considered as a prophylactic against convulsions. Antihypertensive therapy is rarely required.

The containment of overactivity and aggressiveness is a serious problem. The major tranquilizers have had variable success in containing behavioral dyscontrol due to PCP. There is some indication that these drugs potentiate PCP. Therefore, they should be used cautiously during the acute phase. They should be provided for treatment of prolonged psychotic reactions. Control of hyperactivity with paraldehyde or parenteral barbiturates can be considered.

COMMENT

It is clear that the list of adverse effects from PCP makes it the hallucinogen of prime medical concern at this time. It should be recognized that the untoward reactions listed do not occur every time PCP is used. Physicians who see only the undesirable side effects may question why anyone would deliberately consume such an agent.

There are two levels of response to such a question. First, most PCP trips must be pleasant and rewarding with only occasional "bummers" interspersed—and they never require medical attention. Second, the very symptoms we are describing in pejorative psychiatric terminology may be experienced as desirable by some kinds of people. For example, a few individuals experiencing the depersonalization and derealization produced by PCP might come back from the trip relating that they "dissolved into the Eternal" or that the strangeness of their experience was a "New Reality." So the negative aspects of the PCP state could be relished by those seeking out-of-the-body states.

ADDITIONAL READING

1. Bakker, C.B., et al. *Observations on the psychotomimetic effects of Sernyl.* Comprehensive Psychiatry 2:269, 1961.
2. Kessler, G.E., et al. *Phencyclidine and fatal status epilepticus.* New Eng. J. Med. 291:979, 1974.
3. Liden, C.B., et al. *Phencyclidine. Nine cases of poisoning.* J.A.M.A. 234:513, 1975.
4. Luby, E.D., et al. *Study of a new schizophrenomimetic drug—sernyl.* Arch. Neurol. Psychiat. 81:363, 1959.

5. Rainey, J.M., et al. *Prevalence of phencyclidine in street drug preparations.* New Eng. J. Med. 290:466, 1974.
6. Tong, T.G., et al. *Phencyclidine poisoning.* J.A.M.A. 234:512, 1975.

13. PCP (Angel Dust): New Trends in Treatment

PCP (Phencyclidine, Angel Dust) continues to be a widely abused and a troublesome drug. The previous essay described the many and varied clinical states that can be seen when PCP produces adverse reactions. This essay will continue to analyze the situation.

The National Institute on Drug Abuse recently held a two-day conference on phencyclidine. Major investigators of the drug were brought together for presentations and informal discussion. Highlights of that meeting constitute the bulk of this report.

The first problem that arose was one of classification. PCP is so diverse in its actions that it does not easily fit into one of the established pharmacologic groups. It can have depressant, stimulant, analgesic, hallucinogenic, anesthetic, and convulsant activity. Those who approach its study from an anesthesiologist's point of view consider it a dissociative anesthetic like its related compound, Ketalar. This means that a cataleptic state is induced in which pain is not perceived, the individual's eyes are open, but he is unconscious and amnesic for the experience. On the other hand those who have had considerable experience with the psychotomimetic state think of the drug as an hallucinogen that is unique because of the accompanying neurological symptoms, and because of the intense loss of self (depersonalization).

Another noteworthy aspect of PCP is the behavioral dyscontrol that can produce a variety of bizarre activities or violence which, in turn, result in encounters with the police, lawsuits, unusual accidents, strange suicides, and impulsive homicides. This might be attributed to the intense depersonalization, and the inability to understand and evaluate one's situation because at high doses judgment and self-observation are wiped out.

During the 1960s PCP was a universal adulterant provided when mescaline, psilocybin, THC or strong marihuana were requested. Now it is a drug preferred by many. It also is commonly used as a component of a polydrug abuse pattern, and this complicates the clinical picture. Daily PCP use is known, and tolerance develops under such conditions, but a specific withdrawal syndrome has not been described.

THE LOW DOSE PCP EXPERIENCE

The experience is dose-related, with factors such as set, setting, and personality playing a modifying role. At low doses a pleasant floaty euphoria is described, but a few people find even small amounts scary and unhappy. Some of the reports are reminiscent of LSD descriptions: synesthesias, slowing of time, feelings of power, loss of appetite, wakefulness, illusions, and pseudo-hallucinations. Flashbacks apparently occur even more frequently with PCP than with LSD. The amnesia may explain why, even after horrendous experiences, the person may continue to use PCP.

OVERDOSE

Overdose with PCP is manifested by a prolonged eyes-open coma. A sequence of convulsions may occur. Spasm of the larynx and a decerebrate rigidity are occasionally reported. The pupils are small and multidirectional nystagmus is often present. Blood pressure, heart rate, and respirations are increased. Infrequently, a cerebral hemorrhage can result from the blowout of a blood vessel in the brain due to the acute hypertension. The comatose state may alternate with periods of extreme hyperactivity.

TOXIC PSYCHOSIS

If the patient recovers from the overdose a period of agitated delirium can emerge. This is marked by paranoid delusions, hallucinatory experiences, drooling and sweating, grimacing, disorientation, and restlessness. If the dose of PCP was insufficient to induce coma, then the toxic delirium may be the presenting clinical picture. It may last up to a week.

SCHIZOPHRENIFORM PSYCHOSIS

After a single exposure, but more often after many PCP experiences, a schizophrenia-like picture may emerge. Many of those who became psychotic had no prior history of mental illness, and yet they presented a severe, treatment-resistant psychotic reaction that lasted for weeks despite intensive treatment. Others were schizophrenics in remission who were exacerbated into an acute, florid reactivation of their psychosis by phencyclidine.

Such people may show autistic thinking, withdrawn or aggressive behavior, blocking of speech, unpredictability and paranoid delusions, often of self-aggrandizement. These individuals are often admitted to psychiatric hospitals with a diagnosis of acute paranoid or catatonic schizophrenia. They are seen so frequently at present that acute schizophrenics should have a routine urine test for phencyclidine and amphetamines.

It is reported that even after the psychosis improves, certain symptoms may linger. A flattened affect, impaired memory, and a residual paranoid thought disorder may continue for a year or more. Spontaneous relapses have been reported and repeated, PCP-induced psychoses after the first episode are common.

POST-PCP DEPRESSION

Some investigators have noted that after the psychotic state recedes, a substantial depression may intervene. It may last from days to months and usually is amenable to conventional antidepressant therapy. During the period of acute depression suicide precautions may be required.

TREATMENT

The treatment of overdose is based on the principle of ion trapping. Since phencyclidine is a weak base, it is readily excreted in acid fluids. Ammonium chloride in a one or two percent solution can be administered intravenously, or it can be given into a nasogastric tube. When the urine is brought down to a pH of 5.0 to 5.5, a diuretic like furosemide might be given, and a strong diuresis of PCP can be expected.

Another method of removing large quantities of PCP is continuous gastric suction for two to four days. Phencyclidine is excreted into the stomach because of the gastric acidity, and considerable amounts of PCP can be removed in this manner. Ascorbic acid also has been used intravenously for acidification. Naturally, good electrolyte control is needed during the period of acidification and gastric suction.

Tracheal intubation and suction should be attempted only in comatose patients. Hyperstat has been used when the hypertension reaches dangerous levels. Intravenous diazepam or diphenylhydantoin can be used prophylactically to avoid convulsions.

Management of the acute toxic reaction includes sedatives such as diazepam, a quiet environment, and seclusion if necessary.

Treatment of the schizophreniform state is similar to that of any acute functional psychosis. By this time the PCP has been eliminated and the danger of potentiating some of its effects with antipsychotic drugs need not be considered. Any of the antipsychotic drugs can be used—sometimes heroic doses are required.

Management of the violent behavior requires some comment. In a medical situation intravenous diazepam or intramuscular paraldehyde can be considered. When the aggressive behavior is part of an early toxic delirium, bystanders and law enforcement people should be particularly circumspect in their handling of the intoxicated person.

If PCP is suspected as the cause of the odd and unusual behavior, then a non-threatening, reassuring attitude should be adopted. It may be possible to avoid overt violence by achieving a calm relationship with the individual. When physical restraints are necessary, sufficient assistance should be available to apply them. The strength of a PCP-intoxicated person can be impressive, if not incredible.

PREVENTION

Workers in the drug abuse field are quite concerned about the number of untoward PCP complications they are seeing. Some legislatures are considering laws increasing the penalties for manufacture or sale of the drug. School officials and the media have presented material about the dangers that can occur. Large PCP "busts" are regularly announced in the newspapers. In one survey most of the PCP users either had a "bad trip" or knew someone who had reacted adversely to the drug. Nevertheless, supplies are plentiful and not expensive, and there is little indication that usage is diminishing.

The enigma of prevention is especially pertinent to PCP. The real dangers of the drug do not seem to deter more than a few. Indeed, they seem to attract certain individuals. Aside from reducing availability, what can be done to deter people from using or continuing to use this substance?

SUMMARY

As mentioned in the previous essay, it must be remembered that most experiences must be pleasant and devoid of the catastrophic reactions mentioned. What remains to be explained in why, after some frightening or terrifying PCP experience, some people will return to its use. The possibility that they were amnesic for the horrifying period has been mentioned. It might be that they live in hope that the fearful experience will not recur the next time. In some instances they may not even have been aware that PCP caused their trouble. A final possibility is that their self-concept is so miserable that any change in awareness, even an unpleasant one, is considered preferable to their sober condition.

ADDITIONAL READING

1. Aranow, R. and Done, A. *Phencyclidine Overdose: An Emergency Concept of Management*. J. Am. Coll. Emerg. Physicians. 7:56–59, 1978.
2. Bolter, A. *et al. Outpatient Clinical Experience in a Community Drug Abuse Program With Phencyclidine Abuse*. Clin. Toxocol. 9: 593–600, 1976.
3. Cohen, S. *Angel Dust*. JAMA 237:515–516, 1977.
4. Luisada, P. and Brown, B.I. *Clinical Management of the Phencyclidine Psychosis*. Clin. Toxicol. 9:539–545, 1976.
5. Showalter, C.V. and Thornton, W.E. *Clinical Pharmacology of Phencyclidine Toxicity*. Am. M. Psychiat. 134:1234–1238, 1977.
6. Smith, R.J. *Congress Considers Bill to Control Angel Dust*. Science 200:1463–1466, 1978.

14. The Witches' Brews

Since antiquity four plants and related members of the nightshade family have accounted for numerous instances of accidental or deliberate poisoning.

They are belladonna (*Atropa belladonna*, deadly nightshade), strammonium (*Datura strammonium*, Jimson weed, thorn apple), henbane *(Hyocyamus niger)* and Angel's Trumpet *(Datura sauveolens)*.

These toxic herbs were components of the witches' brews of ancient times, the concoctions to be imbibed in preparation for the witches' sabbath. Many of the alleged events that transpired during those arcane rites, such as witches flying on broomsticks, were actually drug-induced hallucinatory experiences. These drugs were also to be found in the recipes of the professional poisoners of the Middle Ages—the Borgia's Saturday Night Specials, for example.

Belladonna derives its name from the practice of some medieval women who enhanced their beauty by dilating their pupils with a drop of a decoction of the leaves. The derivation of Angel's Trumpet is obvious, but it also describes the white, lily-shaped blossoms. Jimson weed, or more properly Jamestown weed, is so named because a troop of English soldiers sent down in 1676 to Jamestown, Virginia, to put down Bacon's rebellion, found some young plants and ate them as greens.

"They turned into natural Fools for several days. One would blow up a Feather, another would dart Straws at it, another, stark naked, sat in a Corner grinning and making Mows, another would fondly kiss and paw his Companions. In this frantik Condition they were confined lest they in their Folly should destroy themselves. They would have wallowed in their own Excrements if they had not been prevented." After eleven days they recovered, not remembering anything that had occurred.

Poisoning from these plants has continued to the present day. In particular, in the United States strammonium has caused problems because it is so widespread. It has a penchant for growing in vacant lots and garbage dumps. The Indians called it the "white man's plant" because of its affinity for their settlements.

Outbreaks of Jimson weed poisoning often affect adolescents whose curiosity leads them to sample the seeds or leaves. Other miniepidemics have been attributed to wheat contaminated by the seeds. Other sources of intoxication have been from the patent medicine Asthmador, which contains 52 percent of strammonium and 4.5 percent of belladonna leaves. Asthmador gained a modicum of popularity during the sixties when venturesome teenagers deliberately ingested larger than recommended amounts and developed the picture of an acute brain syndrome resembling atropine delirium.

Antiparkinsonian drugs in excessive doses can produce a similar picture. The anticholinergic drugs are not in favor at present because of the rather unpleasant aspects of the "trip." Some of the over-the-counter sleeping medications contain scopolamine (hyocine), and instances of intentional and accidental overdose of these medicines are recorded. Of 41 proprietary hypnotics and tranquilizers, 58 percent contained belladonna alkaloids, usually scopolamine hydrobromide. Some of the scopolamine-containing patent medicines include Compoz, Neurosine, Quietabs, Quiet World, Sleep-Eze, and Sominex. In addition, an antihistamine like methapyrilene is included in the formulation.

PHARMACOLOGY

The four plants mentioned contain related alkaloids: atropine, scopolamine, and hyocyamine—all of them powerful inhibitors of acetylcholine. They are the original anticholinergic or antispasmodic drugs used to dilate pupils before eye examinations, reduce salivation before surgery, relax the bronchial muscles in asthmatics, and reduce gastric secretions and peristalsis in those with gastritis or peptic ulcerations.

Scopolamine is about eight times more potent than atropine. The pharmacological action of these alkaloids, however, is approximately similar. Perhaps scopolamine is more sedative and has more central effects than atropine, while the latter has a longer duration of action than the former.

A partial tolerance develops to atropine and scopolamine. Nausea, vomiting, sweating, and salivation have been described on sudden withdrawal of large amounts. Psychological or physical dependence is rarely a problem. Fatalities are infrequent, except in children, despite the critical appearance of some patients. Accidental death seems to be more frequent than death due to poisoning. In one review five of 212 cases died from drowning or falling.

DIAGNOSIS

The clinical picture of poisoning by the alkaloids of the nightshade family is striking. The skin is hot, dry, and red, sometimes a bright scarlet. The pupils are maximally dilated and do not react to light or accommodation. Vision is, therefore, blurred. The tongue, mouth and lips are dry and coated. Complaints of thirst are frequent. Usually the pulse is rapid, and the blood pressure and temperature are elevated.

The mental symptoms tend to fall into one of two patterns. The patient may be in a wild delirium, disoriented, loudly hallucinating, restless and irritable, or he may be in a muttering delirium, confused, stuporous, incoordinated, and quite unable to concentrate or respond appropriately. These two patterns may be dose related, or they may represent phasic differences in the drugs' effects. Medical students have described these classical presenting symptoms in their usual alliterative way: "hot as a hare, blind as bat, dry as a bone, red as a beet, and mad as a wet hen."

The quality of the mental changes are reminiscent of other deliria due to toxic substances, high fevers, or brain injuries. The delusional content is "homely," as a rule ordinary events are involved. A truck driver may imagine that he is driving his vehicle cross country. He will engage in conversations with friends and strangers along the route. Such pedestrian delusional productions are in contrast to the esoteric fantasies induced by the hallucinogenic groups of drugs.

If the diagnosis of atropine-type poisoning remains unclear, a test dose of 0.1 mg of physostigmine salicylate (Antilirium) injected subcutaneously may help. If salivation, sweating, and intestinal hyperactivity do not occur within 20 minutes, then the diagnosis is confirmed. In bygone days a drop of the patient's urine was placed in a cat's eye. Dilation of the pupil indicated atropine-type intoxication. Today, thin layer chromatography is equally revealing and more elegant.

Since the drugs containing scopolamine or atropine are taken to provide

Table I-5: Differences between Atropine and LSD Intoxication

	Atropine-Type	LSD-Type
Skin	Hot, dry, red	Flushed, moist
Mouth, tongue, lips	Dry, coated	Slight dryness
Thirst	Present	Absent
Pupils	Widely dilated, fixed	Dilated, reactive
Heart rate	Increased	Slight increase
Blood pressure	Elevated	Elevated
Temperature	Elevated	Elevated
Urinary retention	Present	Absent
Constipation	Present	Absent
Sleep	Drowsiness	Insomnia
Reflexes	Hyperactive	Hyperactive
Coma	At high doses	Does not occur
Mental confusion	Present	Absent
Periods of lucidity	May be present	Occurs
Illusions	Present	Present
Visual hallucinations	May be present	Usually pseudo-hallucinations
Auditory hallucinations	May be present	Rare
Time distortions	Disoriented for time	Apparent slowing of time
Paranoid thinking	May be present	May be present
Speech	Slurred	Blocked
Synesthesias	Absent	Present
Transcendental experience	Not described	May be present
Recall of experience	Amnesia	Good recall
Response to physostigmine	Effective	Not effective
Response to phenothiazines	Worsening	Improvement

a "psychedelic" experience, the differential diagnosis between atropine-type and LSD-type intoxications are provided in the Table.

TREATMENT

The specific antagonist for anticholinergic drug overdose is physostigmine, the cholinergic drug of choice. A slowly administered intravenous of 2 mg of physostigmine should reverse the symptoms described under

"Diagnosis." Diazepam is used for quieting the patient and treating or preventing convulsions. Phenothiazines are contraindicated because of their anticholinergic effects.

Gastic lavage or induced vomiting should be seriously considered when confronted with strammonium or related drug poisoning. The anticholinergic action of these agents can completely immobilize the gastrointestinal tract so that plant material will remain there for longer than expected. Emesis has been induced as long as 36 hours after ingestion of Jimson weed seeds, and found in the vomitus. This paralysis of peristalsis may explain in part, the prolonged duration of the symptoms.

Cooling measures, oxygen, and a nonstimulating environment are recommended. Catheterization may be needed for the urinary retention, and enemas for the loss of bowel tone. Physostigmine (eserine) eye drops can be used if the pupilary dilation persists longer than the other anticholinergic symptoms.

SUMMARY

For those who seek to alter or obliterate their sober consciousness, the plants that contain scopolamine and atropine offer a not too pleasant way. The recovery of those who come upon these deliriants and consume too much accidentally can be hastened by the cholinergic drugs and proper medical care. Although their past has been fascinating, it will, hopefully, fade away.

REFERENCES

1. Dean, E. S. Self-induced strammonium intoxication, JAMA, 168: 882 (Sept 14) 1963.
2. Hughes, J. D. and Clark, J. A. Strammonium poisoning, JAMA, 112:2500 (June 12) 1939.
3. DiGiacomo, J. N. Toxic effect of strammonium simulating LSD Trip, JAMA 204:173 (Apr 15) 1968.
4. DeYoung, G. and Cross, E. G. Strammonium psychedelia, Can. Anaes. Soc. J. 16:429, 1969.
5. Gowdy, J. M. Strammonium intoxication. JAMA 221:585 (Aug 7) 1972.
6. Hall, R. C. W., et al. Angel's Trumpet Psychosis: A central nervous system anticholinergic syndrome, Am. J. Psychiat. 134:312, 1977.
7. Goldsmith, S. R., et al. Poisoning from ingestion of a strammonium-belladonna mixture. JAMA, 204, 169 (Apr 8) 1968.

8. Greenblatt, D. J. and Shader, R. I. Nonprescription psychotropic drugs. In: *Psychopharmacology in the Practise of Medicine.* Ed. M. E. Jarvik, Appleton, Century Crofts, New York, 1977.

15. Cocaine

BACKGROUND

Cocaine use in this country has been increasing steadily. The cocaine story begins 3000 years ago according to the Incan records found in what is now Peru and Bolivia. One tale, which lacks confirmation, is that the pre-Columbian trephining operations done on the skull were performed with the local anesthetic properties of spittle from chewed coca leaves. Coca leaves (*Erythroxylon coca*) were given by royalty as a highly valued reward for special services. It was a drug of the ruling classes. The Conquistadores later discovered that coca gave the Indians the stamina to work the tin and silver mines and provided it as part of their pay. The chewing of the leaves with some lime added has become a way of life for the present-day, poverty-stricken Indians living in the Andean highlands. For them the "cocada" is the only available answer to the scarcity of food, the back-breaking work in the mines, and the cold, thin air of the two mile high atmosphere. To them a "cocada" means not only a cud of coca leaves, but also a measure of time—approximately 40 minutes—the length of time the chewed leaves are effective. A cocada also is a measure of distance, approximately two or three kilometers. That is the distance that can be covered while chewing a cocada under mountainous conditions. Thus it is used for its anti-fatigue, anti-hunger, and anti-pain properties. Little or no "high" is reported under such conditions. The chewing of coca leaves in the two mile high altitude is so different from "snorting" cocaine at sea level in an urban setting that it might seem as though two different drugs were involved.

One report claims that 90 percent of the adult males and 20 percent of the adult females in the northern Andes are coca chewers. Nine million kilograms of coca leaves are consumed yearly in Peru alone. The plant grows in the foothills but is consumed in the mountains. It is said that mountaineers who came down to the plains to work, give up their coca habit.

The scientific study began when cocaine was extracted from coca over 100 years ago. The leaves contain about 1 percent cocaine. Two prominent names have been associated with the earlier work: Sigmund Freud and

Sherlock Holmes. Freud wrote glowingly of cocaine's ability to cure the morphine and alcohol habits: "Inebriate asylums can be entirely dispensed with." After a few unfortunate experiences, his enthusiasm subsided. Following a suggestion from Freud his colleague Koller discovered its ability to anesthetize the eye. Now that safer and more predictable anesthetics have been developed, the medical use of cocaine is minimal.

The fictional character Sherlock Holmes took cocaine for many years ("Quick, Watson, the needle") apparently for his cyclic depressions. It is not known whether or not his creator Conan Doyle shared the cocaine dependence. Eventually, both disappeared for a three year period, and they returned to their readers cured.

It was William Halstead, the pioneer surgeon from Johns Hopkins, who discovered regional anesthesia by blocking peripheral sensory nerves with cocaine. He, too, became a compulsive cocaine user and struggled for a long time to overcome his habit.

By the beginning of the twentieth century many patent medicines and soft drinks contained a little cocaine. When the Pure Food and Drug Law and the Harrison Tax Act were enacted early in the twentieth century the practise was discontinued. At present the Coca Cola company extracts the cocaine from the imported leaves and turns it over to the government for medical purposes while using the de-cocainized leaves as a flavoring agent.

PHARMACOLOGY

Cocaine is more absorbed from the gastrointestinal tract, but it more rapidly enters the blood stream from all mucous membranes, the nose being a favored site. Subcutaneous, intramuscular, and intravenous routes of administration have been used. Cholinesterases metabolize it rapidly. It is excreted in the urine and can be detected there on testing. The LD_{50} is said to be about 1000 mg. but much smaller doses have caused death, and much larger amounts have been taken without side effects.

Its local anesthetic action is due to a blockade of the transmission of painful stimuli. Its stimulant effect is, in part, the result of prevention of the re-uptake of norepinephrine into the nerve cell in certain areas of the brain. Cocaine is a powerful constrictor of small blood vessels. This accounts for the ulceration of the nasal septum after it has been "snorted" for long periods in high doses.

Tolerance and withdrawal symptoms occur at high doses, therefore it is correct to speak of cocaine addiction. It is the craving to repeat the experience which accounts for chronic cocaine use.

Dilation of the pupils is maximal. Elevations of the heart rate, blood pressure, and respirations are the result of its sympathomimetic effect.

Overdoses produce tremors, convulsions with a temporal lobe seizure pattern, and delirium. Death is due either to cardiovascular collapse or respiratory failure.

THE COCAINE STATE

It may have been the rock musicians who rediscovered and reintroduced cocaine to the drug culture of the late 1960s. They serve as a pattern of prestige for millions of young people and their songs ("cocaine, cocaine running around my brain") spread the word. The quality of the experience ("the highest high of all") is such that craving to repeat the experience can become the only reason for existence, especially cocaine base smoking.

When injected or inhaled, cocaine produces a condition of hyperstimulation. Overalertness, euphoria, and feelings of great power dominate. The excitation and "high" are reminiscent of a high dose amphetamine injection, the major difference being that cocaine is very short acting. Heavy users who want to maintain the elation have been known to reinject cocaine intravenously every ten minutes. For some, the restlessness and hypervigilance becomes too much, and an unpleasant tension associated with paranoid thinking takes over. Consistent use sometimes results in a depressive reaction when cocaine is discontinued. The depression may be due to a depletion of norepinephrine stores because of its prolonged extracellular exposure at the synapse. The depression is "cured" temporarily by the injection of cocaine, thereby contributing to a perpetration of the cocaine "habit."

As with amphetamines, cocaine delays ejaculation and orgasm. It has been used to treat premature ejaculation when it was first introduced into medical practise. It is the prolongation of the sexual act combined with an intensification of sensory awareness that accounts for the claims of an aphrodesiac effect. Some occasional users state that they seek only the above mentioned sexual effects rather than the euphoriant action.

SIDE EFFECTS

Heavy use of cocaine will lead to weight loss, insomnia, and anxiety reactions. Oversuspiciousness and paranoid thinking with hallucinations and delusions are not infrequent. Some insight into the delusional nature of the thought may be retained. Hallucinations that are supposed to be typical of cocaine psychoses include beliefs that bugs are crawling under the skin (cocaine bugs) and of miniaturized visual hallucinations. Violent behavior occurs, but the brief action of the drug is sufficient to prevent sustained aggressive activities. It should be recalled that the stereotype of the crazed, homicidal "dope fiend" was the cocaine user, not the heroin addict. Even for the cocainist, the "dope fiend" stereotype ordinarily does not apply.

TREATMENT

The treatment of acute adverse cocaine reactions is generally unnecessary because they are over before arrival at the point of treatment. If an overdose requires intervention, intravenous barbiturates or phenothiazines may be employed. The respiratory depression which accompanies cocaine poisoning can also be made worse with large doses of sedatives. Anti-convulsants are not believed to be effective in preventing convulsions.

The chronic use of cocaine requires removal of the drug, dealing with the depression that may come forth, and changing the patient's attitudes and life style. Group therapy with recovered stimulant-dependent people may be effective.

PATTERNS OF USAGE

The following patterns of cocaine abuse can be identified.

The Pure "Cokehead"

As a rule, those who use this drug tend to use others in order to supplement or modify the action of cocaine. A small number of pure "cokeheads" are to be found. Some will try to maintain the state during their waking hours. This is an expensive procedure with high quality cocaine selling for about $2000 an ounce. Street cocaine is generally adulterated with lactose, procaine, amphetamine, or strychnine. If any cocaine is to be found, it might be as little as 5 percent. Intravenous injections as often as every ten minutes are necessary to maintain the upper reaches of the cocaine state. This means dozens of injections a day.

Polydrug Users and Cocaine

A common pattern is to try cocaine when it is available, but to employ other agents for everyday use. A fair number of people will try "coke" a few times and return to their customary mind-altering substances because of inability to afford this "rich man's speed" on a regular basis.

In Combination with Heroin

The classical "speedball artist" simultaneously injected cocaine and heroin intravenously. The majority of British addicts until recently were supplied with both drugs. Now a strong effort is being made to eliminate prescriptions for cocaine. Cocaine produces too much jitteryness and excitement for some people, and they prefer to combine it with a narcotic or some other depressant.

In Connection with Methadone Maintenance

It has been found that some patients in methadone maintenance programs are using cocaine. Of course, methadone can reduce the "high" when heroin is used, but it will not prevent cocaine, amphetamine, or sedative "highs." Certainly some clinic patients have used cocaine, but the extent of its usage in this population is not precisely known. At least one methadone program was found that the number of clients using cocaine can be reduced by testing for cocaine metabolites in the urine and confronting those with positive urines.

SUMMARY

Large amounts of cocaine are being smuggled into the United States. At this time the distribution pattern appears to be concentrated in the larger cities, particularly Los Angeles, San Francisco, New York, and Miami. The principal consumers are multiple drug users with only small numbers being exclusively into cocaine. If the black marketplace should become flooded with large amounts of cocaine, it can be predicted that many more people will become involved, more "cokeheads" will appear, and more social problems such as impulsive, violent activities will become manifest.

REFERENCES

1. Bejerot, N. A comparison of the effects of cocaine and synthetic central stimulants. Brit. J. Addictions 65:35–37 (May) 1970.
2. Chambers, C.D., Taylor, W.J.R. and Moffett, A.D. The incidence of cocaine abuse among methadone maintenance patients. Internat. J. Addictions. 7:427–441, 1972.
3. Cocaine. Fact Sheet of the National Clearinghouse for Drug Abuse Information Series 11, No. 1, January, 1972.
4. Gay, G.R., Sheppard, C.W., Inaba, D.S. and Newmeyer, J.A. Co-

caine in perspective: "Gift from the Sun God" to "The Rich Man's Drug." Drug Forum. 2(4) 409–430 (Summer) 1973.
5. Ritchie, J.M., Cohen, P.J. and Gilman, A., eds. The Pharmacological Basis of Therapeutics, 4th Ed., New York, MacMillan, 1970, pp. 371–401.
6. Woods, J.H. and Downs, D.A. The psychopharmacology of cocaine. In: *Drug Use in America: Problems in Perspective.* The technical papers of the second report of the National Commission on Marihuana and Drug Abuse. Vol. 1, pp. 116–139, 1973. U.S. Govt. Printing Office, Washington, D.C. 20402.

16. Methadone Diversion

BACKGROUND

Methadone maintenance programs have expanded very considerably. It is now believed that some 80,000 heroin-dependent people are being treated in about 800 methadone maintenance clinics across the country.

The controversies about methadone maintenance remain. Those favoring the procedure claim that it is the most effective available method of dealing with heroin addiction. They point to the apparent decrease in numbers of addicts as a result of large scale intervention with methadone. Their opponents claim that it is only trading one addiction for another, that it is the establishment way to subjugate minorities, and that the methadone maintenance patients are zombies. No attempt will be made to deal with these issues at this time. Instead, we shall consider the problem of methadone diversion, a matter which should concern both proponents and opponents of methadone maintenance.

WHAT IS METHADONE DIVERSION?

Methadone diversion is the rechanneling of licit methadone into illicit traffic. This may occur when the clients sell or give their methadone to others, through sales by clinic staff, or by robberies and hijackings. Until recently doctors were able to prescribe methadone. A small number of physicians in Miami, New York, and Washington added to black market supplies by carelessly handing out prescriptions for the drug. The source of methadone has dried up since the laws were changed to prohibit prescribing methadone except under special conditions.

Methadone now appears on the street in two major forms. One is in a liquid, usually a synthetic orange juice like Tang. The other is the 40 mg disket. Both forms are used only in methadone programs and are said to be incapable of conversion to intravenous use. The disket brings about $5.00 on the street and the liquid between $6.00 and $10.00. The amount of methadone in the latter varies according to the client's daily dose, which may be from 20 mg to 120 mg.

THE FIVE CITY STUDY

In order to determine the extent of the problem the National Institute of Drug Abuse contracted for a study of methadone diversion with the Institute for Social Research at Fordham University. The study was performed in five cities: New York, St. Louis, Philadelphia, Miami, and San Juan, Puerto Rico. It was done prior to April, 1973, at which time a more restrictive policy on take-home methadone went into effect under FDA regulations. Whether the situation has improved since then is not known. Interviews with 381 street addicts, with 266 addicts mostly in methadone treatment programs, and with local and federal law enforcement officials in the five cities constituted the sources of information. Some of the key questions asked follow.

Table I-6: Specific Survey Questions

	Street Addicts	Addicts in treatment
Did you ever buy or use illegal methadone?		
Yes	61%	71%
Did you buy or use illegal methadone during the past week?		
Yes	45%	31%
How often do you use illegal methadone?		
Less than once a month:	18%	10%
One to nine times a month:	50	41
Ten to 29 times a month:	11	6
Everyday	21	43
Where did the illegal methadone come from?		
Patients in programs	74%	59%

TABLE I-6 (*continued*)

	Street Addicts	Addicts in Treatment
Special dealers	7	16
Pushers	6	16
Doctors	10	19
Friends	8	12
Others in program	6	7
	111%*	129%*

Why did you use methadone?

Detoxify	19%	27%
Limit my habit	7	2
Keep from getting sick	65	70
Get high	12	21
	103%*	120%*

How available is methadone on the street?

Available	72%	51%
Difficult to obtain	15	39
Impossible to obtain	2	10
Do not know	11	0

How available is heroin on the street?

Available	86%	—
Difficult to obtain	13	—
Impossible to obtain	1	—

Note: The New York City respondents stated that methadone was more available (84%) than heroin (63%).

How many clients in treatment sell their methadone?

Everybody	10%	12%
More than half	28	18
Less than half	25	30
Refused to answer	2	—
Do not know	35	39

(* more than one response)

Information Obtained from Law Enforcement Officials

The investigators found law enforcement personnel surprisingly supportive of the rehabilitative efforts of local treatment programs. Objections were expressed about those programs where profit was the main concern, or where careless operations caused problems. Methadone diversion was not viewed as a pressing law enforcement issue, and the heroin distribution system was receiving their full attention at that time.

This position is in sharp contrast with earlier police attitudes, which were strongly opposed to dispensing narcotics to addicts and certainly to giving them methadone to take off the premises. Apparently, the favorable results of methadone therapy have produced a change in the posture of enforcement officers toward the procedure.

In a small survey of 95 heroin addicts in Brooklyn, Chambers obtained results generally comparable to the above. Some 79 percent declared that methadone was available for purchase on the street. When asked whether they had purchased any during the past six months, 56 percent responded "Yes." In their neighborhood the disket form was exclusively seen. The price of a disket averaged $4.00. Methadone patients were the source of supply for 74 percent. The reasons given for purchase were: prevent withdrawal sickness, 41 percent; "clean up," 17 percent; "boost" other drugs, 40 percent; and resell, 2 percent.

Some Conclusions of the Survey

1. Illicit methadone was widely reported as being available by the drug abusers. Information from enforcement officials confirmed this fact. A substantial proportion of addicts not in treatment used methadone every day. An even larger number said that they use it a few times a month. Reasons given for methadone use varied from "to get high" to "to keep from getting sick."

2. The chief source of illicit methadone is the patient attending a methadone maintenance clinic.

3. Methadone has become an important new commodity in the illicit drug subculture.

4. At the time the study was done, enforcement officials were much more involved in heroin control than in the problem of methadone diversion. When arrests for illicit methadone did occur, they were triggered by complaints about notorious treatment programs or by blatantly overdealing activities.

Some Recommendations of the Survey

1. Treatment programs should monitor diversion activities more effectively. As a result of the study, there is sufficient reason to believe that a significant traffic in diverted methadone exists. Take-home privileges should be tightened up for those who do not use their methadone as prescribed.

2. The use of a tracer substance in the methadone (a minute quantity of a vitamin, for example) is feasible for special situations. It is not recommended for universal use. From a tracer police seizures could identify the source of the confiscated methadone.

THE SIGNIFICANCE OF METHADONE DIVERSION

Methadone diversion would be a trivial matter, just another example of "games addicts play," were it not for certain ominous overtones associated with the practice.

Significance for the Client

It seems clear that substantial numbers of methadone maintenance clients sell some or all of their take-home supplies. With the proceeds they seem inclined to buy heroin to "shoot over," or cocaine, barbiturates or amphetamines to "shoot around" their habits. Aside from the possible pharmacologic dangers involved, cheating on the program speaks for a cynical attitude toward their own rehabilitation.

Significance for the Treatment Program

When treatment staff does not know, or does not care what is happening to their clients, a breakdown in their ability to help takes place. The addict who successfully sells his methadone has succeeded in "conning" his therapist, a situation that does not engender respect and mutual openness.

Significance for the Addict Population

Methadone maintenance apologists insist that street methadone has a therapeutic usefulness in that it is used to detoxify or treat withdrawal sickness. This sounds encouraging, but it is only partially true from the data presented. In the five city survey 65–70 percent said that they used illegal methadone to keep from getting sick. Unfortunately, the same question was not asked about heroin usage. Most heroin addicts will respond to such an inquiry by insisting that they use heroin to keep from getting sick. Only small numbers of long-term addicts speak of getting high from street heroin, or if they do, it turns out to mean "feeling normal."

It is well known that during a heroin "panic" a certain small number of addicts will stop using and will not resume when heroin becomes available again. A relative shortage of heroin is supposed to exist on the East Coast now. The presence of a stable, black market supply of methadone assures the ability to continue to remain addicted. The few who may have become discouraged and "cleaned up" are now being tided over with methadone.

Significance to the Community

One major factor in reducing the prevalence of opiate addiction is reducing supplies. It is impossible to eliminate supplies completely, but making it difficult to sustain a habit provides some motivation to stop using. This is what may be meant by the "burnt out" addict who stops using after 20 years or so on heroin. Illegal methadone palpably adds to the pool of available opiates and perpetuates the addiction of those who might become discouraged by the strenuous efforts needed to remain opiate dependent.

The spread of opiate dependence is from the addicted to the non-addicted. The more addicts the greater the dangers of spread. Therefore, if street methadone has kept any number of individuals in an addicted state, that danger is a matter of considerable concern.

Perhaps even more important, the public and press reaction to methadone diversion may result in disenchantment with the treatment. Two years ago the *New York Times* and other newspapers ran many articles on diversion, primary methadone addiction, and accidental deaths due to methadone. We must recall that it was public revulsion that caused the closing of the morphine maintenance clinics in this country during the 1920s. What caused the revulsion? It was the diversion of morphine into illegal channels.

SUMMARY

Methadone maintenance has a role to play in the treatment of the heroin dependent person. Methadone diversion can only do harm and should be reduced to the lowest possible level.

REFERENCES

1. Chambers, C.D. *et al.* Methadone diversion: A study of illicit availability. In: "Methadone: Experiences and Issues." Ed.: Chambers, C.D. and Brill, L., Behavioral Publications, 1973, N.Y., pp. 87–93.
2. Knowles, R.R. Methadone maintenance in St. Louis. In: "Metha-

done maintenance," Ed.: Einstein, S., Marcel Dekker, 1971, N.Y., pp. 66–73.
3. Martin, J.M. *et al.* Methadone diversion: A study of five cities. Institute for Social Research, Fordham University, N.Y., 154 pages.

17. Internal Opioid Compounds

One of the most exciting recent research findings in the field of drug abuse, in fact, in all of neurochemistry, has been the discovery that all vertebrates have built-in, anti-pain compounds in the central nervous system. Furthermore, these compounds act on specific receptor sites at nerve cell synapses, the same binding sites occupied by the drugs we call narcotics.

A lock and key relationship exists between these receptor sites and internal or injected compounds with pain-relieving, euphoriant effects. Slight modifications of the structure of opiates, or of their electrical charges will not permit a "fit" with the receptor molecule, and all narcotic activity will be lost.

Similarly, certain minor manipulations of the spacial configuration of a narcotic can change it from a strong narcotic agonist to a narcotic antagonist that will prevent any narcotic from producing its effects. This occurs because a narcotic antagonist like naloxone (Narcan) can displace or prevent an agonist like morphine from occupying available narcotic receptor sites.

The presence of opiate receptors has been assumed for some time, but the puzzling aspect of the situation has been why they should exist. Now the answer is at hand: endogenous opioids fit the receptor molecule and the narcotic drugs also happen to fit into the same site.

THE ENKEPHALINS

At present two types of internal anti-pain compounds have been identified: the enkephalins and the endorphins. The term "endorphin" is becoming the generic name for the whole group. Enkephalins are small peptides consisting of five amino acids. One amino acid chain consists of tyrosine-glycine-glycine-phenylamine-methionine, and it is called methionine enkephalin. Leucine enkephalin is similar with leucine substituted for the methionine. It may seem strange that such divergent molecules as the phenanthrene, morphine, the phenyl-piperidine, Demerol, the diphenyl-methane, methadone, and the amino acid chain of the enkephalins all fit into the same stereospecific receptor site. When seen spacially, however, there are similarities at one part of all these compounds providing grounds for the assumption that they fit into the opiate receptor at that point.

The enkephalins are distributed in the regions of the brain where opiate receptors are known to be concentrated. These include the substantia gelatinosa, a relay area in the spinal cord for burning, dull pain sensation transmission. From there, the noxious sensations are transmitted along the spinothalamic tract, through the periaqueductal gray matter, and up into the thalamus and the limbic system. It is known that morphine is more effective against burning pain than sharp pain. The latter has a separate transmission pathway that is less involved in the enkephalin mechanism of control.

It appears that the enkephalins are neurotransmitters modulating pain perception and the emotional response to it. In addition, they may play a role in emotionality, producing feelings of pleasure just as opiates induce euphoria. It is speculated that individuals with low enkephalin levels might be susceptible to depression.

Nerve cells that are modulated by enkephalins inhibit the firing of excitatory neurons thus reducing the sensation of pain or of unpleasant emotional affects. Narcotics perform similar functions. They increase the inhibition of the transmission of noxious stimuli by occupying opiate receptor sites that the enkephalins leave vacant.

When a drug like morphine is given in large doses over a period of weeks, enkephalin formation is reduced or eliminated by feedback mechanisms from the receptor sites that are totally occupied. It may be that the enkephalins are involved in the withdrawal syndrome upon sudden discontinuance of a narcotic. The complete absence of the enkephalins may evoke some symptoms of early abstinence. Repeated injections of enkephalins have produced tolerance and withdrawal effects in mice. The narcotic antagonists precipitate withdrawal in animals made tolerant to the enkephalins.

The well-known antitussive and gastrointestinal slowing effects of the narcotics are also possessed by the enkephalins. Concentrations of opiate receptors can be identified in the solitary nucleus, which is involved in the cough reflex and in reducing gastrointestinal secretion and motility.

THE ENDORPHINS

Three endorphins have been identified: alpha, beta, and gamma. They are long-chain peptides consisting of 16 to 91 amino acids. All of them contain the methionine enkephalin sequence. The pituitary gland is one source of the endorphins. Their action is blocked by the narcotic antagonist naloxone. The long peptide chain prevents rapid degradation so that they are longer acting and more potent than the enkephalins. The endorphins are as much as 48 times more active than morphine when injected into the cerebral ventricles and are three times more active intravenously despite the fact they cross the blood-brain barrier poorly.

THE ROLE OF NARCOTIC ANTAGONISTS

The fact that naloxone immediately reverses the effects of endorphins, enkephalins, and all the known narcotics is very suggestive that all of these substances act on a common site of action. The more potent the narcotic, the greater affinity it has for the specific opiate receptor.

It has been found that sodium ions increase narcotic antagonist binding and reduce agonist binding. Since sodium ions are readily available, antagonists are ordinarily capable of displacing agonist molecules that have previously located themselves on the specific receptor. Therefore, antagonists are able to quickly reverse the symptoms and signs of narcotic agonist overdose.

One of the most impressive experiences in emergency medicine is the restoration of breathing and consciousness in a moribund patient who had taken an overdose of some opiate. Narcotic antagonists also have provided the means for the breakthrough in identifying the properties of endogenous opioids.

Stimulation of electrodes implanted in the periaqueductal gray matter of six patients with intractable pain provided complete relief in five and partial analgesia in one. When the electrical stimulation was very frequent, tolerance developed to further stimulation and also to narcotics. Naloxone reversed the pain relief provided by electrical stimulation. It is tempting to assume the stimulation was mediated by an endogenous opioid.

When administered to a person who has not recently taken an opiate, the pure antagonists like naloxone produce no visible effects. Theoretically, they should increase pain sensitivity, and preliminary work indicates that this is a possibility. Since enkephalin levels are reported to be elevated in acute schizophrenics and to return to normal as clinical improvement occurs, naloxone has been tried in a small number of hallucinating schizophrenics. In the initial study improvement seems to have occurred, but a later, controlled study was unable to confirm the finding. Very recently, another blind study showed essentially no change in schizophrenic patients and in those with affective disorders indicating that acute blockade of opiate receptors is not associated with global improvement in psychotic symptomatology.

ACUPUNCTURE

A recent investigation into the mechanism of acupuncture analgesia has been performed in anesthetized cats. Pin prick stimuli applied to a limb caused an increased firing in dorsal horn cells as measured by recording electrodes, indicating that painful sensations were being transmitted. A needle was placed in the correct acupuncture point, and electrical stimulation was induced. The increased firing in the dorsal horn cells ceased. No block of the firing occurred when the acupuncture needles were placed in "dummy" positions.

From the time course of the inhibition of the firing it seems likely that enkephalins mediated the acupuncture effect. The inhibition of firing was reversed by naloxone, providing further evidence that some internal opioid acting over the opiate receptor sites must have been responsible for the acupuncture effect. The work has been replicated in rats, but further testing of the above hypothesis is needed before definite conclusions can be reached.

DISCUSSION

The identification of opiate receptors at specific neuronal synapses and of naturally occurring peptides that have analgesic, and perhaps euphoric properties, has many implications—some of which are not yet clearly discernible. We are at the threshold of applying these important pieces of knowledge. A few of the implications that are perceptible now will be discussed.

1. The long held hope that a non-addictive pain-reliever might be constructed receives new support. Two possibilities arise. The synthesis of an amino acid chain with long-acting narcotic properties that can cross the blood-brain barrier is one conceivable direction. A second is that with the current, simpler modes for testing narcotic effects, a drug with just the right combination of agonist and antagonist properties can be developed that provides narcosis with little or no abusable potential. Larger than average doses would produce a reversal of the narcotic reaction because the antagonist would neutralize the narcotic effect.

2. Is it possible that the enkephalins-endorphins are more than antinociceptive agents? Could they also play a role in mood disorders considering the concentration of opiate receptors in limbic system structures? This area is just beginning to be explored.

3. Now that we know that all vertebrates have a built-in method for

dealing with pain and other noxious emotions, our ability to help those in distress will be based on more solid grounds than in the past. Analgesics and pain-relieving methods can be more precisely tested, as exemplified by the study of acupuncture described earlier.

4. The issues of tolerance and withdrawal to narcotics must be re-opened and our traditional notions reexamined. It is tempting to believe that the new knowledge will provide assistance in the treatment of opiate addiction.

5. The fact that the presence of specific opiate receptor sites has been proven means that their physiology and biochemistry will be intensively scrutinized. Questions of enkephalin blocking, reuptake, turnover and in-hibition of the metabolizing enzymes are being studied. The sensitization and blockade of the receptor site will be closely investigated by the many groups involved in opioid transmitter and receptor site research.

SUMMARY

Instead of summarizing what has been written, it seems worthwhile to mention some of the investigators who provided the initial research in the field of endogenous opioids and their receptors. They and their associates are to be congratulated on their contributions. They are listed below in alphabetical order.

Avram Goldstein, *Addiction Research Foundation, Palo Alto, California.*

Roger Guillemin, *Salk Institute, La Jolla, California.*

John Hughes, *University of Aberdeen, Scotland.*

Choh Hso Li, Eddie T. F. Wei and Horace H. Low, *University of California, San Francisco, California.*

Solomon H. Snyder, *Johns Hopkins University, Baltimore, Maryland.*

ADDITIONAL READING

1. Davis, G. C., Bunney, W. E. *et al. Intravenous naloxone admini-stration in schizophrenia and affective illness.* Science. 197:74–77, 1977.

2. Feinberg, A. P., Creese, I. and Snyder, S. H. *The opiate receptor.* Proc. Nat. Acad. Sci., U.S.A. 73:4215–4219, 1976.
3. Goldstein, A. *Opioid peptides (endorphins) in pituitary and brain.* Science. 193: 1081–1086, 1976.
4. Guillemin, R. *Endorphins, brain peptides that act like opiates.* New Eng. J. Med. 296: 226–228, 1977.
5. Hosobuchi, Y., Adams, J. E. and Linchitz, R. *Pain relief by electrical stimulation on the central gray matter in humans and its reversal by Naloxone.* Science. 197: 183–186, 1977.
6. Marx, J. L. Neurobiology: *Researchers high on endogenous opiates.* Science. 193: 1227–1229, 1976.
7. Pert, C. B. and Snyder, S. H. *Opiate receptor: Demonstration in nervous tissue.* Science. 179: 1011–1014, 1973.
8. Pert, C. B. and Snyder, S. H. *Properties of opiate receptor binding in rat brain.* Proc. Nat. Acad. Sci. U.S.A. 70: 2243–2247, 1973.
9. Pomeranz, B. *Naloxone blockade of acupuncture analgesia: endorphin implicated.* Life Sciences. 19: 1757, 1977.
10. Snyder, S. H. *Opiate receptors and internal opiates.* Scientific American. 236: 44–67, 1977.
11. Snyder, S. H. *Opiate receptors in the brain.* New Eng. J. Med. 296: 266–271, 1977.
12. Volavka, J., Mallya, A. *et al. Naloxone in chronic schizophrenia.* Science. 196: 1227–1228, 1977.
13. Walker, J. M., Berntson, G. C. *et al. An analog of enkephalin having prolonged opiate-like effects* in vivo. Science. 196: 85–87, 1977.
14. Wei, E. and Low, H. *Physical dependence on opiate-like peptides.* Science. 193: 1262–1264, 1976.

18. Polydrug Abuse

Polydrug abuse is a new name for an old practice: the use of two or more mind-altering drugs for non-medical purposes.

The "speedball artists" of bygone days had discovered the intensification of the "high" when heroin and cocaine were injected in the same syringe. Combined amphetamine-barbiturate abuse has been reported for many years. About 15 years ago Cohen and Ditman described, among other complications associated with LSD, and phenomenon they called "multihabituation."(1) This consisted of the frequent consumption of a bewildering variety of hallucinogens, stimulants, narcotics, and sedatives taken together or sequentially. The practice seemed to be a way of life in certain subgroups. Individuals were observed who would take any substance, known or unknown, in any quantity. Their associates called such persons "garbage cans."

The concept of polydrug abuse (if we ignore the unholy marriage of a Greek prefix with an Old French noun) is a good one. It is becoming increasingly difficult to find abusers of a single drug.

CLASSIFICATION

A number of types of polydrug abusers can be classified.

1. Those who have a basic dependence upon one drug but who use additional agents when they are available. Cocaine is expensive and is the basic drug only for the affluent. Many users of other substances will snort cocaine whenever someone makes it available to them.

2. Those who move from one class of psychochemical to another, trying various combinations to either intensify the effects, or to diminish certain of the side effects. In the latter instance some stimulant abusers take a sedative in combination in order to take the edge off the feeling of tenseness that amphetamines or cocaine can cause.

3. Those who cycle their drug use: tranquilizers during the day, sedatives at night, and stimulants in the morning.

4. Those whose basic drug is in short supply or who are in drug deterrent programs. During a heroin "panic," cough syrups, alcohol, or other depressant drugs will be used to intoxicate or to reduce the severity of withdrawal symptoms. People in methadone maintenance or narcotic antagonist programs know that shooting ordinary amounts of street heroin will have little or no effect. Some of them will "shoot around" their treatment drug by using barbiturates or cocaine, or they will turn to alcohol. The claim is made that when marihuana was in short supply during Operation Intercept, users moved to other, more damaging substances.(2)

5. Those who will consume anything at hand.

Prevalance

In an effort to obtain marihuana-sophisticated volunteers for a marihuana research project, Carlin and Post interviewed 106 men who responded to a newspaper advertisement.(3) They were questioned about their drug-using practices. Psychedelic drugs were used by 74 percent. Six percent had tried heroin or morphine, with none currently addicted. Opium had been smoked by 27 percent. Amphetamine usage was admitted by 60 percent, primarily in cramming for school examinations. Tranquilizers were taken by 47 percent and barbiturates by 44 percent. In general, the multiple use of drugs in this particular group involved no tendency for them to graduate to dependence on more dangerous drugs.

On the other hand, a survey of suburban adolescents referred by a juvenile court revealed more serious patterns of multiple abuse of solvents, alcohol, pills, cannabis, and narcotics that were considered destructive.(4) The incidence of psychiatric disorders was high in this population.

The most common basic drug is alcohol, next in popularity (if tobacco be excluded) is marihuana. Only a few years ago some counterculture members alleged that marihuana would be their recreational agent, with alcohol performing that function for the Establishment. Unfortunately, cannabis users are now also into the dominant culture's beverage.(5) The opposite is also happening. The National Commission on Marihuana and Drug Abuse report of 1972 indicated that 6 percent of people over 50 interviewed had smoked marihuana.(6) Of those, 45 percent were Republicans and 55 percent were Democrats. Professionals, salespeople, bankers, and similar groups were represented.

TREATMENT

Detoxification

The problem of the detoxification of mixed addictions to alcohol or the sedative-hypnotics in combination with heroin or methadone has occurred with some regularity. In many instances gradual detoxification with methadone and a barbiturate can be done simultaneously. Sedative-hypnotic toxicity should be taken more seriously than opiate toxicity in view of the quality of street heroin. It will require a longer time to become drug free from a barbiturate or non-barbiturate sedative than from heroin. As an alternative, a maintenance amount of methadone can be given while diminishing quantities of the barbiturate are used. After the sedative dose has reached zero, methadone detoxification can commence.

The abstinence syndrome can be avoided in cases of mixed alcohol, tranquilizer and sedative-hypnotic dependence by using a single drug, phenobarbital or secobarbital, for example. Since these central nervous system depressants all show cross tolerance with each other, any member of the group can be used for gradual detoxification.

It is not necessary to detoxify with stimulants in treating combined stimulant-depressant dependence. Utilizing recommended depressant methods for detoxification will amply take care of the stimulant problem.

Overdose

In instances of combined heroin-barbiturate overdose, the mainte-nance of an effective heart action, blood pressure and respiratory gas ex-change is the first consideration. The injection of a narcotic antagonist like naloxone (Narcan) will increase the rate of breathing and level of con-sciousness if the intoxication is primarily due to the narcotic. If it is not, no harm will be done.

Pupil signs may be variable in multiple drug overdose. Even if the pupils are not constricted, a trial intravenous injection of a narcotic an-tagonist should be considered. Otherwise, the question of what kind of drug has caused the coma, respiratory depression, and cardiac arrest need not be answered immediately. The critical task is to support the vital func-tions until recovery occurs.

Long Term

The long-term management of polydrug users is universally considered to be more difficult than one drug abusers. The impression is that the former is a "sicker" group that tends not to remain in treatment. Group therapy or involvement in a therapeutic community is the usual treatment mode. The ultimate goal is to provide a viable alternate life style that is gratifying and meaningful to the patient.

Some work has been done with heroin-alcohol addicts using a metha-done maintenance-Antabuse regimen.(7) Daily methadone and Antabuse has been successful in a small number of cases. The drugs do not cause ad-verse reactions when used together. Some people, vulnerable to become dependent on drugs, may decompensate mentally if access to their alcohol or other drug is interdicted by chemical blockade. They had abused one or more substances in an effort at self-treatment. Without access to some anxiety reducing agent, they have been known to become overtly psycho-tic. This possibility should be considered in drug deterrent therapy.

Issues

One of the frequently asked questions about marihuana is: "Does it lead to harder drugs?" Aside from the question of the appropriateness of calling some drugs "hard" and others "soft," the answer has to be quali-fied. Most marihuana users also indulge in alcohol and hallucinogens. They are apt to be involved with stimulants, depressants, and opiates more frequently than cannabis abstainers.

There is no pharmacologic reason, however, for the use of the other classes of drugs. It appears that once one illicit drug is used, it is easier for the individual to become involved in others. This spreading into other cat-egories of drugs is primarily a peer group phenomenon of socialization. Naturally, psychologically troubled people will tend to try and continue the use of an array of drugs, if relief of anxiety and depression is achieved.

The description of alcoholics as oral characters may be a simplification of a much more complex problem. Nevertheless, heavy drinking is positively correlated with heavy smoking. This combination is now being charged with causing increased numbers of malignancies of the mouth, larynx, pharynx, and esophagus. Heavy drinking or heavy smoking alone do not seem to produce the unexpectedly large numbers of cancers in this region.(8) For example, if the risk of oral cancer in nonsmokers and nondrinkers is placed at 1.00, the risk for those who smoke 40 or more cigarettes a day and do not drink is 2.43. For the 40 or more cigarettes a day consumers who also take more than 10 drinks a week, the risk is 15.50.

In an alcohol-heroin polydrug user with liver dysfunction, it is sometimes difficult to determine whether one drug or both have contributed to the liver injury.(9) Chronic alcoholism produces fatty infiltration of the liver cells, an inflammatory reaction in the portal triads, and eventually their scarring (cirrhosis). This is apparently a direct toxic effect of the alcohol plus the associated nutritional deficiency. Heroin addiction produces a hepatitis often with a high Australian antigen titer due to injection of the virus along with the heroin. When both factors are combined, the liver damage is greater, and the onset of hepatic insufficiency is more rapid.

A few years ago, before methaqualone (Quaalude) was placed in Schedule II (triplicate prescription required), its combination with alcohol was rather popular. "Luding out" as the practice was called, relied upon the synergistic action of the sedative-hypnotic and alcohol for its effects.

Not all polydrug use involves abusable drugs exclusively. When Mandrax [methaqualone plus diphenhydramine (Benadryl)] was marketed in England, it became more popular than methaqualone alone. Apparently the mild sedative action of the antihistamine added to the quieting effect. Another combination of an antihistamine [tripelannamine (Pyribenzamine)] was also popular, both here and in England at one time. In combination with camphorated tincture of opium [Paregoric] it was strained and injected intravenously. It went by the name of Purple Velvet.

SUMMARY

The overuse of many drugs rather than a single one causes problems for both the patient and the treater alike. The use of secondary agents to modify or enhance the subjective effects of a primary substance can be hazardous because of potentiation or enzyme inhibition. Treatment is often difficult because of atypical clinical signs and altered responsiveness to standard management.

NOTES

1. Cohen, S. and Ditman, K. S. Complications associated with lysergic acid diethylamide. J.A.M.A. 181:161, 1962.
2. McGlothlin, W., Jamison, Kay and Rosenblatt, S. Marihuana and the use of other drugs. Nature. 228:1227, 1970.
3. Carlin, A. S. and Post, R. D. Patterns of drug use among marihuana users. J.A.M.A. 218:867, 1971.
4. Dodson, W. E., *et al.* Pattern of multiple drug abuse among adolescents referred by a juvenile court. Pediatrics. 47, 1033, 1971.
5. Tec, N. A clarification of the relationship between alcohol and marihuana. Brit. J. Addiction, 68:191, 1973.
6. National Commission on Marihuana and Drug Abuse. Marihuana use in American society. Vol. 1, 249–339, U.S. Gov't Printing Off., Washington, D.C. 20402.
7. Pascarelli, E. F. Disulfiram (Antabuse) in the treatment of methadone maintenance alcoholics. In Dupont, R. L. and Freeman, R. S., eds. Fifth National Conference on Methadone Treatment. 1973, Napan, N.Y., pp. 316–323.
8. Alcohol and Health. II Report, 1974, U.S. Gov't Printing Off., Washington, D.C. 20402, p. 69.
9. Stimmel, B., *et al.* Hepatic dysfunction in heroin addicts. Alcohol vs. viral etiology. Gastroenterology, 60:754, 1971.

19. Alcohol-Drug Combinations

Now that alcohol-containing beverages have become basic mood-altering substances upon which a variety of other drugs are overlaid, some consideration should be given to the implications and impacts of such multiple drug use.

The difficult problems of studying one drug are multiplied when two or more substances are used together, and definitive investigations in this area are not yet available. Some circumscribed work can be mentioned; the rest of our information on drug-alcohol combinations is derived from clinical impressions.

REASONS FOR ALCOHOL-DRUG USE

When drugs are taken together it is usually for one of four reasons.

**1. Additional Drugs Are Used to Intensify the Effect of
the Primary Substance**

Since combining depressants are either additive or potentiating, they are frequently added to alcohol. When the marihuana or the heroin is weak, alcohol is added to reinforce the effects. When sleeping pills do not work, a quantity of ethanol is consumed along with them. If a few drinks don't seem to unwind the tense individuals, tranquilizers might be added.

**2. Multiple Drugs May Be Used to Reduce the Undesirable
Side Effects of the Primary Agent**

Barbiturate-amphetamine combinations are popular because some people dislike the "wired up" feeling of large amounts of amphetamines. Alcohol has been employed by amphetamine abusers for similar purposes. In addition, they use large amounts of alcohol when coming down from an amphetamine binge to help induce sleep. Kipperman reports on a group of heavy drinkers who used moderate amounts of amphetamines to keep from passing out so that they could continue to drink. This practice could be hazardous because the built-in safeguard against overdosing with alcohol, namely unconsciousness, is evaded.

**3. One or More Drugs May Be Used to Substitute for the
Preferred Drug When It Is in Short Supply or Unavailable**

When a heroin "panic" is on, narcotic addicts will drink large amounts of codeine cough syrup or alcohol, or swallow any available sedative. These drugs will not prevent all of the symptoms of the abstinence syndrome but they will keep the user relatively comfortable.

**4. In Some Instances a Hodge-podge of Chemicals Is Taken Together
without Particular Rationale or Interest in How They Will Interact**

This is the "garbage head" syndrome, still occasionally seen among those who have little concern for their physical or mental health. It is difficult to understand the random ingestion of assorted psychochemicals. One suspects that the self-concept of such individuals must be quite low. The statement that they make with their omnivorous drug taking seems to be: "Anything is better than what I am."

EFFECTS OF ALCOHOL-DRUG USE

That alcohol taken in conjunction with other mind-altering drugs can be a serious matter, is confirmed by the Drug Abuse Warning Network summaries. DAWN obtains reports from emergency rooms, crisis centers, and medical examiners in 24 urban areas on the frequency of drug mentions.

Alcohol alone is not included, but alcohol-in-combination with other drugs is. For the latest month available, April, 1977, alcohol-in-combination was the leading item in medical examiners' mentions. It was second in emergency room and crisis center mentions. Ethanol-sedative and ethanol-opiate combinations were the most frequent causes of death reported by medical examiners, exceeding deaths due to heroin alone.

SOME COMBINATIONS

If the use of alcohol and caffeine is set aside, the joint use of alcohol and tobacco is the most frequent combination. Heavy drinkers tend to be heavy smokers, in fact, in one survey, they smoked more than mental patients, drug addicts, and a normal control group. Objectively, there is little to recommend this combination. Performance is not improved as compared to alcohol alone, and some investigators have even found a decrement on performance tests. It must be that subjectively something satisfactory happens. An alternative explanation is that heavy smoking and drinking are conditioned behaviors and have little to do with feelings of satisfaction.

Now that some recent data indicates that cancers of the head, neck, and esophagus are more frequent in alcoholics who smoke excessively than in alcoholics who do not, or in heavy smokers who do not drink inordinately, this abuse combination assumes added importance. The speculation offered for the increased incidence of upper digestive tract cancers in this population is that alcohol may increase the solubility of the carcinogen in tobacco.

ALCOHOL AND SEDATIVE-HYPNOTICS

Many of the alcohol-sedative adverse interactions can happen in patients who drink only moderately, and are, by no means, limited to the chronic alcoholic. A fatality can occur at BAC (blood alcohol concentrations) of 0.1 mg percent (4–5 ounces of whiskey) combined with a blood barbiturate level of 0.5 mg percent of pentobarbital in a non-tolerant person. Ordinarily, the lowest levels of blood barbiturate that can be associated with death is about 1.0–1.5 mg percent of a hypnotic barbiturate. Much less alcohol and hypno-sedatives are also needed to produce severe states of intoxication.

This group contributes substantially to the "accidental suicide" by overdosing out of confusion, memory impairment or a lack of information about the synergistic effect of the depressant drugs. After a night of heavy drinking it may not be a good idea to take four or five sleeping pills in order to get a good night's rest. The rest may be unexpectedly long.

ALCOHOL AND MINOR TRANQUILIZERS

A lack of public awareness exists about the decremental effects of combined minor tranquilizers and alcohol on alertness and psychomotor skills. Benzodiazepines may increase alcohol blood levels, and add their depressant effect to those of moderate to large amounts of alcohol. Driving skills with meprobamate and alcohol are impaired over and above the drowsiness and inattention that occurs.

It is clear from the experimental studies of performance and from actual accident reports that have been studied utilizing blood testing for psychotropic drugs, that combinations of alcohol and the minor tranquilizers are more disruptive of driving and related behavior than either drug alone. Nor is the practice of driving under the influence of such a combination rare. Finkle's study showed that 10 percent of arrested drivers had both alcohol and a minor tranquilizer in their blood stream.

ALCOHOL AND OPIATES

This combination of consciousness-changing drugs is important for several reasons.

1. Patients on methadone maintenance are known to abuse alcohol, in fact, about a quarter of them have substantial problems with alcohol. The death rate of methadone maintenance patients who drink heavily is as much as 10 times as great as those methadone maintenance patients who abstain.

2. Both alcohol and heroin damage the liver. Heroin use introduces hepatitis B through contaminated injections. Alcohol excess induces alcoholic hepatitis and cirrhosis. The combination can lead to fulminating liver disease. More than 20 percent of New York City heroin addicts showed evidence of chronic alcoholism at autopsy.

3. The depressant effects of alcohol and opiates are additive, if not supra-additive, and this can be deadly. If a person has become addicted to both narcotics and alcohol, the treatment of withdrawal becomes much more complicated.

4. From studies of double addicted people, it seems that their prognosis for recovery is worse. They are a more disturbed and antisocial group, and their behavior is more aberrant.

ALCOHOL AND MARIHUANA

Although both of these drugs worsen performance, recent studies reveal that together an additional decrement in manual dexterity, vigilance, information processing, temporal organization, and perceptual control occurs. Pot and pop wines or beer have become a frequently used mixture. This particular combination also increases the heart rate to the point that people with borderline cardiac function may decompensate while under the influence.

ALCOHOL AND STIMULANTS

The common assumption that strong black coffee antagonizes the intoxicating effects of alcohol is not completely true. Caffeine does improve reaction time, but other tests of manual dexterity, mental arithmetic, perceptual speed, verbal fluency, etc., were either uninfluenced or were performed worse after caffeine. Caffeine also has no effect on the BAC. It is possible that a drinker may feel more alert after three cups of hot coffee (300 mg of caffeine) and will attempt to drive. But he will remain handicapped in many areas of psychomotor coordination, in search and recognition activities, and in other complex tasks.

Some mention has already been made of possible joint uses of amphetamines and alcohol. Cocaine and alcohol combinations are used in a similar fashion: to make the heavy drinker more alert and to help the cocaine user reduce the tension and edginess of that stimulant.

ALCOHOL AND OTHER DRUGS

Now that antidepressants such as amitriptyline (Elavil) and doxepin (Sinequan) are becoming abused drugs, the effects of their combination with alcohol should be noted. They potentiate the depressant effects of alcohol. Operating machinery or driving a car while under the influence of the combination may be hazardous. The effects of the major tranquilizers and the sedative antihistamines are enhanced by alcohol beverages in a similar manner. The over-the-counter sleeping potions contain scopolamine and an antihistamine. These drugs can lead to more CNS depression than expected when used with alcohol.

A common combination consists of the use of alcohol together with analgesics like aspirin. This joint use does not seem to lead to additional behavioral impairment. However, the effect of salicylates on the clotting mechanism, and the irritant effects of both substances on the stomach lining have caused gastric hemorrhages, some of which have been life-endangering.

Volatile solvent inhalers also are known to drink wine or beer while sniffing. Alcohol is chemically closely related to some solvents, and it adds to the anesthetizing effect of all of them.

DRIVING AND ALCOHOL-DRUG USE

The presumptive level of driving while intoxicated has been a BAC of 0.1 mg percent. Certain countries and states are looking into the adverse effects of lower BACs on driving performance, levels between 0.05 and 0.1 mg percent, and some are considering a lowering of the BAC presumptive of intoxication.

In a recent report from California as many as 22 percent of drivers who were stopped for driving under the influence had detectable marihuana or marihuana and alcohol levels. This is the first study of its kind because roadside testing for THC has only recently become available.

Combinations of alcohol with sedatives, tranquilizers, narcotics, antihistamines and marihuana can only worsen driving performance because the depressant effects of the combinations are, at least, additive. Combinations of stimulants with alcohol may not improve the operation of a car. Although reaction time may be reduced, other, more complex functions necessary for the driving situation, are either unchanged or less satisfactorily performed.

Even when drugs are used in therapeutic doses and not in the amounts taken by abusers, their joint use with alcohol can be hazardous. A Scandanavian study examined the blood levels of 74 drivers in accidents who required hospitalization for their injuries. They were compared with 204 drivers who were not in traffic accidents.

Of those hospitalized, 41.8 percent had measurable blood alcohol concentrations, 9.5 percent had detectable diazepam (Valium) levels, and 10.8 percent had both drugs in their bloodstream. The control group revealed that 1.5 percent had alcohol, 2 percent had diazepam, and none had both drugs on testing.

SUMMARY

We appear to have entered a second, more complicated, phase of drug abuse. Although pure alcoholics and addicts still can be found, the use of multiple drugs is becoming more frequent. In fact, it is becoming a sort of cottage industry to figure out new mixtures of chemicals and spread the word by means of the underground press.

We are witnessing a potpourri of drug-taking by barefoot psycho-pharmacologists whose trial and error chemical blends never have been tested for safety. The result has been a more precarious form of drug-taking than when single drugs were abused.

20. Drug X: The Most Dangerous Drug on Earth

We are justifiably concerned about the effects of mind-altering drugs upon ourselves, our families, our community, and our society. We wonder whether a day will come when some drug will appear that will destroy the fabric of our social, economic, and political structure by its disintegrating effects upon the person and the community.

What would happen if a drug came into use (let's call it drug X), and it turned out to have these wide-spread and devastating effects? The adverse effects would be exerted not only upon the individual, but also on those around him, and upon the entire social system. They would be extensive enough to make sociologists and economists wonder whether we will be able to afford the human and financial costs of X abuse in years to come.

Drug X is here.

What have been the documented results of the drug X pandemic in this country? Only some of the proven noxious effects can be mentioned; the entire list is too long to be detailed in this space.

1. Ten million people, including increasing numbers of teenagers are dependent upon it, and their use of it is out of control. With one person in twenty in the land a problem Xaholic, it means that 40 million people (the afflicted and their families) are directly involved with the sequellae of destructive X usage.

2. X happens to produce a lengthy intoxicated state. This means that for many hours before coma sets in, or recovery occurs, judgement is impaired, controls over behavior are diminished or absent, and motor skills are reduced. As a result, intoxicated people are accident prone, not only to themselves, but also to those in their vicinity. To cite only one example of

their lethality, over 25,000 traffic deaths and hundreds of thousands of injuries occurred last year in connection with excessive X use.

3. Aggressiveness as a result of the impairment of the control over one's behavior has made X the most violence-producing of all drugs. Some 90 percent of all assaults, and 50 to 60 percent of all homicides take place while the aggressor was under the influence of X. In at least two studies it was also found that half of the victims had significant blood levels of X. Most homicides occur on weekends, a period when most X is consumed.

4. Police statistics across the nation consistently report that a third to a half of all arrests are related to this drug. Police, court, jail, and probation costs are enormous.

5. Half the rapes are committed while the rapist is under the influence of X.

6. In one study 67 percent of all sexually aggressive attacks against children were committed after X had been consumed by the perpetrator. X is also strongly related to the initiation of incestuous activities with minor children.

7. The suicide rate among X addicts is 6 to 20 times higher than in the general population. Even suicide attempters have high Xism rates with figures ranging from 13 to 50 percent above non-user levels. The role of the drug itself as an agent to commit suicide should be noted. Although it is possible to cause death from the use of X alone, the more common pattern is to combine other depressant drugs with the consumption of X. The potentiating effect of X upon sedatives, depressants, and tranquilizers is well established. Potentiation also accounts for fair numbers of accidental deaths in individuals who happen to consume sublethal quantities of X plus other depressants without suicidal intention.

8. Hundreds of thousands of families are disrupted by divorce, desertion, or separation, primarily because one or both partners are Xaholics. The children of such marriages are particularly affected by the neglect, persecution, and physical attacks to which they are exposed over many years. From studies of battered children it is becoming clear that many of the parents are chronic Xaholics. The children whose family life was made chaotic by X may, themselves, take to this same drug in the search for relief from their distressing situation.

9. Industry loses five billion dollars a year and government estimates

that their X dependent employees cost a half billion dollars each year. Poor job performance, lateness and absenteeism, illness, waste of materials, and bad decisions are only some of the causes of the losses to production and operations. The price of general inefficiency and the loss of key, trained personnel are incalculable. The total cost to society is put at more than 15 billion a year.

10. Chronic Xism causes brain damage that eventually becomes irreversible. It also causes damage to the nerves, the liver, and the pancreas. It interferes with the uptake of vitamins and other essential nutritional factors while requiring more of certain nutrients for its own metabolism. Every cell of the body is affected by these deficiencies. Resistance to infection is diminished, and death due to pheumonia and tuberculosis is common. Fractures and other trauma are normal hazards for the X-intoxicated person. The life span of the chronic user is shortened by 11 years.

11. Although tension and depression may lead to problem Xism, the protracted use of this chemical produces tension and depression. Estimates vary and statistics tend to be inaccurate because of cover-up diagnoses, but a fifth to a quarter of admissions to psychiatric hospitals are directly or indirectly caused by acute or chronic X ingestion.

12. The morning after a bout of X consumption many people will complain of headache, nausea, anorexia, shakiness, and muddled thinking. This unpleasant condition appears to deter no one from going on another bout.

13. After a prolonged binge of heavy X usage a characteristic withdrawal syndrome may be precipitated. It consists of grand mal convulsions, a toxic psychosis with hallucinations, and difficult-to-control tremulousness and agitation. The withdrawal syndrome carries a definite mortality risk. This frightening condition deters hardly anyone from going on another spree.

14. Despite heated debates about drug A being a steppingstone to drug B and so on up the drug ladder, in every survey drug X usually is the first intoxicating drug used by adolescents. If we were really serious about a steppingstone theory leading to heroin addiction, we would be concerned about the role of drug X. But a discussion of which drug leads to which drug is pointless. The harm that comes from X is much greater than the dangers of heroin in all respects.

Considering the harmful and disagreeable aspects of the agent it may be difficult for those not familiar with X to understand why its popularity continues to increase each year. They may properly ask why people continue to use the substance long after they have lost their health, their jobs, their family, their assets, their friends, and their self-respect. An answer is not easy to come by. First of all, even though 10 percent of the using population are in trouble with the drug, 90 percent are not, at least, not at present. All those who use X socially have the firm conviction that they are in the 90 percent group, and most of the people in the 10 percent group think that they are also in the 90 percent group. Therefore, a major problem is the complete lack of insight into one's own condition with regards to his X habit. This permits a denial of the reality situation for a long time, often for a lifetime.

Additional factors include the "pushing" and "dealing" activities of the supplies and users, and the strong cultural acceptance of the drug. Regarding the latter point, we symbolically equate the use of X with manliness (and womanliness) and with friendliness and social enjoyment. Certain behaviors like fighting, not approved while sober, are more apt to be tolerated if the individual is intoxicated with X. The mass media portrays X-taking as a pattern of prestige, and we all laugh at the sloppy, X-onked-out character on the screen. In this country it is difficult to be an X abstainer, although there are a few of these.

A further reason for the enormous consumption of X must be mentioned. In low doses many people report feelings of relaxation, well being and gregariousness. In addition, some will assert that they enjoy the taste of X. It is these low dose properties which make X attractive, and they account for its role as a social lubricant. Unfortunately, society has not found a way to prevent the transition to the social, psychological, physiological, and economic toxicity of the chronic, high dose state.

All sorts of legal policies have proven ineffective. Prohibition of X is hardly considered these days in view of the disasterous experience with a prohibition experiment of half a century ago. It is currently freely available and openly sold. In some states only the original packages can be purchased, but in most parts of the country it can be bought by the single dose or by the car load. A meal can hardly be ordered, a plane flight taken, a conference attended (even those on Xism), to say nothing of a visit to friends without being invited to down some form of X. People have been known to feel rejected or insulted when the invitation is refused. Controls over sale extend only to minors, Indians, and Election Day closing of X stores. The situation is so grotesque that X is not even considered a drug, and a package insert is not included with each purchase.

Prevention and education efforts have, in general, been ineffective. Attempts to teach the facts about X are received with disinterest and apathy. Scare tactics about X are unnecessary, because the facts are scary as they are.

What seems to be needed is an entirely new cultural attitude toward X in which it is recognized for what it is—a dangerous drug, dangerous for 10 million people, their families and those around them. How this new attitude can be achieved, is, unfortunately, obscure.

X has to be an imaginary drug. It is inconceivable that an advanced society would put up with the tragedy of X.

SELECTED REFERENCES

1. Amir, M. Patterns in forcible rape. University of Chicago Press, Chicago, 1970.
2. Bennett, R.M., *et al.* Alcohol and human physical aggression. Quart. J. Studies Alcohol. 30:870, 1969.
3. Blum, R.H. Presidents Commission on Law Enforcement and Administration of Justice, Task Force Report, Washington, D.C. Government Printing Office, 1967.
4. Blum, R.H. National Commission on Causes and Prevention of Violence, Staff Report. Washington, D.C. Government Printing Office, 1969.
5. Goodwin, D.W. Alcohol in suicide and homicide. Quart. J. Studies Alcohol. 34:144, 1973.
6. Shupe, L.M. Alcohol and crime. J. Crim. Law and Criminal. 44:661, 1964.
7. Tinklenberg, J.R. Alcohol and violence in Fox, R. and Bourne, P. (eds.) Alcoholism: Progress in Research and Treatment, Academic Press, 1973.
8. Wolfgang, M.E. Patterns in criminal homicide. Science Editions. New York, John Wiley and Sons, 1966.

21. Drug X: Another Point of View

The following essay was contributed by Dr. Robert A. Moore, Medical Director of the Mesa Vista Hospital, San Diego, California.

In the preceding essay Dr. Sidney Cohen refers to drug X as "the most dangerous drug on earth." Quite obviously, Dr. Cohen is referring to alcohol and the many tragic consequences of excessive alcohol use.

He presents compelling data and conclusions about the many sad consequences of alcohol use: impaired health, early death, family breakups, highway traffic fatalities, homicide, suicide, sexual assaults, and huge losses in industry from impaired productivity. Hard to measure are the harmful effects upon children raised in a family where one or both parents are alcohol abusers because it affects both their image of themselves as potential adults and their attitudes towards alcohol use for the future. Hospitals and jails find their clientele heavily represented by alcohol abusers. One certainly cannot dispute the major impact of these conclusions, and it would be foolhardy to defend alcohol abuse as a socially desirable behavior.

There is a less clearly stated point of view in the presentation: that there is an inherent risk in drinking alcohol, even in moderate or low dosage, because of the implication that everybody considers himself or herself a normal drinker, but perhaps all drinkers are vulnerable. There is a tone resembling "the myth of social drinking" presented by Dr. Max Hayman several years ago.

While Dr. Cohen recognizes attempts at legal prohibition in the past was not effective, he wonders if a new cultural attitude could be developed towards alcohol, recognizing it "for what it is—a dangerous drug." He then ends by saying "how this new attitude can be achieved, is, unfortunately, obscure."

There is ample literature with quite adequate documentation outlining all the ill effects of alcohol abuse. There is much research showing the effects of alcohol on the various body systems, upon such societal institutions as marriage and the family, and such indirect lethal actions of alcohol as traffic fatalities. Still, the literature pours in. New grant applications are produced to further study the ill effects of alcohol. One wonders at the need to be constantly producing more arguments as to the evils of "John Barleycorn," as if by an orgy of "bad news" we will be able to undo this epidemic "that will destroy the fabric of our social, economic, and political structure by the disintegrating effects upon the person and his community.'' (Cohen) Our traditional treatment programs for alcoholics include lectures and films on the ill effects of alcohol upon the body. Perhaps there is an assumption inherent in this that the general public, as well as people suffering from the ill effects of alcohol, are unaware of this information and if we can simply convince them of the truth, the problem will be brought under control, both for the individual and for society. It appears the assumption is that alcoholics drink through ignorance of what they are doing and the harm they are producing. Having been better informed, they will mend their ways.

Similar education programs have been traditionally used in traffic safety: "If you drink, don't drive! If you drive, don't drink!" And, if you don't follow this admonition, you will be arrested and punished.

Despite this outpouring of "bad news," which has been increasing in volume in the past few years, there was a 32 percent in per capita absolute alcohol consumption in the United States between 1958 and 1971 (1) and it appears that there has been continued growth in consumption since then. This is not a phenomenon limited to the United States since, during a roughly comparable period of time, there has been a 61 percent increase in West Germany, a 54 percent increase in Denmark, and an 83 percent increase in the Netherlands. And so it goes. About the only reassurance we find in the hope that education will reverse the trend is in France, where, during a comparable period of time, there has been a 9 percent decrease in alcohol consumption per capita, primarily a decrease in wine use (18 percent) offsetting a 20 percent increase in distilled beverage consumption during the same time.(1)

Drinking alcohol is hardly a new idea. "Alcoholic beverages were presumably discovered, rather than invented, in prehistoric times. Their origin is buried in antiquity, though the presence of wine and beer is well attested in archaeological records of the oldest civilizations and in the diets of most preliterate peoples."(2) Very early, man discovered beneficial effects from alcohol and developed a primitive system of production. "The near universality of alcoholic beverages imposes an irresistible inference: Man from earliest times appreciated the mood changing effects of these fluids, regarding them as useful and beneficient. In his attempts to appease or manipulate the divine or magical powers that he perceived as determining his fate—in his early groping for relatedness to the mystical forces of nature—man offered up to these forces something precious"(2) "Alcoholic beverages were obviously more suitable than any others for evoking these moods of release, mystification, and ecstasy that were sought as a way to communicate with and relate to powers that were invincible and beyond knowing. In particular, alcoholic beverages facilitated the rights of orgyastic communicants. Small wonder that Dionysus/Bacchus became the most popular of the gods among the Greeks and Romans." (2)

Much could be said about the continued use of alcoholic beverages in religious and social rituals but it was also secularized into common use because of the pleasure it produced. A quantum step forward occurred in the fifteenth century with the discovery of the process of distillation, producing the "spirit of wine" leading us now to refer to distilled beverages as "spirits."

In our own country, it is worthy of note that total absolute consumption per capita of people 15 and older remained at a reasonably steady rate from 1850 to the mid 1960s, with the exception of a turn-down during the period of Prohibition (3). If one were to comment in the late 1960s about alcohol consumption, one would have said that there has been no significant increase in alcohol use in our country, a rather surprising statement considering many alarming comments about the increasing epidemic. As indicated earlier, one cannot make that statement at this point in time since there has been now a rather precipitous upturn in alcohol consumption in the last few years. (1). Of particular concern is the increase in drinking among minors. (4). At the present time, various surveys, such as the Alcoholic Drinking Practice Survey in 1964 and 1965 and the Harris Survey in 1972–1974 showed that the majority of people 21 and older are drinkers. A 1974 Gallup Survey indicates that 68 percent of the population over 18 drinks. The Harris Survey shows that 58 percent drink more than once a month with 31 percent drinking less than .22 ounces of absolute alcohol a day, 18 percent drinking from .22 to 1.0 ounces of absolute alcohol a day, and 9 percent drinking over 1 ounce of absolute alcohol a day (5).

Since alcohol has been used so long and everywhere, and since a high proportion of our adult population and now a high proportion of our teenage population are drinkers, isn't it time that we looked more into the question of why?

All the research—no matter how sophisticated and detailed—that delineates the evil effects of alcohol tells us very little about why alcohol is so popular. Yet, we continue to fund such research in a desperate hope that knowledge of the ill effects of alcohol will somehow conquer this problem. A physiological model has been developed by Virginia Davis to attempt to explain the phenomenon of addiction—suggesting that there may be the development of an abnormal alkaloid metabolite resulting from effects of acetaldehyde upon catecholamine metabolism and that this metabolite might have some addictive effect (6)—but otherwise we find little work directed towards the "why." While there are varying rates of alcohol consumption and abuse among ethnic groups in this country, social classes, perhaps even personality types, the ubiquitousness of alcohol consumption and the large number of abusers in all groups suggests that alcohol has some overriding quality to it that crosses class lines, ethnicity, genetics, and personality development.

Thus, one is led to the conclusion that alcohol must do something very good, that it is a highly desirable compound for a majority of our population, and that understanding these good and wonderful qualities of alcohol may be much more important to us in trying to comprehend this phenomenon and develop some methods of control.

For example, it is much easier to gather data about the ill effects than the good effects. Marital disruption where alcohol plays a part is more measurable than marriage retention where alcohol has played a part. Are some marriages maintained partially through the influence of alcohol in softening disputes? It is easier to measure the number of children who are in emotional difficulty with drinking parents than it is to find the opposite. Are some parents softer figures as a result of alcohol in their relationship with their children? It is easier to measure how many rapists, exhibitionists, murders, and assaulters committed their acts under the influence of alcohol than the opposite. Does alcohol help some individuals avoid loss of control? Suicide rates are quite high among alcoholics but would this same group of people have an equal or higher suicide rate if alcohol was not available? In no way is this an attempt to dismiss the very serious effects of alcohol abuse, but rather it is an attempt to pose the opposite question to give a proper perspective.

We need to know what the "payoff" is in alcohol use. The greater the payoff or the greater the need for such a payoff, the greater the consumption will be. Thus, we may find that excessive use of alcohol is a result of payoffs that differ only in degree from those received by the normal and controlled drinker. It would be simplistic to say that many people drink because "it's expected" or because there is peer pressure. While this may be a factor, the fact that the drinking continues suggests that once having met "drug X" a love affair is easily developed.

One area of study that may give us more knowledge of the "pay off" is attempting to better understand how we learn early in life to experience strong emotions. Krystal in his theoretical attempts to wed psychoanalytic and neurobiologic findings, suggests that affect intolerance may play a role in addictive disorders.(7, 8, 9) Alcohol may dampen strong affect in some and in others allow some expression by providing "dutch courage." This affect intolerance or the inability even to recognize its existence (alexithymia), may be a regression due to early infantile trauma or could be a biological error in the "affect thermostat" related to endogeneous opiates. If there is a genetic factor predisposing to alcoholism, perhaps this is where it is operative.

Whatever the true state of affairs may be, the drinker experiences alcohol as a very rewarding substance that brings him or her back repeatedly even after hearing of the "bad news." Alcoholics have a very difficult time explaining what alcohol does for them that is so rewarding. This is not surprising since problems of alexithymia and affect intolerance were established in the time of life before a cognitive capacity to explain them had developed.

Lastly, maybe some "good news" needs to be presented for the sake of a balanced view. The Second Special Report to the U.S. Congress on Alcohol and Health of 1974 reports on some interesting data from the Tecumseh Health Study being conducted in Tecumseh, Michigan by the University of Michigan Medical School. It appears that light drinking (four ounces of absolute alcohol a week or less) and heavy drinking do not appreciably affect the coronary heart disease rate in men aged 45–59 as measured by death by coronary or confirmed myocardial infarction. More startling, previously light and heavy drinkers who have stopped have an increase in coronary heart disease rates in the range of 3:1. Even correcting for such issues that would predispose towards coronaries as hypertension, heavy smoking, and high cholesterol, this trend remains.(8). Studies of mortality and alcohol do not show a clear effect of alcohol use. Certainly, heavy drinking is associated with higher mortality. The report summarizes: "All-in-all, the data on general mortality suggests that for amount of drinking, apparently unlike amount of smoking, there may be some kind of threshhold below which mortality is little affected. In the absence of further evidence, in fact, the classical "Anstie's limit" seems still to reflect the safe amount of drinking which has not substantially increased the risk of early death."(9) It is interesting to note that Dr. Anstie defined his "limit" in 1864, and that "limit" is one and a half ounces of absolute alcohol a day which would be equivalent to between three and four ounces of whiskey, a pint of wine, or about a quart of beer.

In summary, Dr. Cohen has made some very important points about "drug X," points that need wide distribution and understanding. This is not in any way a rebuttal or dispute with Dr. Cohen and his facts but an attempt to present a balanced picture. Without the balanced view, we may be disappointed in our attempts to establish effective rehabilitation programs and, more importantly, modifications in drinking styles in our country generally referred to as "responsible drinking."

NOTES

1. Second Special Report to the U.S. Congress on Alcohol and Health. U.S. Department of Health, Education, and Welfare. June, 1974, p. 6.
2. First Special Report to the U.S. Congress on Alcohol and Health. U.S. Department of Health, Education, and Welfare. December, 1971, p. 5.

3. Ibid. p. 15.
4. Second Special Report. pp. 8–12.
5. Ibid. pp. 8–12.
6. Davis, V.E. and Walsh, M.J. Alcohol, amines and alkaloids: a possible biochemical basis for alcohol addiction. Science 167: 1005-1007, 1970.
7. Krystal, H. The genetic development of affects and affect regression. *The Annual of Psychoanalysis*, Vol. II. New York, International Universities Press, 1974.
8. Krystal, H. Affect tolerance. *The Annual of Psychoanalysis*. Vol. III. New York, International Universities Press, 1975.
9. Krystal, H. Alexithymia and psychotherapy. American Journal of Psychotherapy, 33: 17–31, 1979.
10. Second Special Report. pp. 91–96.
11. Ibid. pp. 104–121.

22. Sleep and Sleeping Pills

THE NATURE OF SLEEP

What we call sleep is a composite of at least five distinct, incompletely understood, cyclic states. The newborn spends 18 hours a day in this condition of reduced consciousness. Young adults average about 7 to 8 hours. Aging people require still less, 4.5 to 6.5 hours a day. Rare cases are known of normal people who slept only 3 hours a day for years while maintaining an active and productive physical and mental existence.

The need for sleep is a biologic requirement, but total wakefulness over a two or three-day period has no known harmful effects. The notion that lack of one or two night's sleep is debilitating is without basis. Attention span, reaction time, and physical dexterity may be minimally impaired, but the major debilitating factor is related to the worry about not having slept.

Two kinds of sleep can be identified: REM (rapid eye movement) and non-REM. The latter is divided into four stages, which range from dozing (Stage I) to deepest sleep (Stage IV). The EEG shows a progressive slowing and an increase in amplitude from stages I to IV. Non-REM sleep is associated with little mental or physical activity although muscle tone is retained. By contrast, REM sleep (dreaming or paradoxical sleep) is characterized by a loss of muscle tone except for the eye muscles, which perform scanning movements, apparently in response to the dream content. The

EEG shows even more low voltage, fast wave activity (arousal) than during the waking state. Most dreaming occurs during this period, which occupies about 25 percent of total sleep time. Narcolepsy is a REM state malfunction. The sleep disorders listed in the Table as dyssomnias occur during the non-REM condition.

THE NATURE OF INSOMNIA

The biologic rhythm of waking and sleep is a powerful one, but it can be disturbed by physical, mental or situational factors. The disorder called insomnia is a subjective condition in which the individual complains of chronic, insufficient or poor sleep along with fatigue or even drowsiness during his waking hours. Three kinds of sleep loss can be delineated, but many confirmed insomniacs will complain of all of them.

1. Difficulty in falling asleep (increased sleep latency) is often noted. It consists of spending an hour or hours awaiting the onset of unconsciousness. Mentally overstimulated people tend to have an increased sleep latency. They may require considerable time to unwind, or more correctly, to dampen the activity of their reticular formation, the brainstem area regulating alertness.

2. Broken sleep consists of multiple awakenings during the night with difficulty in falling asleep again. Such people may be oversensitive to external sounds or internal discomforts. However, brief periods of waking during the night are normally observed on all night EEG recordings, especially during major body movements such as turning from side to side.

3. Early morning awakening is a bitter complaint, especially of older persons. Awakening at three o'clock in the morning and not being able to fall asleep again is a distressing event. The time until morning is spent worrying about what happens to people who do not sleep enough. Early morning insomnia is supposed to be a symptom of depression, and it is. Nevertheless, such individuals are not invariably depressed or even insomniacs. Some simply have a physiologic requirement for sleep which is less than average.

A preoccupation about getting insufficient sleep usually turns out to be caused by an individual's expectation that exceeds the minimum daily requirement. One may almost speak of a "sleep neurosis," a compulsive drive to avoid being awake during the night and early morning hours. People tend to be fearful of lying in bed for hours and of ruminating about their troubles, real or imagined. Some elderly people, in particular, seem obsessed with their insomnia and persistently brood about it during their waking hours. Sleep neurosis accounts for many of the problems some people have with sleeping medication and with their well being. Dement estimates that a third to a half of all insomniacs actually get as much sleep as those who are unconcerned about their repose. He recommends an all-night sleep recording as the best treatment for insomnia because it will help convince the patient that his beliefs about not sleeping enough are erroneous.

A fair amount of geriatric insomnia relates to ignorance about the fact that advancing years are accompanied by a normal reduction of the sleep requirement. The overconcern leads to overmedication in the unnecessary effort to achieve the magical eight hours of slumber a night. A further cause of pseudo-insomnia is the fact that aging is associated with a sharp reduction of Stages III and IV sleep. Therefore, the feeling of having slept, really slept, is missing. These people may claim that they never "sleep a wink." In fact, they spend hours in Stages I and II sleep, as proven when all-night electroencephalograms are taken. They may be awake to hear the church bell ring every hour, but in between they doze and nap. Another trick played upon light sleepers is that they may dream they are awake and therefore insist that they never closed an eye.

But true insomnia also exists, and its causes are many. Chronic pain or aches, depression, tension, nocturia, the restless leg syndrome, and nocturnal muscle cramps are a few of its causes. Certain drug dependencies to be described also produce hyposomnia (reduced sleep time). It would be rational to educate the patient if his sleep problem is due to misinformation about sleep requirements. If the insomnia is secondary to some of the causes mentioned, it should be approached by dealing with the cause. Even so simple a matter as providing a mild analgesic at bedtime or avoiding fluid intake after dinner will permit unbroken sleep in those with musculoskeletal aches or with a need to void a number of times during the hours of sleep. When sleep appears to be actually reduced below the physiologic minimum, then measures to correct the situation are indicated. These measures do not consist of automatically prescribing hypnosedatives, at least not initially.

THE ROLE OF DRUGS IN INSOMNIA

Certain drugs that are prescribed or taken by the patient cause insomnia. Amphetamines and weight control drugs are well known to produce a prolonged hyperalertness. Other sympathomimetic agents such as ephedrine or methylphenidate (Ritalin), which may appear in cold remedies or tonics, keep a few people sleepless. Some coffee drinkers who have not acquired tolerance to the stimulant effects of caffeine are kept wakeful by a night time cup of coffee. Sensitivity to the excitatory effect of caffeine is an infrequent, but well documented condition. Even cola drinks, which contain about 50 mg of caffeine, (a cup of coffee or tea has 100–150 mg of caffeine) are overstimulating for the few people. On the other hand over-fatigued people claim that tea acts as a sleep inducer for them.

LSD and other hallucinogens, except cannabis, induce a hypervigilant state that can last for an entire day. Cannabis has a sedative quality, and it is occasionally used at bedtime to produce sleep. Alcohol has a variable effect, producing relaxation and sleep for most consumers, but wakefulness for many others. It is widely used as an hypnotic under non-medical conditions (the night cap).

The withdrawal and CNS depressants results in insomnia. Lowering or eliminating the customary amount of barbiturates or other sedatives is associated with a restless inability to fall asleep. The same is true in the alcohol, the heroin, the methadone, or the minor tranquilizer dependent person. Almost all depressants cause a reduction in REM sleep. When they are abruptly discontinued, a REM rebound occurs, which accounts for the frightening nightmares and chaotic sleep patterns of the DTs and lesser withdrawal syndromes.

A CLASSIFICATION OF THE SLEEP DISORDERS

Insomnia may be the worst treated of ailments because the short term cure is so simple and effective—sleeping pills. A detailed study of the causes is rarely undertaken, and individualized treatment is not often practiced. To indicate how often insomnia is based on causes that can be treated with other than sleeping medication, a table outlining the sleep disorders appears on page 116.

THE MISUSE OF SLEEPING MEDICATION

The casual overprescribing of barbiturate and non-barbiturate hynosedatives can produce a number of undesirable effects. When used rationally, these are valuable agents, but they have some built-in hazards that require a thoughtful approach to the problem of the insomniac.

Sleeping Pills as a Suicide Agent

The barbiturates are a popular manner of attempting or achieving suicide particularly in females. Since insomnia is often associated with de-

Table I-7: The Sleep Disorders

---

1. Insomnia (Hyposomnia)

    1. Physiologic hyposomnia of the aged
    2. Pseudoinsomnia (sleep neurosis)
    3. Primary (idiopathic)
    4. Secondary, due to:

    Physical Factors:

        a. Pain while lying prone or supine
        b. Itching
        c. Angina decubitus
        d. Sleep apnea
        e. Hypermetabolic states as hyperthyroidism and hypoglycemia
        f. Pregnancy
        h. Restless legs syndrome
        i. Impending delirium tremens
        j. Nocturia

    Situational Factors:

        a. Discomfort due to bed, noise, heat, humidity, etc.
        b. Sleeping pill withdrawal
        c. Stimulant ingestion

    Psychological Factors:

        a. Depression
        b. Tension states and worry
        c. Mania
        d. Paranoid states

11. Hypersomnia (Excessive Sleep Patterns)

        a. Idiopathic
        b. Narcolepsy with or without cataplexy
        c. Daytime sedative or tranquilizer use

III. Dyssomnia (Abnormal Sleep Patterns)

        a. Somnambulism
        b. Night terrors
        c. Excessive bruxism and snoring
        d. Enuresis

pression, providing large quantities of these drugs makes self-destruction easy. Even the practice of giving no more than a week's supply is no guarantee that the determined patient will not save up sufficient supplies to acquire a lethal amount. Psychological autopsies of some suicides have revealed that they had obtained sleeping prescriptions from a number of doctors prior to their death. As little as ten 100 mg secobarbital or pentobarbital capsules might be deadly in a non-tolerant person, and even fewer are needed when they are combined with other CNS depressants. The tranquilizers have a much more favorable ratio between the effective dose and the lethal dose.

Sleeping Pills as a Producer of Insomnia

Daily intake of the barbiturates and related drugs eventually produces tolerance. This occurs by an increased induction of those enzymes used in the oxidative breakdown of barbiturates. As the dose is increased to maintain an hypnotic effect, enzyme induction increases. Meanwhile, REM time is chronically decreased. If the drug is suddenly cut off, a severe inability to sleep occurs, and if it finally is achieved, the REM rebound induces vivid nightmares that awaken the patient. Kales has done work that demonstrates that insomniacs on hypnotics for many months or years sleep no better than insomniacs not receiving medication. The removal of someone from moderate or large amounts of sleeping medication should proceed gradually by reducing a dosage unit every few days in order to reduce the severity of REM rebound.

Sleeping Pills as Drug of Abuse

Hypnosedatives are the favored drugs of abuse by the aging adult. Usually, they are legally obtained, but the directions on the bottle are disregarded, and larger than ordinary amounts are consumed. This happens over time as one capsule becomes ineffective, then two, then more. Eventually, very large amounts of these drugs are ingested in the pursuit of sleep, and the person has become physically and psychologically dependent on his medication.

A second form of abuse is the consumption of sleeping pills as daytime sedatives. This develops in individuals with high anxiety levels. A calming effect occurs, but tolerance development soon requires additional amounts. One or two dozen sleeping capsules may be consumed every 24 hours. These people are in a precarious position: a sudden increase of a few more capsules may produce poisoning; on the other hand, a sudden drop in their daily intake may provoke the delirium tremens.

A third type of problem resides in the presence of these agents in the home. Young people have been known to explore the medicine cabinet for mind-altering substances to sample. Medically prescribed sedatives can initiate drug-taking practices which are later continued with black market "sleepers."

THE USE OF SLEEPING MEDICATION

The non-chemical techniques of sleep procurement always should be considered first, and if insufficient, used in conjunction with chemotherapy. The goal is to develop a pattern of conditioned behavior that encourages the onset of sleep. During the hour or two prior to sleeptime a slumber routine should be worked out and regularly followed. The ritual can include hot drinks, warm baths, a set of relaxation exercises, and boring reading materials, according to the patient's inclinations.

It is unnecessary to commence the chemical pursuit of sleep with the sleeping pills. Certain of the antihistamines, muscle relaxants and minor tranquilizers like diazepam (Valium) are as potent and effective as any sleeping potion. Even if the hyposedatives become necessary, they ought to be used intermittently rather than interminably. In the instance of a chronically ill insomniac living in a sleep disrupting situation, short courses of the hypnosedative alternating with an antihistamine, a tranquilizer or a placebo, will avoid the development of tolerance and maintain the effectiveness of the various medications. The swallowing of any pill becomes a part of the conditioning process. At least a part of its effectiveness must be attributed to the conditioning in addition to its pharmacological action. It is difficult to imagine that a single dosage unit of some sleeping medicine taken nightly for years, will still retain a pharmacologic effect. Any of the barbiturates or non-barbiturate sedatives can be used in brief courses of a week or two. The benzodiazepines like Dalmane (30 mg) or chloral hydrate (1.0–2.0 Gm) may be preferred agents because they inhibit REM activity least.

SUMMARY

The diagnosis and treatment of the hyposomnias is a neglected area of medicine. Perhaps this is so because the barbiturate and non-barbiturate sedatives are so successful in procuring sleep over the short term. When used consistently, certain adverse effects can arise. Therefore it is preferable to treat sleeplessness by a search of its causes.

Many complaints of insomnia seem related to the nature of modern urban existence, which ignores biological rhythms and requires that we live by the clock. Other complaints arise from unreal anxieties and misinformation about sleep needs. Re-education and reassurance of the patient may be as helpful as any pill.

REFERENCES

1. Brebbia, D.R., *et al.* Medical Challenge, pp. 62–75, May, 1974.
2. Dement, W.C., *et al.* Sleep Disorders: The State of the Art. Hosp. Practise, 8:57–71 (Nov.) 1973.
3. Kales, A. *et al.* Hypnotic drugs and their effectiveness: All night EEG studies of insomniac subjects. JAMA, 213: 2229, 1970.
4. Kales, A. *et al.* Chronic hypnotic drug use. JAMA, 227: 513–517 (4 Feb) 1974.
5. Marder, L. Non-narcotic drug dependency. Drug Therapy, pp. 87–95, June, 1974.
6. Modell, W. Geriatrics. 29:126–132 (Feb.) 1974.

23. The Barbiturates: Has Their Time Gone?

Seventy-five years ago the first of a long series of barbiturates was introduced. It was barbital (Veronal), and it has since disappeared from the marketplace. It was followed 10 years later by phenobarbital (Luminal), a hardy perennial, still widely used. Hundreds of barbituric acid derivates have been tested, and dozens have been approved for daytime sedation and nocturnal hypnosis.

Dr. Peter Bourne of the White House Office of Drug Abuse Policy and Dr. Robert DuPont, director of the National Institute on Drug Abuse, have recently called for a reevaluation of the barbiturates in the light of their risk/benefit ratio. In particular, the moderately-rapid-acting hypnotic barbiturates are causing concern for reasons to be mentioned.

The very rapid-acting barbiturate anesthetics and the slower-acting phenobarbital are not believed to pose a great social hazard. As an anticonvulsant and inexpensive anti-anxiety agent, phenobarbital retains some usefulness in medicine. However, certain of the disadvantages of the hypnotic barbiturates also applies to it.

WHAT'S WRONG WITH THE BARBITURATES?

After all, since these drugs are effective sleep producers and fairly successful sedatives, why should their medical use be brought into question? The reason why authorities are questioning the large scale use of barbiturates is, in part, their pharmacologic problems, but mainly it is for public health reasons. It is unlikely that their medical use will be prohibited at this time, rather an educational effort probably will be initiated to remind physicians of the possible dangers and side effects involved. The reasons why some public officials are dubious about barbiturates are evident when their drawbacks are examined.

Public Health Problems

1. The barbiturates are the most frequent chemical agents used to commit suicide. Although the number of deaths due to these drugs has decreased since 1970, more than a thousand people succeeded in suiciding with them in 1975.

2. Accidental deaths due to sublethal combinations of barbiturates and alcohol are well known to coroners and medical examiners.

3. These agents are an important part of the street drug scene. No generation gaps exist in the abuse of barbiturates. From grammar school to the geriatric crowd, from overwrought businessmen to bored housewives, the misuse and abuse of barbiturates alone or in combination with other chemicals, are visible problems. The possibility of violent behavior unleashed by these disinhibiting drugs, of accident proneness due to psychomotor clumsiness, and of unplanned overdosage, is real.

4. The barbiturate abstinence syndrome is a serious medical emergency, more life-endangering than that of all other drugs of abuse. Lives are lost despite the availability of skillful medical intervention.

Pharmacologic Problems

In addition to these cogent public health reasons, a number of pharmacologic points must be mentioned, some of which may be very important to physicians and their patients.

1. The barbiturates shift sleep patterns, particularly decreasing total rapid eye movement (REM) sleep. After chronic use, stopping these drugs results in a REM rebound with its nightmarish, sleep-disrupting dreams. Patients then demand re-institution of their sleeping medication, and a difficult management problem over the long term can develop. Over days or weeks tolerance evolves, requiring either increasing amounts of the soporific or a loss of its efficacy.

2. The barbiturates tend to depress the respiratory center. Patients with marginal pulmonary reserve may become apneic when full doses are used for their insomnia.

3. People with acute intermittent porphyria, sometimes an undiagnosed entity, may sustain a life-endangering reaction when they ingest average amounts of a barbiturate. The sudden increase in porphyrin synthesis can cause a paralysis that may include the muscles of respiration.

4. A much more common disadvantage of barbiturate therapy is their induction of hepatic microsomal drug-metabolizing enzymes. The presence of phenobarbital and other barbiturates induces liver enzymes that accelerate the barbiturates' biotransformation into inactive compounds. This is the basis for tolerance development, but the overabundance of available enzymes also causes many other substances to be more rapidly degraded. In some instances the ineffectiveness of certain drugs can be traced to concomitant barbiturate use. A partial list of the various drugs affected by enzyme induction is provided in the Table on page 123.

At times the interference with the action of these drugs is minor, in other cases it can be critical. For example, barbiturates reduce the effectiveness of certain anticoagulants. Therefore, more of the anticoagulant must be given to maintain the desired prothrombin time. When the barbiturate is discontinued (usually on leaving a hospital), the patient might bleed out.

On the other hand, in the instance of phenytoin (Dilantin)—phenobarbital interactions, a very commonly used combination, multiple mechanisms are involved. Plasma levels of phenytoin tend to decrease, but they might also increase or remain unchanged when phenobarbital is added, depending on the net result of multiple enzyme shifts. (1)

The liver microsomal drug-metabolizing enzyme system also involves endogenous substances. Bilirubin is one of the number of naturally-occurring chemicals so affected. This provides the rationale for use of phenobarbital to reduce jaundice in neonatal hyperbilirubinemia.

ARE THERE ALTERNATIVES TO THE BARBITURATES?

There may be no objection to prescribing small amounts of the hypnotic barbiturates for acute stress situations that result in sleeplessness. Their long-term use is much more difficult to justify. Insomnia is such a pervasive complaint that the question immediately arises: What alternatives do we have for dealing with the symptom of insomnia?

Before a pharmacologic response is given, we should remind ourselves that much of what is called insomnia is not primary insomnia. It represents instead:

1. Misinformation about physiologic sleep requirements.

2. Overconcern about insomnia caused by that misinformation.

3. Secondary insomnias due to physical, emotional or environmental factors. These causative factors should be corrected rather than treating the symptom of insomnia.

4. The decreased sleep need, and the loss of Stage IV sleep with the aging of the individual.

The act of falling asleep is conditionable, and sleep rituals, individualized for each person, are helpful. These consist of a sleep routine beginning an hour or so before sleep time, and practiced daily. Physical exercise during the day also has been shown to improve sleep duration.

When hypnotics are needed, it has been shown that 30 mg of flurazepam (Dalmane) is equivalent to 100 mg of pentobarbital in decreasing sleep latency and increasing total sleep time. The advantages of the benzodiazepines over the barbiturates include less tolerance, withdrawal, and REM sleep effects, lesser abuse potential, greatly reduced lethality, essentially no interference with the metabolism of other drugs, and no effects upon the respiratory center in hypnotic doses. The disadvantage is increased cost.

The benzodiazepines have a wide span between their lethal and their therapeutically effective doses. In the cat it is about 200:1 for flurazepam. In the same animal the therapeutic index for pentobarbital is only 9:1. Other species show a similar range of differences in therapeutic indices. Recent reports maintain that when taken without other depressants, accidentally or for suicidal purposes, benzodiazepine overdose does not cause death.(2, 3, 4, 5, 6, 7) Others have mentioned isolated instances of benzodiazepine deaths. (8, 9)

Another possible alternative is chloral hydrate, an hypnotic that even antedates the barbiturates. One gram is not quite as effective as 100 mg of pentobarbital. Chloral has some problems of interference with the metabolism of other drugs including the anticoagulants.(1) The combination of chloral and alcohol may be especially toxic. Tolerance and physical dependence has occurred, and gastric irritation must be expected if it is given on an empty stomach. It disturbs the REM sleep cycle less than the barbiturates.

Certain antihistamines have a sedative quality that can be exploited for sleep induction. Benadryl, Phenergan, Vistaril, and Dramamine are only a few of the antihistamines with sedative properties. Clinical experience has indicated that when average amounts of these drugs are combined with other sedatives a satisfactory hypnotic effect often results.

The other non-barbiturate hypnotics confer no greater safety margin over the barbiturate group. They seem to produce tolerance, dependence, and withdrawal as often as the barbiturates. Overdose is even more difficult to treat because some of these compounds do not dialyze well. They may interfere less than the barbiturates with the biotransformation of other classes of drugs.

If a patient has been stabilized on one of the major tranquilizers or tricyclic antidepressants, another solution to the problem of insomnia may be at hand. All or a large part of these drugs could be given at bedtime and their sedative action exploited. These long-acting drugs will be effective through the next day.

An ideal hypnotic would be one that has a wide safety margin, is effective, does not produce tolerance or physical dependence, and has little or no hangover. The ideal hypnotic is probably a long way off, although improvements over the current ones are to be expected.

SUMMARY

A trend away from the barbiturate hypnotics and toward the benzodiazepines is clearly perceptible in England, Australia, the United States, and other countries. Barbiturate suicide deaths are decreasing, and a rise in benzodiazepine deaths is not taking place.

In Australia and England the suicide rate is falling, but the rate in the

Table I-8: Effect of Barbiturates on Drug Activity

Drug or Drug Class	Altered Drug Effect	Cause
Phenothiazines	Decreased tranquilizer effect	Enzyme induction
Tricylic Antidepressants	Decreased antidepressant effect	Enzyme induction
Anticoagulants	Decreased anticoagulant effect	Enzyme induction
Corticosteroids	Decreased steroid effect	Enzyme induction
Quinidine	Decreased quinidine effect	Enzyme induction
Tetracyclines	Decreased antibiotic effect	Enzyme induction
Phenytoin	Decreased anticonvulsant effect	Enzyme induction
Digitoxin	Decreased cardiac effect	Enzyme induction
Alcohol	Decreased sedative effect during chronic alcohol intake	Enzyme induction
Alcohol	Increased CNS depression during acute alcohol intoxcation	Reciprocal, potentiation, or additive action

United States is rising slightly. It would seem desirable to have the use of barbiturate hypnotics continue to diminish, not only because fewer completed suicides will result, but also for the other reasons outlined.

NOTES

1. Goodman, L. S. and Gilman, A. *The Pharmacologic Basis of Therapeutics,* V edition, Macmillan, New York, 1975.
2. Matthew, H. Letter. Lancet 1:224, 1974.
3. Blackwell, B. Rational drug use in the management of anxiety. J. Pharmacol. Exp. Therap. 9:1-7, 1975.
4. Greenblatt, D.J. and Shader, R.I. *Benzodiazepines in Clinical Practice.* Raven, New York, 1974.
5. McBay, A. J. and Hudson, P. Drug deaths in North Carolina, N.C. Med. J. 35:542-544, 1974.
6. Gray, N.J. and Froede, R.C. Evaluation of deaths from overdose: A clinicopathologic study. Am. J. Clin. Path. 61:778-784, 1974.
7. Holland, J. et al. Drugs ingested in suicide attempts and fatal outcomes, N.Y. State J. Med. 75:2343-2348, 1975.
8. Davis, J. M. and Termini, B. A. Attempted suicide with psychotropic drugs: Diagnosis and treatment. Med Counterpoint 1:43-49, 1969.
9. Dinovo, E. C., et al. Analysis of results of toxicologic examinations performed by coroner's or medical examiner's laboratories in 2,000 drug-involved deaths in nine major U.S. cities. Clin. Chem. 22:847-850, 1976.

24. The Methaqualone Story

Table I-9: Methaqualone

Trade Name	Manufacturer	Methaqualone Dose Unit
Quaalude	Rorer	150 & 300 mg
Sopor	Arnar Stone	75, 150 & 300 mg
Parest	Parke Davis	200 & 400 mg
Optimil	Wallace	200 & 400 mg
Somnafac	Cooper	200 mg
Somnafac Forte	Cooper	400 mg
Dimethacol	Pennwalt	40 mg (with methscopolamine)
Biphetamine-T	Pennwalt	40 mg (with amphetamines)

HISTORY

During the past few years illicit supplies of methaqualone, particularly in the forms known as Quaalude and Sopor have been plentiful in the streets and schools of the United States. They compete with the barbiturates as the most popular "downer" on the black marketplace. A review of methaqualone's brief history may help us learn how to deal with the present situation and to avoid similar drug "explosions" in the future.

During a screening program for antimalarials in India in the early 1950s, methaqualone was found to have hypnotic properties. It was studied here and abroad and found to be a relatively safe hyposedative about half as potent as secobarbital by weight. By 1960 it had been introduced for sale in England, Japan, and other countries. It was sold over the counter and became popular, not only as a sleeping pill, but also among young people for its intoxicating effects. A combination of methaqualone with diphenhydramine, an antihistamine marketed in England as Mandrax, was particularly highly regarded and abused. In Japan, Hyminal, their brand name for methaqualone, quickly became the most abused sedative, especially by juveniles.

Information about the abuse of methaqualone in Japan and England was known to observers of the drug scene in this country when Quaalude was approved in 1965. Nevertheless, the drug was placed in Schedule V (minimal abuse potential) whereas equivalent agents like the barbiturates were in Schedule III (moderate abuse potential). It is difficult to learn why this underscheduling of methaqualone occurred despite the knowledge of problems with the drug in other countries. It is now in Schedule II (high abuse potential). This is also the recommendation of the National Commission on Marihuana and Dangerous Drugs in their recent second report.

> For the most part, the social cost of the nonbarbiturate sedatives is significantly lower than that of the other CNS depressants. However, there is one important exception—methaqualone—which is not even classified as a controlled substance and, therefore, is subject only to a minimal level of control. The risk potential of methaqualone is roughly equivalent to that of the short-acting barbiturates. Moreover, recent evidence indicates that illicit use of this too easily obtained substance is increasingly common among adolescents and has become a significant problem in a number of locations. Since, unlike the barbiturates, methaqualone does not have large-scale medical uses, the Commission recommends that it be placed in Schedule II, along with the amphetamines.

Why was one of the streets in Miami called "Quaalude Alley" during the presidential convention of 1972? Why is there enough Quaalude to "pave the streets in Columbus"? Why are they "carried by the bagful in College Park, Maryland"? According to Daniel Zwerdling of the Washington Post, who wrote an excellent article on the subject, it is the hottest selling sedative hypnotic. Physicians who use it believe that it is safe, causes no hangover, and is not addicting. Unfortunately, none of these are true. In addition to a brisk prescription business, quantities of the drug are supposed to have been stolen from manufacturers, truckers, and wholesalers.

PHARMACOLOGY

Methaqualone is a quinazolone. As such it differs a little from other hypnosedatives chemically. Actually, its central ring is similar to the malonylurea ring of the barbiturates. It is similar to the barbiturates in its physiologic and psychologic effects. Tolerance develops, and cross tolerance to other central nervous system depressants has been verified. An abstinence syndrome identical to that seen upon withdrawal from barbiturates, other sedatives, tranquilizers, and alcohol is being described with increasing frequency. Convulsions, tremors, deliria, nightmares, severe headache, and abdominal pain are seen upon sudden discontinuance of chronic use of 2.0 gram or more a day. Deaths have been mentioned in a few cases. Physical dependence occurs much more than "rarely," as described in the 1973 Physicians Desk Reference. Cross dependence (the ability of a drug to prevent the abstinence syndrome from appearing when it is substituted for the regularly used drug) is present between methaqualone and the drugs with which it manifests cross tolerance.

Death from acute overdose is known. The lethal dose varies. One death occurred following ingestion of 24-300 mg tablets in a non-tolerant person. Much less is needed when methaqualone is combined with alcohol, cannabis, or other depressants. It is metabolized in the liver, and this should be remembered when prescribing it to patients with hepatic insufficiency.

SIDE EFFECTS

Nausea, weakness, and indigestion are not uncommonly associated with methaqualone usage. Numbness and tingling are also mentioned. Rashes occur as frequently as with barbiturates, and they may be of the same type as barbiturate skin reactions. Bone marrow aplasias are most infrequent but can occur. Hangover following a single tablet taken for sleep is complained of occasionally. This consists of feelings of heaviness, grogginess, dizziness, and headache.

TREATMENT

Acute Overdose

As with all sedative overdose states, the maintenance of the airway, with or without assisted respiration as needed, is the prime consideration. Support of the cardiovascular system with cardiac massage and intravenous pressor agents may be required. Gastric lavage is desirable to retrieve any residuals of methaqualone in the stomach. Dialysis, where available, should be considered in persisting coma. The use of stimulants such as picrotoxin, amphetamines, or metrazol are not recommended.

Withdrawal from Chronic Methaqualone Use

Chronic methaqualone use in large amounts resembles similar states induced by sedatives or alcohol. Clumsiness, unsteadiness, impaired psychomotor dexterity, defective judgment, and difficulty in concentrating are usually present. Nystagmus, memory defects, and epigastric pain are other manifestations of chronic usage. Recommendations for the detoxification from metaqualone include the following.

(1) Hospitalize if the patient has been taking six or more dosage units daily. (A methaqualone dosage unit is 200 mg.) Remember that various methaqualone preparations come in 40-400 mg strengths.

(2) For each dosage unit give 100 mg of secobarbital, 30 mg of phenobarbital, or 200 mg of methaqualone. The total dose should be divided into four doses given every six hours during the first 24 hours. Reduce by one dosage unit a day until the patient is drug-free.

(3) If the patient appears intoxicated (nystagmus, slurred speech, ataxia) when the next dose is due, reduce that dose by half. If the patient shows signs of withdrawal (tremulousness, weakness, hypotension, delirium) the dosage of the sedative must be increased.

(4) Convulsions are a special symptom of withdrawal because of their life-threatening property. Intravenous Valium or Amytal should be administered in an effort to control the seizures.

FABLES

A number of newly generated myths are prevalent in the drug subculture about methaqualone, and they should be exorcised.

"Methaqualone Is an Aphrodesiac"
What has been rediscovered is the disinhabiting effect of all depressant drugs upon ego controls permitting sexual acting out under conditions in which it may not have occurred. Sexual performance may actually be impaired by methaqualone.

"Methaqualone Is a Safe Downer Since it is Not a Barbiturate"
Methaqualone is no safer than other sleeping pills. Deaths from overdose, during withdrawal and from alcohol-methaqualone combinations attest to this.

"Methaqualone Is Not Addicting"
It produces all the characteristics of physical addiction: tolerance, withdrawal, and psychological dependence.

" 'Luding Out' is a Safe Way to Get High"
"Luding out" (from Quaalude) is the use of methaqualone and an alcoholic beverage to get "stoned." This can be a dangerous matter because of the addictive effects of the two drugs.

DISCUSSION

This is not the first time that the abuse potential of a new drug has not been recognized. It is not even the first time that claims about the non-addictiveness of sedatives have turned out to be incorrect. Essig has pointed out that gluethemide (Doriden) and methylprylon (Noludar) were considered to be nonaddicting, nonbarbiturate sedatives when they were first offered for sale. Bridge and Ellinwood propose, quite reasonably, that all non-barbiturate sedatives be considered to have an addiction potential unit proven otherwise. Prior to their approval sedatives (and also stimulants and narcotics) should demonstrate evidence of lack of abuse liability, or they should be classified in a schedule which restricts their easy availability.

The widespread misuse of Quaalude confirms the belief that easy availability of mind altering substances creates a consumer market for them. If Quaalude had been properly restricted at the time of its introduction, its abuse would have been negligible. We had an opportunity to avoid a Quaalude epidemic by learning from the experience in other countries, but failed to do so.

REFERENCES

1. Addiction Research Foundation. Methaqualone: A new high. The Journal. 1:12 (Dec.) 1972.
2. Bridge, T. P. and Ellinwood, E. H. Quaalude Alley: A one way street. Am. J. Psychiatry 130:217, 1973.
3. DeAlacron, R. Methaqualone. Br. Med. J. 1:122, 1969.
4. Essig, C.R. Addiction to non-barbiturate sedatives and tranqualizing drugs. Clin. Pharmacol. Ther. 5:334, 1964.
5. Gerald, M. C. and Schwirian, P. M. Nonmedical use of methaqualone. Arch. Gen. Psychiatry. 28:627, 1973.
6. Kales, A. et al. Allnight EEG studies of chloralhydrate, flurazepam and methaqualone. Arch. Gen. Psychiatry. 23:219, 1970.
7. Kato, M. Epidemiology of drug dependence in Japan. Int. J. Addict. 4:591, 1969.
8. Kessell, A. Methaqualone: Efficacy as a hypnotic and side effects. Med. J. Aust. 1:531, 1971.
9. Kunnes, R. Methaqualone addiction. Contemporary Drug Problems. 2:47, 1973.
10. Madden, J. S. Dependency on methaqualone. Br. Med. J. 1:122, 1969.

11. Matthew, H. Methaqualone. Efficiency as a hypnotic and side ef-
     fects. Med. J. Aust. 2:546, 1971.
12. Methaqualone and REM sleep. Med. Letter Drug Ther. 11:65,
     1969.
13. Roman, D. Schizophrenia-like psychosis following Mandrax
     therapy. Brit. J. Psychiatry. 12:619, 1972.
14. Schnoll, S. H. and Fiskin, R. Withdrawal syndrome with metha-
     qualone. J. Psychedelic Drugs. 5:79, 1972.

25. Valium: Its Use and Abuse

Valium (diazepam) is the most frequently prescribed drug in the United States with 75 percent of the prescriptions written by non-psychiatrists.

A number of recent popular articles have been made strong, even alarming statements about the drug. These articles make a review of the proper and improper uses of the agent timely.

PHARMACOLOGY

Valium is a benzodiazepine minor tranquilizer. Other marketed benzodiazepines include: Librium (chlordiazepoxide), Dalmane (flurazepam), Serax (oxazepam), Tranxene (chlorazepate), and Clonapin (clonazepam). Valium has a half life in humans of between 20 and 50 hours. The safety index, that is, the spread between the effective and the lethal doses, is unusually large. The mode and locus of its anti-anxiety activity remains unestablished. A selective depression of limbic system activity is postulated, perhaps through a reduction of serotonin turnover in that area.

THE USES OF VALIUM

The reasons why Valium has come to be so widely used have been summarized by Hollister.(1)

1. *"The benzodiazepines are virtually suicide proof. Massive overdoses have been taken with very little difficulty in managing patients and with no fatalities in the absence of other drugs."*

In cases of death due to suicidal or accidental overdoes of Valium, other depressants almost invariably were ingested along with it. In fact, it is so safe that physicians have been less vigilant than they should have been in their prescription discipline.

2. *"Metabolic tolerance to the benzodiazepines is a lesser problem than with meprobamate or phenobarbital, both of which rapidly induce drug-metabolizing enzymes. Therefore the benzodiazepines are less likely to lose their clinical effects on chronic dosage."*
They also are less likely to interfere with the metabolism of other drugs since they only minimally affect microsomal enzyme induction.

3. *"The duration of action of the benzodiazepines is somewhat longer than that of meprobamate . . . Doses need to be given less frequently, and clinical benefits are more sustained."*

4. *"The relative lack of tolerance to the drug, and the long duration of action make it a poor candidate for the production of physical dependence. Physical dependence occurs, but only with high doses over long periods of time. Well documented cases of withdrawal reactions associated with the clinical use of benzodiazepines have been difficult to find."*
Since Hollister wrote the above, additional instances of withdrawal reactions have been reported.

5. *"Various sleep laboratories report that benzodiazepines produce remarkably little change in normal sleep patterns as compared with most other sedative-hypnotic drugs."*
Although Valium is used primarily as an anti-anxiety agent, it has a number of other valuable actions. It is a muscle relaxant and is employed in various muscular dystrophies and spastic states. As an anticonvulsant, it has some usefulness in *petit mal,* myoclonic seizures, eclampsia, alcohol and barbituate withdrawal states, and in *status epilepticus.* It is not an effective in *grand mal,* psychomotor discharges, and focal seizures.

Many psychosomatic disorders and physical diseases associated with considerable tension are benefited. It is often given as a preanesthetic and prior to cardioversion. Both physicians and street people consider it the drug of first choice for hallucinogen-induced panic and anxiety reactions.(2)
Moderate or severe anxiety, not lesser feelings of unease or discomfort, are indications for such a drug. When the anxious feelings produce an inability to cope, or if they incapacitate the individual, then Valium or

a similar drug may permit the patient to deal with the problem without panicky feelings, a disturbed attention span and ineffective mental functioning.

SIDE EFFECTS AND COMPLICATIONS

Drowsiness, unsteadiness, and weakness are the most frequently reported adverse effects. Paradoxical reactions in which the patient becomes more excited and upset are not frequent but they must be kept in mind, otherwise more Valium will be administered. High doses produce all the signs of intoxication that other CNS depressants induce. This is especially true in the elderly. Patients should not engage in activities requiring mental vigilance while under the influence. The possibility of potentiation of other depressants is a real one, and the concurrent ingestion of alcohol, sleeping pills, and other sedatives should be avoided.

The Food and Drug Administration has released a bulletin report on the risks of minor tranquilizer usage during pregnancy with subsequent cogenital malformations.(3) The studies cited did not provide conclusive evidence that minor tranquilizers caused fetal abnormalities. Some association, however, was suggested.

Meprobamate was the agent most likely to be involved in such defects. Salicylates exceeded the anti-anxiety agents in percentages of malformations by far. The first trimester is the period when the risk is greatest. There is rarely a compelling indication for the use of the minor tranquilizers during early pregnancy. They should certainly be avoided along with all other nonessential drugs during this vulnerable period.

The scientific literature contains many articles mentioning that death following the ingestion of Valium alone does not occur. Suicide attempts with more than 200 times the average does have failed. An Australian article ascribes the substitution of benezodiazepines for barbiturates in prescribing practices as a part of the explanation for the fall in the suicide rate between 1962 and 1973.(4)

In England between 1965 and 1970, 12,354 barbiturate deaths, or 133 per million prescriptions were recorded. During the same period nitrazepam (Mogadon), the major benzodiazepine in use there, accounted for 90 deaths or 11 per million prescriptions. Of the 90 deaths only 36 were ascribed to nitrazepam alone.(5, 6)

In this country recent newspaper and magazine articles mention increasing numbers of fatalities allegedly due to Valium. Which information is correct? The great majority of Valium related deaths are associated with other drugs and alcohol. On the other hand it is hardly likely that any drug, especially a depressant, is absolutely incapable of being lethal at some dosage level.

THE OVERUSE OF VALIUM

Its very popularity makes the question of overuse pertinent. If overuse exists, it is in the area of prescribing Valium for minor anxiety states or for other trivial indications. Lesser degrees of anxiety-tension, which may have been endured in the past, are often treated concurrently by one of the minor tranquilizers because the patient insists upon relief. Relief usually occurs, and when this is reported back to the physician, his subsequent liberal use of the drug is reinforced.

Blackwell makes the point that: "Once the question of overuse is entertained, it often becomes a scapegoat issue in which the physician is blamed for prescribing, the patient for asking, and the industry for advertising. There is little evidence for such viewpoints."(7)

Instead, the enormous use of Valium and other anti-anxiety agents may be a consequence of a recent shift in cultural values. It may no longer be a virtue to "tough out" noxious emotions as in the old days. Using chemicals for relief is currently an acceptable alternative for large segments of the population.

THE MISUSE OF VALIUM

Valium suffers from success. It is so safe and generally effective that physicians prescribe it for lesser indications and without adequate supervision. For example, mild tension or appropriate situational anxiety is not an indication for any psychochemical. The patient should learn how to deal with such unpleasant states by learning appropriate psychological maneuvers.

Prescriptions are written for large quantities of Valium tablets. The physician proceeds to lose touch with his patient for long periods and misses opportunities to readjust or discontinue the medication. Patients with Valium in their medicine cabinet have been known to prescribe it for others who have tension headaches or similar disorders. In busy hospital clinics patients have been able to go from one clinic department to another collecting scripts for Valium and stockpiling, giving away, or selling their supplies.

A few pharmacists use relaxed standards about dispensing Valium because of its large safety factor. It is a Schedule IV drug, and renewals should not exceed five within the six months following the first prescription. This requirement is sometimes not heeded.

THE ABUSE OF VALIUM

For the past 10 years Valium has been a sort of folk medicine in the drug subculture to treat complications of illicit use. Psychedelic takers always had a few tablets around in case of a "bummer." A "speedfreak" might keep a "stash" of Valium to ease the "crash" at the end of an amphetamine binge. Methadone maintenance patients have been known to take their private supply of Valium when anxiety-provoking life situations were encountered. These types of usage, while by no means recommended, evoked little concern.

For the past two years street supplies of Valium have been on the increase. In July, 1975, all benzodiazepines were placed in Schedule IV after a long period of negotiation between the federal agencies and the manufacturers. Insufficient time has elapsed to determine whether nonmedical supplies will be reduced by the rescheduling.

As of November, 1975, Valium ranked second in frequency of "mentions" from crisis center and emergency room reports constituting about 10 percent of all drug "mentions." In general, these were part of a polydrug abuse pattern. Alcohol, and sedative-hypnotics were consumed in combination with Valium.

Valium, alone, in doses of 100 to 500 mg a day produces an intoxicated "high."(8) At such excessive levels over prolonged periods, sudden withdrawal has resulted in an abstinence syndrome similar to other sedatives. A proper question, but one which cannot be answered is: What would the abusers of Valium be using if it were unavailable? If they are using Valium instead of barbiturates the trade-off is not a bad one for them. If, in the absence of Valium, they would use no other drug, then its abuse is certainly undesirable.

In order to ascertain the ratio between legitimate use and the misuse or abuse of some of the common sedatives, the number of prescriptions (per 100,000) has been correlated with the number of "mentions" in the Drug Abuse Warning Network (DAWN).(9) The figures provided below are for the 13 month period ending April 1, 1975.

Sedative	Mention per 100,000 Prescriptions
Valium	41.54
Librium	28.21
Doriden	44.94
Placidyl	72.34

When compared to its level of medical use, the misuse-abuse of Valium appears to be of the same order of magnitude as other common sedatives.

SUMMARY

Drugs should be taken to prevent or relieve illness or to enhance health. Their use to achieve intoxication or avoidance of life and its realities can be harmful psychologically and physically. At what point stress becomes distress is an issue society seems to be re-evaluating at present.

With particular reference to Valium, certain measures ought to be taken to reduce its availability to those who misuse-abuse it.

1. Increased attention should be focused on the safeguarding of supplies from the manufacturing through the distributing and to the retailing levels.

2. Large amounts should not be prescribed, and prescriptions should be written so that the quantity prescribed cannot be tampered with.

3. Doctors should prescribe Valium and similar drugs for proper indications. Patients on these drugs ought to be supervised. Many patients who experience anxiety relief should have their dosage reduced or eliminated under supervision. Most instances of anxiety are not perpetual emotional states.

4. Caution should be observed when prescribing benzodiazepines for dependency-prone individuals.

5. The contents of the medicine cabinet should be safeguarded from juvenile and adult drug seekers.

NOTES

1. Hollister, L. E. *Clinical use of psychotheraputic drugs.* C. C. Thomas, Springfield, Ill., 1973, pp. 129-131.
2. Solursh, L. P. and Clement, W. R. *Use of diazepam in hallucinogenic drug crises.* JAMA 206:644 (Aug 26) 1968.
3. FDA Drug Bulletin. 5 (4):14 (Nov-Dec) 1975.
4. Whitlock, F. A. *Suicide in Brisbane 1956 to 1973: The drug death epidemic.* Med. J. Australia 1:737 (June 14) 1975.
5. Barraclough, B. M. *Are there safer hypnotics than barbiturates?* Lancet, 1:57 (Jan 12) 1974.
6. Editorial: *Barbiturates on the way out.* Brit. Med. J. 3:725 (Sept 27) 1975.
7. Blackwell, B. *Minor tranquilizers: Use, misuse or abuse? Psychosomatics.* 16:28, 1975.

8. Patch, V. D. Letter, New Engl. J. Med. 290:807, 1974.
9. DAWN III. Statistical Summary DEA and NIDA. Contract No. DEA-75-22. IMS America, Ltd., Ambler, Pa. 19002.

26. The Major Tranquilizers

The major tranquilizers are also known as antischizophrenics, antipsychotics, and neuroleptic drugs.

More than 20 years have passed since the first reports appeared on the effect of reserpine and chlorpromazine on psychotic states. Now it is possible to evaluate the impact of these agents and those that have followed them upon chronically psychotic patients and upon the practice of hospital psychiatry.

It would be well to remind ourselves what the practice of psychiatry was like in large, public psychiatric institutions before the 1950s. It is difficult to imagine how it was unless it was experienced. Some large mental hospitals were more reminiscent of Eighteenth Century Bedlam than of modern psychiatry facilities.

The major problem was violence. It was the violence of beat-up patients, beat-up staff, rooms torn apart, windows broken, toilets stuffed, clothes torn off, excrement thrown around, and the all-day dehumanization of everyone. It was a time when knives and forks could not be provided at meals—when curtains, wall pictures, and anything but nailed-down furniture were not possible to use. There were the "pack" rooms with their row on row of slabs and tubs for what was euphemistically called "hydrotherapy." There were the seclusion rooms furnished with nothing but a mattress and an out-of-reach light bulb where a creature, nude or in rags, paced like a caged animal, shouting back at his hallucinations. There was the insulin suite, the lobotomy ward—and always the interminable locking and unlocking of every door in the place. In such a chaotic situation, the "good" patients were the mute, posturing catatonics.

What has brought about the vast changes from the turbulent days of 20 years ago? Why have so many of the megahospitals reduced their census sharply downward or closed entirely? There is no one reason. But those of us who have lived through this striking transformation know how much the neuroleptic drugs have contributed.

Lest there be some misunderstanding on the point, the efficacy of the antipsychotics is not based upon sedative action. Sedatives had been available long before the neuroleptic era, and they did nothing except transiently stupify the raging psychotic. The effect of neuroleptics is more specific. Every effective neuroleptic blocks dopamine receptor sites. Some evidence indicates that disorders like the schizophrenias could be due to excessive firing of dopaminergic neurons in the limbic system.

In retrospect we can speak of a revolution in the management of the psychotic patient. Nobody pretends that the revolution is over.

The drugs that contributed to the revolution were the phenothiazines, the rauwolfia alkaloids, the butyrophenones, and the thioxanthines. Of these, the phenothiazines have played the dominant role. They are the best understood with reference to their effectiveness and their side effects. The phenothiazines must be considered the standard antipsychotic agents against which newer compounds must be compared. The following terms are used synonymously:

Aliphatic phenothiazines—*Thorazine type drugs*
Piperidine phenothiazines—*Mellaril type drugs*
Piperazine phenothiazines—*Stelazine type drugs*
Butyrophenones—*Haldol type drugs*
Thioxanthines—*Navane type drugs*

With one or two exceptions every marketed major tranquilizer seems to be effective. There is no best drug. The best drug is the one that is best known to the prescriber and is best suited to the particular needs of the patient. It is in the area of side effects that these drugs differ significantly. The question that really should be asked is: "Which potential side effects are least noxious or less likely to develop in this special patient?"

It is not possible to deal with all the special considerations and unresolved problems in one essay. Only a few issues of current importance will be dealt with here.

DEPENDENCE ON PSYCHOACTIVE DRUGS

Abuse of sedatives and stimulants in adults is as distressing as the more publicized adolescent drug abuse. Agents such as the minor tranquilizers, sleeping pills, and amphetamines have been prescribed too casually without the supervision they require. As a result susceptible patients have become dependent upon them. In a person with a history of drug or alcohol dependence who needs an antianxiety drug, consideration should be given to those that neither produce a "high" nor induce physical dependence. The major tranquilizers in small doses are appropriate in such instances. No one, for example, becomes "hooked" on the phenothiazines.

The tense and jittery dried out alcoholic will inevitably overuse his sedative-tranquilizer if it provides him with a feeling of being "stoned." He may progress from alcohol dependency to barbiturate or meprobamate dependency and not be a bit better off. Actually, he will be worse off because his physical dependence will be masked, and his withdrawal syndrome will be at least as serious with these agents as with ethanol.

NEUROLEPTIC POLYPHARMACY

There is still no good evidence that two or more neuroleptics do more or are safer than equivalent doses of one. In fact, some drugs interfere with the metabolism of others and difficulties can arise from such interactions. The more drugs prescribed, the greater the chances of error by the patient or other dispensers of his medications.

Anti-Parkinsonian drugs are still being prescribed routinely when major tranquilizers are ordered as a "propylactic" against emergence of the extra-pyramidal syndrome. They reduce blood levels of the neuroleptic, thereby reducing its effectiveness. Studies have shown a majority of patients on anti-Parkinsonian drugs do not need them. Placebos have been substituted without development of a movement disorder in most patients. These agents do not prevent tardive dyskinesia—there is a possibility they increase the likelihood of its development.

After a proper maintenance level of an antipsychotic drug has been reached, a single daily dose will be satisfactory for most patients. If that dose is given at bedtime, sleeping medication will be unnecessary (barbiturates increase neuroleptic breakdown), and some side effects will be slept through. After the patient has reached a satisfactory clinical state, drug holidays can be tried under supervision.

INSTITUTING ANTIPSYCHOTIC THERAPY

A family or personal history of response or idiosyncrasy to specific neuroleptics can be very useful. The metabolic patterns of blood relatives tend to be similar. When time permits, starting with low doses and increasing the dose every few days will avoid certain side effects (hypotension, drowsiness). Eventually, an individualized dosage level will be achieved that can be manipulated up or down according to the clinical need.

Gradual increments in dose are not possible when hyperactivity must be contained *now*. In such instances the starting dose must be measured against the level of hyperactivity while still attempting to keep it on the low side of elderly patients.

The absence of an adequate, baseline, pre-medication physical examination is sometimes regretted. Some of the complications blamed on neuroleptics existed before they were started but were diagnosed only when they were deliberately sought after. Extrapyramidal motion disturbances, skin rashes, non-specific T-wave changes and ocular opacities are picked up after long-term treatment and reported as drug-induced when, in fact, the condition sometimes preceded the pharmacotherapy.

NEUROLEPTICS FOR SPECIFIC CLINICAL SITUATIONS

The hope that certain antipsychotic drugs would be found to be specifically effective in specific psychiatric syndromes has not been fulfilled. Studies have not determined a theoretically appropriate drug to be predictably suitable for certain clinical or computer-derived symptom complexes. When such studies happened to turn out positive, they could not be replicated. There are impressions that the piperazine phenothiazines are preferable for non-paranoid or core schizophrenics, while the piperidines are more suitable for the paranoid, hostile schizophrenics, but exceptions to the impression are numerous.

For the patient who is unreliable about swallowing his prescribed medication, the injectable depot fluphenazines are helpful. These long acting drugs have certain disadvantages, but they are not as important as the certainty that a person who needs the drug, gets it.

Although these agents are called antipsychotics, they are valuable for some patients with psychosomatic disorders. In the small doses used, side effects are minor and they can provide both psychological and autonomic tranquilization.

DRUG-INDUCED PSYCHOSIS, AGITATION, AND DEPRESSION

Although major tranquilizers reduce agitated, psychotic behavior, they can sometimes exacerbate it. A toxic delirial state may develop quite different from the psychosis under treatment. Instances of psychiatric decompensation have been described following the use of long acting, intramuscular fluphenazines. These are akasthisias (restless legs syndrome) with their frightening body image changes and associated anxiety about not being able to control one's body. Intramuscular injections of an anti-Parkinsonian drug will reverse the condition.

Drug-induced depression is well known with reserpine. It also occurs, but less frequently, with other antischizophrenic drugs. In some instances it is due to shifts in the biogenic amines. It may represent the uncovering of a previously submerged affect after the paranoid psychotic symptoms have receded. Certain patients, whose thought disorder has improved to the point that they achieve insight and awareness of how mentally ill they have been, may become depressed. The so-called stimulating neuroleptics can cause depression as often as the sedative neuroleptics such as chlorpromazine.

NEUROLEPTICS AND CARDIAC FUNCTION

Major tranquilizers have a fairly consistent effect upon the EKG, with the piperidine and aliphatic phenothiazines producing the changes more frequently than other groups. The alternations consist of flattening, notching or lowering of the T-waves, sometimes associated with a small lengthening of the Q-T interval. Apparently, these changes are benign and represent a modification of ventricular repolarization. They disappear when the drug is reduced or discontinued. They can be abolished during treatment by co-administering postassium salts. Whether these changes can, in a few instances, lead to a cardiac arrhythmia cannot be conclusively stated. However, in doses exceeding the recommended maximum limit, drugs of the thioridazine group have presumably induced heart block and ventricular fibrillation.

NEUROLEPTICS AND SUDDEN DEATH

Case reports of sudden, unexpected death in patients on large amounts of neuroleptics are recorded in the literature. What is sometimes forgotten is that chronic psychotic patients die suddenly either from physical exhaustion due to their hyperactivity, or from an ill-defined thalamic syndrome associated with extreme hyperpyrexia in the absence of infection. They also are at least as liable to expire from coronary occlusions, subdural hematomas, or other catastrophic illnesses as nonpsychotic individuals.

All of the neuroleptics, but particularly the aliphatic phenothiazines, produce an orthostatic hypotension initially, or when the dose is suddenly increased. In a person with narrowing of the coronary or cerebral arteries, a serious vascular insufficiency may result from the drop in blood pressure on arising. Another possible cause of death is the aspiration of a bolus of food into the airway. A dysfunction of the swallowing mechanism can result from neuroleptics with or without anti-Parkinsonian medication. The occasional convulsion that occurs with neuroleptics may result in asphyxia or severe head injury. Rarely myocardial changes have been described that could conceivably caused death.

SUMMARY

It is evident that we have not utilized the neuroleptics to the full extent of their potential. Dosage schedules during maintenance are not flexible enough, some patients are overdosed, others are undermedicated. The early identification of side effects remains to be learned. Even with the drugs available, better results could be obtained by using the neuroleptics more skillfully and thoughtfully.

27. Tardive Dyskinesia

The following terms are used synonymously:

Neuroleptic—*major tranquilizer or antipsychotic drug*
Aliphatic phenothiazines—*Thorazine type drugs*
Piperidine phenothiazines—*Mellaril type drugs*
Piperazine phenothiazines—*Stelazine type drugs*
Butyrophenones—*Haldol type drugs*
Thioxanthenes—*Navane type drugs*

WHAT IS TARDIVE DYSKINESIA?

Tardive Dyskinesia (TD) is a complication that can occur in connection with the long-term use of the major tranquilizers and certain other drugs. It consists of slow, sometimes stereotyped, involuntary movements of the nose, tongue, mouth or face, and sometimes other parts of the body. The movements are writhing, purposeless, occasionally irregular, and may or may not be continuous. Sucking, licking, lip pursing, blowing, and chewing motor acts are commonly seen.

The patient may not be aware of the glossal-buccal movements. They occur after years (sometimes months, rarely weeks) of treatment with neuroleptic drugs. Not all dyskinesias are drug-induced. They also occur spontaneously as one of the movement disorders of the extrapyramidal syndrome.

WHO ARE VULNERABLE TO THE COMPLICATION?

Elderly women with senile or other brain impairment, or who have been on large doses of certain neuroleptics for long periods of time are most likely to develop TD. All ages and sexes, however, can be involved —including children.

WHAT IS THE EARLIEST SIGN OF TD?

Abnormal tongue movements may be the first evidence of the syndrome. Therefore, patients on extended treatment with neuroleptics should be routinely examined for this symptom. The tongue should not be protruded for examination.

IS THERE A RELATIONSHIP BETWEEN THE DRUG-INDUCED EXTRAPYRAMIDAL SYNDROME (EPS) AND TD?

Yes. People who have had Parkinsonism or other manifestations of the EPS at the onset of drug treatment, or those who would have had the EPS if they had not been treated with prophylactic anticholinergic medication, are liable to develop TD later. Treatment of the EPS with anticholinergic drugs does not reduce the possibility of TD setting in at a later date. In fact, there are opinions to the contrary.

DO ALL THE MAJOR TRANQUILIZERS CAUSE TD?

Yes, but some cause it more frequently than others. The piperazine phenothiazines, the butyrophenones and the thioxanthines will induce TD and the EPS more frequently than the aliphatic and piperidine phenothiazines.

HOW FREQUENTLY DOES TD OCCUR?

The American College of Neuropsychopharmacology estimates that 3 to 6 percent of a mixed psychiatric population on neuroleptics will show evidence of TD. Chronic, older patients may have a 20 percent rate. Reports on TD in the literature vary from 0 to 86 percent. This wide variance depends upon one's diagnostic sensitivity, the nature of the population reported upon, the drugs used and the dosage levels employed.

HOW LONG DOES TD LAST?

It is frequently diagnosed soon after lowering the dose or after discontinuing the causative drug. It may subside after a few months, or it may be permanent. Much seems to depend upon the susceptibility of the individual patient, and the intensity of the dopamine receptor blockade (to be explained later).

ARE THERE ANY SPECIAL FEATURES OF THE TD IN CHILDREN?

Yes. A condition called WES (Withdrawal Emergent Symptoms) has been described in schizophrenic children whose neuroleptic medication was discontinued. Involuntary movements resulted in half of them. They were most pronounced in the extremities, trunk and head. Ataxia, incoordination hypotonia and tremors of all extremities were observed. The WES disappeared after reinstitution of neuroleptics. The facial symptoms, more common in adults, are rare in children who can manifest choreiform movements of the entire body. The condition appears even after short-term treatment of the children, but the course is more benign.

The WES seems to be the same syndrome as TD with a somewhat different localization since it occurs in growing children with their special neurophysiological makeup.

HOW DO THE NEUROLEPTIC DRUGS WORK IN PSYCHOSES?

In order to understand the way tranquilizing agents may cause TD, something must be said about their presumed mode of action in the psychotic states. The firing of nerve cells across the microscopic gap (synapse) between them is accomplished by a chemical (neurotransmitter) flow.

Each neuron has a specific neurotransmitter (also called a biogenic amine). In the brain some of the more common biogenic amines are acetylcholine, serotonin, norepinephrine, and dopamine. Dopamine and norepinephrine resemble each other chemically. Dopamine, in fact, is a precursor of norepinephrine.

The current theory on the biochemical basis of schizophrenia is that the limbic system, and more specifically, the nucleus acumbens, a center for emotionality, is involved. Neurons in the region of the nucleus acumbens are dopaminergic; that is, dopamine is their transmitter chemical. An excessive firing activity of neurons in this region might lead to defective emotional responsivity.

The causes of such malfunction might be a genetic vulnerability, severe psychological trauma during childhood, current stress, or what is more likely, combinations of these factors. The emotional disturbance, in turn, may lead to disorders of thought and perception resulting in what is called schizophrenia.

All the effective neuroleptic drugs act by blocking the receptor sites for dopamine on the postsynaptic neuron, the nerve cell receiving the impulse from the presynaptic neuron. No doubt feedback mechanisms to the presynaptic neurons have important effects on dopamine synthesis there. In effect, then, dopaminergic transmission in this area is blocked and schizophrenic symptoms are reduced or eliminated.

WHY DO NEUROLEPTIC DRUGS PRODUCE THE EPS?

In addition to producing a dopamine receptor blockade in the limbic system, other dopaminergic nerve fibres elsewhere in the brain are affected. The caudate nucleus of the extrapyramidal tracts also contains dopaminergic cells and their blockade causes the movement disorders known as the EPS days or weeks after treatment starts. The EPS tends to disappear as treatment continues, probably because tolerance to the dopamine blockade in the caudate nucleus occurs.

The reason why anticholinergic drugs are beneficial in the EPS is because cholinergic activity in the caudate nucleus opposes dopaminergic activity. When dopaminergic activity is blocked, cholinergic activity dominates, resulting in the EPS. When cholinergic activity is also blocked by anticholinergic medication, the balance between the two systems is re-established and the EPS improves.

WHY DO NEUROLEPTIC DRUGS PRODUCE TD?

If the dopaminergic blockade in the caudate nucleus is intense over a long period of time, structural damage to the neurons may ensue. It is a phenomenon of nerve cell physiology that injuring a nerve cell can make it hypersensitive to the injuring agent. The damaged postsynaptic cells become highly sensitive to dopamine. While the major tranquilizer is still being taken, the dopamine blockade it produces will suppress the sensitivity because no dopamine is entering the cell at the receptor site. But when the drug is reduced or discontinued, then even small amounts of dopamine produces excessive firing and that results in the clinical picture known as TD. It is for this reason that reinstituting treatment with the neuroleptic may improve the TD.

WHAT IS THE TREATMENT FOR TD?

Treatment of TD remains a problem. The reinstitution of major tranquilizer therapy may produce a remission but that may mean that the patient is locked into the drug for a lifetime. Reserpine and tetrabenazene deplete brain dopamine and they have been effective in a few cases. Amantadine (Symmetrel), an antiviral drug that is claimed to have an effect in some cases of the EPS, has been recommended. Deanol, a cholinergic drug, also is considered helpful. Diazepam and lithium have been used with variable success. Anti-Parkinsonian drugs and L-dopa are contraindicated since the former increases dopamine dominance and the latter increases dopamine levels.

WHAT ABOUT THE PREVENTION OF TD?

Consideration might be given to the use of a piperidine-type phenothiazine in a patient who will need long-term treatment, and who is a good candidate to develop TD (elderly women or children). All patients on chronic neuroleptics should receive the lowest dose that provides the most symptom relief. Drug holidays have been suggested but these should be under supervision so that therapy can be restarted if the patient begins to slip. As soon as the diagnosis is made, the major tranquilizer should be stopped to determine whether the condition will subside.

SHOULD NEUROLEPTIC THERAPY BE WITHHELD BECAUSE OF THE POSSIBILITY OF PERMANENT TD DEVELOPING?

No. The major tranquilizers are valuable drugs in the treatment of psychotic states. A patient who needs them should not be denied the opportunity to improve that these drugs provide. TD and other complications can occur, but consider the alternative. A good knowledge of the drug's effects and side effects and careful supervision of the patient will avoid many of the adverse reactions to these drugs. New drugs are being tested that appear to be effective anti-psychotic agents, and that are unlikely to produce TD.

SUMMARY

Tardive dyskinesia following the use of antischizophrenic drugs has been known for the past 10 to 15 years. It is a distressing condition, not so much to the patient as to the family, friends, and physician. The abnormal movements may disappear after a few months, or they may persist. Treatment has been only occasionally satisfactory. Skilled and devoted medical practice will prevent tardive dyskinesia except in patients highly sensitive to the neuroleptic.

ADDITIONAL READING

1. Anonymous: *Neurologic Syndromes Associated with Antipsychotic-Drug Use.* N. Engl. J. Med. 289:20-23 (July 5) 1973.
2. Cole, J. O. and Stotsky, B. A.: *Improving Psychiatic Drug Therapy. A Matter of Dosage and Choice.* Geriatics 29: 74-78 (June) 1974.
3. Crane, G. E.: *Clinical Psychopharmacology in its 20th Year. Late, Unanticipated Effects of Neuroleptics May Limit Their Use in Psychiatry.* Science 181: 124-128 (July 13) 1973.
4. Crane, G. E. and Smetts, R. A.: *Tardive Dyskinesia and Drug Therapy in Geriatric Patients.* Arch. Gen. Psy. 30: 341-343 (Mar.) 1974.
5. Hussey, H. H.: *Editorial: Tardive Dyskinesias. JAMA 228: 1030* (May 20) 1974.
6. Jacobson, G., et al: *Tardive and Withdrawal Dyskinesia Associated with Haloperidol. Am. J. Psy. 131: 910-912 (Aug.) 1974.*
7. Klawans, H. L., et al: *Neuroleptic-Induced Tardive Dyskinesias in Nonpsychotic Patients.* Arch. Neurol. 30: 338-339 (Apr.) 1974.
8. Simpson, G. M .: *Tardive Dyskinesia.* Br. J. Psy. 122:618 (May) 1973.
9. Snyder, S. *et al: Antischizophrenic Drugs and Brain Cholinergic Receptors.* Arch. Gen. Psychiat. 31: 58-61, (July) 1974.

28. The Abuse of Amphetamines

THE AMPHETAMINES AND THEIR STREET NAMES

Amphetamine is phenylisopropylamine, the racemic mixture being Benzedrine and the d-isomer being Dexedrine. Methamphetamine (Methedrine, Desoxyn) and phenmetrazine (Preludin) are two variants of the amphetamine structure.

Pep pills or "uppers" are also known as "bennies," "dexies," or "bombitas." Methedrine is called "meth," "speed," "crank," "splash," or "crystal." There is a tendency to call all amphetamines "speed" at present.

TYPES OF ABUSE

Many kinds of amphetamine misuse and abuse exist.

Sporadic Use of Average Amounts

The occasional use of amphetamines to remain alert or enhance one's performance is widespread. Students cramming for exams, drivers on extended non-stop trips, athletes attempting to excel, and military personnel on prolonged operations are some of the groups involved. Amphetamines do seem to improve the performance of tired individuals who are involved in prolonged tasks if the drug does not make them jittery. Skilled judgments may be adversely affected. On rare occasions hallucinatory episodes and sudden death (due to hyperthermia?) have occurred even at small dosage levels.

Average Oral Doses Used Indefinitely

Some people who have been given amphetamines for fatigue, depression, or obesity by doctors or friends continue to take them indefinitely. They claim that attempts to decrease or eliminate the medication result in a lethargic depression, or that they are unable to function without their stimulant. Some feel quite guilty about being dependent on their pills. The dose range is 20-40 mg daily.

Large Oral Doses

Certain patients started on amphetamines, or those who enjoy their exhilarating effects find that tolerance develops, and increasing amounts must be taken in order to obtain a stimulating or euphoric effect. The dosage increase may take place over a few days or a few months. Eventually, they level off the dosage at 50-150 mg daily.

Large Inhaled or Injected Doses

Individuals who relish the amphetamine "high" discover that "snorting" or injecting the substance intravenously provides a faster and more intense "flash." Another favored technique is "balling" the material, i.e., instilling it into the vagina prior to intercourse. For these purposes blackmarket crystalline "crank" is preferred, perhaps because the impurities add to the initial "rush." During a "speed run" as much as 1,000 mg may be injected intravenously in a single dose, and up to 5,000 mg injected in a 24 hour period. This is the "speedfreak" phenomenon.

In Combination with Barbiturates

Certain individuals feel too tense from amphetamines alone and prefer combinations with a sedative. Dexamyl (purple hearts) is an example of a marketed preparation that combines Dexedrine and Amytal.

In Combination with Heroin

The original "speedball" was cocaine and heroin. The poor man's "speedball" is methamphetamine and heroin injected together. Another pattern of use is to employ heroin to come down from an amphetamine binge. When the "speed" scene becomes too depleting, some users go over to exclusive heroin use.

THE "SPEED RUN"

Five years ago a sudden sharp increase in the "mainlining" of astonishing amounts of methamphetamine occurred. Since it was a relatively new practice in this country, it is this phenomenon that will be described here.

The "speedfreak" starts his "run" with small amounts of methamphetamine or other stimulants, gradually increasing the dose. He values the immediate "rush" or "flash" even more than the prolonged feeling of being hyperalert, powerful, and full of energy. When he notices that he is coming down, he re-injects. During the "speed run" he is disinclined to eat or sleep and ignores ordinary body care. Ten pounds or more may be lost in a week.

During the "run" he is almost invariably overactive and impulsive, and demonstrates defective reasoning and judgement. Eventually he develops paranoid ideas, usually of being persecuted, and his suspiciousness is well known in the drug culture. In the beginning he retains insight into the delusional nature of his thinking and does not act upon his false ideas. Appropriate hallucinations can accompany the delusional system. The combination of hyperactivity, poor impulse control, and paranoid delusions make for irrational behavior during which he may hurt himself or others in his path. Some inexplicable, bizarre accidents and homicides are traceable to people with amphetamine psychoses. The amphetamine psychosis mimics paranoid schizophrenia and can occasionally last well beyond the period of amphetamine indulgence. The thought disorder is most resistant and can be elicited long after the hallucinations have cleared.

Certain other aspects of amphetamine intoxication are remarkable. Stereotyped behavior is often observed. This may consist of skin picking, bead stringing and unstringing, pacing or interminable chattering. It is worth noting that all mammalian species will perform sterotyped activities under the influence of amphetamines.

When the dosage is raised too rapidly, a peculiar condition, called "overamped" on the street, occurs. The individual is conscious but unable to move or speak. He has an extremely rapid pulse, elevated temperature, increased blood pressure, and, occasionally, chest distress. Death due to overdosage is infrequent in the tolerant person.

Orgasm and ejaculation are delayed or impossible to achieve. As a result marathon sexual activity is described by some "speedfreaks." Others report a complete absence of sexual interest.

After a few days or a week of a "speed" binge, the person becomes so exhausted or so delusional that he or his friends decide that he must "crash." The withdrawal snydrome to amphetamines consists of a long period of sleep, a marked depression, apathy, a variety of aches and pains, and a ravenous appetite. The depression is so severe that it may initiate another "speed run." Reinjection of amphetamines relieves the distressing symptoms.

SIDE EFFECTS OF CHRONIC HIGH DOSES

Cerebral hemorrhages and cardiac arhythmias are infrequent complications of the amphetamine hypertension and tachycardia. A necrotizing angiitis has been described in "speedfreaks." Good evidence for parenchymal liver damage and brain cell injury is at hand. The high caloric requirement due to hyperactivity, along with anorexia combine to produce malnutrition or cachexia in consistent speed users. Severe abdominal pain mimicking an acute surgical abdomen is an occasional diagnostic problem. Dyskinesias, including jaw grinding, have been seen. The diseases of unsterility are added to those of the drug when needles are used so that the liver disorder may have features of a viral and toxic hepatitis.

The paranoid state comes, sooner or later, to all high dose users. After its appearance, it will predictably develop during subsequent "runs." The tendency is for the paranoid state to come forth earlier and earlier if amphetamines continue to be used. Eventually the first dose will precipitate the paranoid reaction. Some "speedfreaks" will stop using because of the excessive suspiciousness and unpleasant delusions of persecution.

Suicide may occur during or after the amphetamine "run." The experience can become terrifying and overwhelming. The person's controls are reduced, and he may impulsively attempt and complete suicide. A greater risk exists during the withdrawal phase where the depression is so prolonged and unrelieved that suicide is elected.

TREATMENT OF AMPHETAMINE ABUSE

Phenothiazines are physiologic antidotes with chlorpromazine the most frequently used antidote. Phenothiazines should not be used if anticholinergic drugs were taken in addition to amphetamines. Street amphetamines are unreliable in quality, therefore barbiturates or certain tranquilizers are safer under ordinary conditions. Diazepam in initial doses of 10-20 mg intramuscularly or orally is a satisfactory sedative. For the depression associated with amphetamine withdrawal the tricyclic antidepressants have been used. It is not necessary to gradually reduce the dose of amphetamines.

The long-term management of the chronic amphetamine abuser is difficult, and relapse is frequent. Group therapy that includes "ex-speed-freaks" has had some success. The chronic amphetamine abuser tends to be a disturbed person who has treated his mood disorder with a highly rewarding euphoriant. His defective life style and inadequate coping mechanisms must be restructured if he is to remain drug free.

TRENDS

1. Federal legislation has tightened controls over amphetamine manufacture, transportation, and distribution, but street supplies remain plentiful.
2. A few county medical societies have asked their members to discontinue prescribing amphetamines except for narcolepsy and hyperkinetic children.
3. Efforts to provide a drug that depresses the appetite regulatory centers without producing central stimulation have been partially successful. We can look forward to a non-stimulating appetite suppresant.
4. The mechanism of action of the amphetamines has been tentatively clarified. They increase the release of catecholamines into the synaptic cleft and retard their reuptake back into the neurone. A so-called false transmitter has been isolated from the spinal fluid following amphetamine administration. It is p-hydroxynorephedrine, but its significance remains to be determined.
5. A recent study indicates that children given amphetamines until adolescence for hyperkinesis do not tend to abuse amphetamines when they grow up.

SELECTED REFERENCES

1. Ellinwood, E. H. and Cohen, S. Amphetamine abuse. Science 171:420, 1971.
2. Ellinwood, E. H. Assault and homicide associated with amphetamine abuse. Am. J. Psychiat. 127:9, 1971.

3. Edison, G. R. Amphetamines: A dangerous illusion. Ann. Int. Med. 74:605, 1971.
4. Halpern, M. & Citron, B. P. Necrotizing angiitis associated with drug abuse. Am. J. Roentgen, 111:172, 1971.
5. Bell, D. S. The precipitants of amphetamine addiction Brit. J. Psychiat. 119:171, 1971.
6. Lynn, E. J. Amphetamine abuse: A "speed" trap. Psychiat. Quart. 45:92, 1971.

29. Ritalin and Preludin

Ritalin and Preludin have in common only that they are both stimulants, they are manufactured by the same pharmaceutical firm (Ciba-Geigy), and they are capable of being abused. Their abuse history is quite different, as are the indications for their use, despite many pharmacological similarities.

RITALIN

Ritalin (methylphenidate) is a stimulant widely used in medicine for mild depression, minimal brain dysfunction (MBD) in children, narcolepsy, and sedative-induced lethargy. It is manufactured in 5, 10, and 20 mg tablets, and in a multiple dose vial containing 100 mg. Ritalin would be just another medically useful drug were it not for two problems that have become associated with its availability.

1) The question whether Ritalin (and amphetamines) are being over-prescribed for MBD and related states.

2) The abuse of Ritalin by drug dependent people.

Ritalin and MBD

The idea that stimulants can be helpful in a condition manifested by hyperactivity seems paradoxical. It may be that the hyperactivity is a release phenomenon. When inhibiting neuronal pathways which should dampen the hyperkinetic activity are stimulated, quieting would occur.

The controversy revolves around the issue whether overactive children without definite neurological deficits should be treated with stimulants. In a few schools more than 10 percent of the pupils have been diagnosed as MBD and given medication.

The actual incidence may be about 3 percent. Those who liberally use stimulants for MBD assert that (1) a therapeutic trial does no harm, and definite behavioral improvement is noted within a few days in those who will respond favorably, and (2) children with hyperkinetic activity, reduction in attention span and learning decrements may not show "hard" neurological signs, and therefore cannot be diagnosed only by neurological and laboratory examinations. Those who are conservative about placing a child on stimulants until he reaches puberty suggest that (1) many of these children are overactive because of personality or situational factors (2) giving children medication when it is not clearly indicated fosters the idea that behavior in general should be "normalized" and controlled, and (3) the youngsters may be conditioned to use psychotropic drugs in years to come. On the last point one survey found that youngsters who were given phenobarbital for epilepsy or stimulants for MBD were no more prone to abuse drugs in adult life than a group not required to take medication.

Ritalin may be the stimulant of choice for MBD since it produces less jitteriness, anorexia, and insomnia than the amphetamines. Tranquilizers are preferred for some patients, and these may be one of the phenothiazines or one of the benzodiazepines. It is generally agreed that the syndrome becomes manifest at about 5 years of age and recedes at 12.

The conclusions of the Conference on the Use of Stimulant Drugs in the treatment of Behaviorally Disturbed Young School Children (January, 1971) were as follows.

1. Diagnosis should be by a doctor, and the patient closely supervised. When carefully diagnosed, the hyperkinetic child can be brought to an improved level of attention, learning, and social abilities. There is no evidence that the use of amphetamines in this age group leads to subsequent addiction in later life.

2. Diagnosis should take into account the child's environment and family relationships as well as other factors. Many children suffer from problems with behavior control attributable to hunger, emotional stress, poor teaching, and overcrowded classrooms. *The use of amphetamines is clearly not called for in these cases.*

3. No stigma should be attached to a child who has been prescribed medication for behavioral disorders.

4. While it is entirely proper for school personnel to draw parents' attention to an individual child's behavior problems in school, teachers and school administrators should scrupulously avoid any attempt to

force parents to accept any particular treatment. With parental permission they should collaborate with the physicians in the total program for the child.

5. Manufacturers of stimulant medication should promote their products solely through the appropriate medical channels and should not seek the endorsement of such products from school personnel.

6. No child should be given the responsibility for taking his own medication. In most cases it is not necessary to bring the drug to school. The same precautions should be taken against the misuse of the medication as with all stimulants.

7. While there is no need for sensational alarm about the health or safety of the child under careful, supervised treatment, abuses and misuses must promptly be called to the attention of the proper authorities. Physicians, educators, parents, and the news media share this responsibility.

The Abuse of Ritalin

The abuse of Ritalin has been sporadic until recently. Just over eight years ago the Pacific northwest, particularly Seattle and Portland, had an unusual spread of high dose, oral and intravenous abuse. This local epidemic may have begun with the proselytizing activities of a single individual who obtained access to a large supply.

Supplies were acquired by forging stolen prescription blanks, robbing drug stores and hospitals, and "ripping off" jobbers and wholesalers by shipment diversion and warehouse theft. Black market Ritalin was never found to be privately manufactured.

Eventually a number of cities across the country reported Ritalin abuses. The effects of large amounts of Ritalin are similar to those of the amphetamines. An initial "rush" is followed by an exuberant feeling of well being that terminates in a droopy "down," the depressed state acting as a goad to inject more Ritalin. As with the amphetamines, paranoid states and impulsive overactivity can develop.

One special problem for the intravenous user is that Ritalin is manufactured using talcum as a filler and binder. Talc is an insoluble, irritant crystal which can produce abcesses when it is injected under the skin. If it is instilled into a vein, the lung capillaries prevent its further passage. Pulmonary abcesses and fibrosis are occasional results of multiple injections, and lungs have had to be removed for large abcesses. A septic thrombophlebitis adds to the danger of lung infection. A dozen deaths are supposed to have occurred in the Seattle area during 1971 due to the use of intravenous Ritalin. Ritalin has been combined with heroin and methadone to produce a more intense high. There is some anecdotal evidence that it prolongs the action of heroin.

Now that Ritalin, Preludin, and the amphetamines have been transferred to Category II (requires a narcotic-type prescription which cannot be renewed) their availability for non-medical use should be reduced. Nevertheless sporadic cases and an occasional focal outbreak of abuse can be expected.

PRELUDIN

Preludin (phenmetrazine) is a stimulant almost exclusively prescribed for weight control. It is marketed as a 25 mg tablet and as 50 and 75 mg Endurets (prolonged action tablets). Sweden's experience with Preludin and other central stimulants may be worth recounting since it illustrates certain points in the epidemiologic spread and in the evolution of a drug abuse epidemic.

Stimulant Abuse in Sweden

Amphetamine abuse was recorded in Sweden only a year or two after it was introduced in 1938. At first it was sold over the counter, but when reports of dependency were recorded, it was placed on the prescription list. By 1944 it was necessary to restrict it on the same basis as narcotics. This measure was only temporarily helpful. By 1959 some 33 million doses were prescribed despite its restricted status. During 1965-1967 an experiment that permitted prescribing of legal amphetamines for those dependent upon them ended in failure without any benefit to the users, and with additional people becoming involved. Finally, in 1968 prescriptions for central stimulants could be filled only if they were approved by a special commission. This has led to a marked reduction of stimulant prescribing with only a few dozen narcoleptic or MBD patients being approved for use of the drug.

Preludin was introduced in 1955, and it rapidly became preferred by those abusing stimulants. By 1959 it was classed with the narcotics, and the requirement for approval of prescriptions by a commission followed 10 years later. These restrictions were ineffective. The drug was smuggled in from other countries where it was easily available. Illicit laboratories are also producing the material. Preludin remains the drug of preference, but all stimulants were used, including Tenuate (diethylproprion). The Swedish experience indicates that all stimulants have an abuse potential.

The pattern of Preludin abuse consists of oral use of above average amounts initially with some of those involved escalating to intravenous injections. Swedish sociologists who have attempted to understand the nature of the outbreak relate that a single individual developed and popularized the intravenous use of Preludin tablets. The tablets are dissolved and strained, or black market phenmetrazine powder is used. Eventually, hundreds or thousands of milligrams are injected at a time. In 1968 an estimated 8,000 to 10,000 Swedish intravenous stimulant abusers existed. Since then the numbers may have stablized or decreased following intensive control and treatment measures. Sweden has a population of eight million.

Lessons from the Swedish Experience

Although Preludin has been occasionally misused in other countries, only in Sweden did it become a serious public health problem. It may be worthwhile to examine the causes of this situation.

Preludin abuse was preceded by amphetamine abuse in Sweden. Thus, a non-medical market for stimulants had already existed when Preludin was introduced. The ease of obtaining Preludin when amphetamines were more tightly controlled made it popular. It is doubtful that Preludin is a better euphoriant than dextroamphetamine, in fact it is less so on a weight basis.

It seems that the ability of a drug dependent group to find new substances when their favorite drug comes into short supply is phenomenal. If interdiction is to be of any value, all comparable substances in the class must be interdicted. Furthermore, control of illicit materials must accompany the control of those originating in medical channels.

The increasing legal restrictions on Preludin improved the situation only temporarily. As medical supplies were eliminated, black market supplies took their place. We should learn from this experience that when a demand exists supplies will somehow become available. The legal countermeasures were necessary and desirable, but they could not be expected to solve the problem in themselves.

An experiment to institute "amphetamine maintenance" in Sweden was a catastrophe and had to be abandoned. The thought behind providing amphetamine abusers with the drug was that the profit factor would be eliminated, and pure material would keep the complications of unsterile injections down. Unfortunately, the patients on the study abused the situation. New amphetamine abusers were generated when patients sold part of their supplies, and the project collapsed. It has become evident that when a maintenance program is not carefully supervised, or when illicit supplies are easily available, the maintenance program may do more harm than good. The American "morphine maintenance" of the 1920s failed because of sloppy administration. The "British system" of "heroin maintenance" failed and had to be completely redesigned.

Our current methadone maintenance program will fail unless it is carefully administered, and supplies of heroin are substantially curtailed.

The intravenous use of Preludin apparently originated from a single abuser. Many epidemics in communities that never had problems with drugs have started from a single focus. It is almost impossible to be sufficiently alert and respond rapidly enough to forestall an outbreak. Nevertheless, this would be an ideal way to deal with the situation.

Some of the factors we assume to be causative in drug abuse do not apply to the Swedish situation. Sweden has no poverty, no ghettos, no race problem, and no wars for the past 170 years. There is little crowding, the population is fairly homogeneous, and political or social repression does not exist. Why should Sweden have a problem with stimulants, and more recently with other drugs?

RECENT REFERENCES

1. Hearings: Subcommittee to Investigate Juvenile Delinquency. Amphetamine Legislation, July 15 & 16, 1971. U.S. Government Printing Office, Washington, D. C., 1972.
2. Inghe, G. The present state of abuse and addiction to stimulant drugs in Sweden. In, Abuse of Central Stimulants. Sjoqvist, F. and Tottie, M. Almqvist & Wiksell, Stockholm, 1969.
3. Lucas, A. R. and Weiss, M. Methylphenidate hallucinosis. J.A.M.A. 212:1079, (Aug. 23) 1971.

30. On the Smoking of Cigarettes

The introduction of tobacco into the Old World from the New unleashed social and political reverberations that have continued until today. Almost five hundred years ago the plant was brought to Spain from the West Indies. It was quickly put to use as a miracle medicine and as a recreational agent.

Because of its exotic origin in the newly discovered Americas, tobacco was considered a panacea for many diseases. But its medical usage waned by the seventeenth century, except for an alleged efficacy during cholera epidemics. Meanwhile, the social use of tobacco as snuff and pipe tobacco spread rapidly throughout Eurasia, usually in connection with wars and maritime activities. The upper classes were usually the first to acquire the habit, but it soon was taken over by all classes.

It should not be assumed that the dissemination of tobacco use occurred without considerable opposition. The arguments were even more heated then than those at present. Rulers and religious leaders distrusted its alien origin. There was concern that the tobacco houses were becoming centers of political unrest. In Turkey and in at least one city in Germany, Nuremberg, smoking in public was punishable by death. Two Popes excommunicated tobacco users. In Russia castration was a possible sentence for repeated offenders. All of these draconian measures failed, as did prohibitions.

Eventually, the taxes gained through national monopolies or on import duties became so desirable that almost all of the interdictions were abolished. One of the major concerns of the time was of the fires caused by careless smokers. In those days fire was a serious hazard in the combustible dwellings, and whole city sections might be incinerated from a single blaze. Non-smokers also found the practice of smoking, chewing, and snuffing objectionable. In the books of the time health hazards are mentioned, but they were not the primary basis for the objections to tobacco.

American tourists brought cigarettes home from England during the 1850s. When these were made from imported flue-cured Virginia tobacco they were mild enough to inhale. These slim, white tubes filled with golden leaf cuttings were attractive, not only to men but also to women and children. They gradually increased in popularity until at present more than 4,000 cigarettes are consumed per capita each year in the United States.

TOBACCO AS A PATHOGEN

The statistical evidence linking cigarette smoking with lung cancer and a variety of other malignancies, coronary artery disease and obstructive pulmonary diseases is very convincing. Smokers have a higher incidence of cancers of the mouth, larynx, esophagus, pancreas, and urinary tract than non-smokers. Lung cancer is on the increase in women paralleling their increased smoking of cigarettes. As early as 1936 Fleckseder[2] noticed that 94 percent of those who had died of cancer of the lung were smokers. It was the more definitive work of Wynder, et al.,[8] Hammond,[3] and Ochsner et al.,[5] that made the connection between the amount of smoking and the appearance of pulmonary neoplasms evident.

The causative ingredient in tobacco that produces the cancers, bronchitis, and emphysema is the coal tars. Tobacco smoke contains a series of tumor initiators, co-carcinogens, and cilia-toxic agents. All three of these components act together in the genesis of carcinomas, and the cilia-toxic agents produces the mucous blockages and infections that underlie the chronic, obstructive respiratory diseases. Because of the impairment of cilia movement and the inability of lung macrophages to remove dust from the alveoli and bronchial tree, tobacco encourages occulsion of the air sacs and their eventual disruption.(1)

Nicotine and carbon monoxide appear to be the percursors of coronary artery disease and atherosclerosis.

THE RISKS INVOLVED

If the risk of developing lung cancer for a non-smoker is placed at 1, a linear progression is present according to the numbers of cigarettes used. For male smokers who consume 30 or more cigarettes a day the relative risk is 80. In women a similar but lesser rise to 25 in those smoking more than 30 cigarettes daily is found. For men smoking 30 or more filter cigarettes the risk is 70, while for women no difference is discernible between filter and non-filter cigarettes. The progression curve for cancer of the larynx is similar but lower. Filter cigarettes appear to offer a greater degree of protection to both sexes.(9)

The rewards of non-smoking are considerable. A third of a million people would not die prematurely each year. There would be 85 to 90 percent fewer deaths from cancers of the upper airway and lungs and from chronic respiratory diseases. Half of those who die from cancer of the bladder, and a third who die of atherosclerotic heart disease and arteriosclerosis would be spared.(7) The national costs of smoking in 1975 from direct health care costs, fire, property damage, lost earnings, and the retail cost of tobacco was estimated at 41.5 billion dollars.(4)

The carcinogenic activity of tobacco is reversed soon after discontinuing smoking. The incidence of lung cancer in ex-smokers falls after a short period of time to equal that of non-smokers. With regard to the cardiovascular changes, tobacco discontinuance will not reverse the process, but it may slow the progression. Pulmonary emphysema will also not be reversed, but the process may be halted.

PREVENTION

Primary Prevention

The smoking habit is generally acquired during early adolescence, often on the basis of peer mimicking. The number of regular male smokers 15 to 16 years of age has stayed at about 18 percent between 1968 and 1974. Unfortunately, regular smoking in girls of similar age doubled from 10 to 20 percent during the same period. This has happened despite fairly general knowledge of the linkages between smoking and disease.

As with prevention efforts for all drugs of abuse, it has been found that teaching young people about the hazards of smoking is no more than modestly successful. Deterrent prevention campaigns that speak to the psychosocial detriments of smoking and teach methods of resisting the pressure to smoke, seem to have greater effectiveness.

Secondary Prevention

Up to a quarter of former smokers have been able to give up the practice by their own devices or with the assistance of a variety of anti-smoking programs. Men are twice as successful as women in this regard. Success correlates positively with education in the ability to give up the habit. Among the 54 million people in the United States who still smoke, college graduates use filter cigarettes more often than grammar or high school graduates.(9)

Since millions cannot or will not desist from smoking, the development of a less harmful—but not to be understood as safe—cigarette is justified. This is done by selective breeding of the plant to produce low tar, low nicotine leaves, and the interposition of suitable filters and aerators. Less than 9 mg of tar, 0.6 mg of nicotine, and low levels of the other known hazardous substances should be achieved. Even with reduced amounts of the toxic agents, a smoker may counteract any benefits of the less harmful cigarette by inhaling it deeply, smoking more units, or smoking each cigarette more completely.

Since it is the nicotine that is desired, reducing that alkaloid to the lowest possible level may not be desirable. In fact, a very low tar, moderate amount of nicotine might be preferable, except in those people vulnerable to cardiovascular disease. All in all, non-smoking is the preferred practice whenever possible.

Tertiary Prevention (Treatment)

The most commonly employed techniques for the cessation of smoking include individual and group counseling, hypnosis, and learning theory approaches such as conditioned avoidance techniques. In general short-term success rates are excellent, but when the clients are followd for one year the abstainers average about 25 percent.

It is believed that periodic reinforcement and contacts over a follow-up period would improve the number of favorable outcomes. A comparison among the various therapies is difficult for many reasons, but the impression is that group therapy yields the best results and is the most cost effective.(9) Even with assistance from one of the clinical approaches, those trying to stop smoking will do best with positive reinforcement from family, friends, and counselors, especially during the first months of abstinence.

A number of aversive techniques is in vogue. Electrical shocks, unpleasant odors, warm stale smoke, and imagined noxious experiences are used. A number of studies has been carried out that require the rapid smoking of large numbers of cigarettes in order to make the user physically uncomfortable from the tobacco overload. They have not been more successful than other measures. Sensory deprivation has been tried with excellent initial results, but not so favorable longer-term outcome. Contingency contracting can be used with all of the various efforts to eliminate smoking. It consists of a formal written agreement between client and counselor and sets down each person's duties and expectations. It has not been fully evaluated to determine whether outcome is improved.

Occasional use is made of chemical approaches. If nicotine is the habituating substance, it is reasonable to provide the smoker with nicotine chewing gum or lobeline, a related alkaloid. Such nicotine substitues do not seem to be helpful alone, but when combined with other techniques, may add to the improvement rate. In some countries smoking deterrents such as silver nitrate or potassium permanamate mouth washes are used to make subsequent smoking unpleasant. These are rarely helpful alone.

There is a real need for a low cost, widely disseminable antismoking method. One that has recently come forth is a mass media, usually television, effort accompanied by kits and smoking diaries. Sometimes, entire communities become involved in a sort of vast group counseling effort. Large scale relaxation exercises are taught. All these measures and more are reviewed by Schwartz.(6) About two-thirds of all smokers say that they would like to quit. Most make a number of efforts to do so. If more low cost, informal opportunities to stop were available, more might succeed.

For most people abrupt discontinuance of smoking is preferable to gradually cutting down to zero cigarettes. When someone decides to try to eliminate smoking, the motivation is high. If a long withdrawal process is carried out, by the time cigarettes must be given up, motivation may be fading. A very heavy smoker could reasonably cut down over a period of a week before cessation, but very gradual cutbacks or continuing to smoke at a much reduced rate usually ends in a return to previous smoking patterns. The withdrawal symptoms are unpleasant and uncomfortable but they are not life-threatening and they can be ameliorated by symptomatic management.

Perhaps the problem of stopping is analagous to heroin addiction. One of the easiest procedures in medicine is the detoxification of the heroin addict. Detoxification should not even be considered a treatment, merely an opportunity to start treatment. Just so, anti-smoking programs usually stop when they should be starting—after the smoker has been detoxified. Treatment of the smoker should persist for months if not years after abstinence has been achieved.

SUMMARY

We will become a nation of preponderant girl and woman filter tip cigarette smokers if present trends continue. It is regrettable that, since tobacco-related diseases are among the most preventable, young women are smoking more than ever.

Tobacco usage is another example of the point that the facts are not much of a deterrent to practices that have become habitual. Knowledge does not make people free, it merely makes them guilty about doing something harmful to themselves.

The facts about the dangers of some habitual practice will only infrequently alter the habit, especially if the dangers will develop not now, but later. We probably shall never collect the mass of evidence about the hazards of the illicit drugs of abuse that have been accumulated about tobacco. Still, millions persist in smoking cigarettes for what seems to be trivial gratifications.

That most smokers want to stop but are unable to do so reflects upon the problems of all addicted people. Changing the established behavior patterns is difficult. When rewarding pharmacologic agents also are involved, the life-style changes are even more difficult to accomplish.

NOTES

1. Cohen, D., *et al.* Smoking impairs long-term dust clearance from the lung. Science. 204:514-516, 1979.
2. Fleckseder, R. On bronchial cancer and some causative factors. Munch, Med. Wschr. 83:1585-1588, 1936.
3. Hammond, E. C. The place of tobacco in the etiology of lung cancer, CA, May, 1952.
4. Luce, R. B. and Schwertzer, S. O. The economic costs of smoking-induced illness. In: Research on Smoking Behavior, Eds: Jarvik, M. E., et al. NIDA Research Monograph 17, U.S. Govt. Printing Office, Washington, D.C. 20402, 1977.
5. Ochsner, A., *et al.* Bronchogenic carcinoma—its frequency, diagnosis and early treatment. JAMA 148:691-697, 1952.

6. Schwartz, J. L. Smoking cures: Ways to kick an unhealthy habit. In: Research on Smoking Behavior. Eds: Jarvik, M. E. *et al.* NIDA Research Monograph 17, U.S. Government Printing Office, Washington, D.C. 20402, 1977.

7. Van Lancker, J. L. Smoking and disease. In: Research on Smoking Behavior. Eds: Jarvik, M. E., *et al.* NIDA Research Monograph 17, U.S. Government Printing Office, Washington, D.C. 20402, 1977.

8. Wynder, E. L. and Graham, E. A. Tobacco smoking as a possible etiologic factor in bronchogenic carcinoma—A study of 684 proved cases. JAMA 143:329-336, 1950.

9. Wynder, E. L. and Hoffman, D. Tobacco and health. A societal challenge. New Eng. J. Med. 300:894-903, 1979.

II
EPIDEMIOLOGY AND TREND ANALYSIS

1. Drugs: The Global Situation

GENERAL

In our preoccupation with local problems, we tend to disregard the global nature of drug abuse. The latest upsurge in drug-abusing activities is worldwide, and any attempt to explain the phenomenon must account for its international dissemination.

Striking similarities, but also important differences, are to be found between our drug problems and those in other lands. Drug pandemics have occurred in the past, but the nature of modern existence makes the current one particularly diffusible. Never before have we been capable of transmitting news instantaneously to all parts of the world. International travel is rapid and within the reach of millions. Vast migrations, urbanization, and wars have introduced drug-using customs to cultures who have never been involved. Modern technology is capable of producing and delivering large quantities of mind-altering substances at low costs to any city on earth. These "advances" coming at a time of fairly universal unrest, turmoil, anxiety, and loss of established values, make the global overuse of chemical changes of consciousness quite understandable.

A few years ago when traveling in other countries, it was not uncommon to hear the comment that the drug abuse epidemic was an "American disease." The phrase was meant to express the notion that American youth set the international pattern in dress, music, and drug-taking. Perhaps, the notion was supported by recognizing our easily identifiable young people hanging loose anywhere from Katmandu to Pago Pago. Actually, though we have made certain contributions to the problem, so also have other cultures.

COMMON FACTORS ACROSS NATIONAL BOUNDARIES

Certain universal trends can be identified throughout the world.

1. The penetration of alcoholic beverages into almost every culture is the most impressive single event. Alcohol is displacing kava in Melanesia and betel nut in the East Indies. It is inexpensive, ubiquitous, and effective in providing certain kinds of altered states of consciousness. Unfortunately, for too many people it is dependency-producing and with a considerable, proved ability to cause tissue damage. Youthful alcohol abuse is a growing problem on every continent.

2. Multiple drug abuse is a common phenomenon. Alcohol and cannabis are generally the basic intoxicants with sedatives, stimulants, hallucinogens and opiates laid on according to the mood, occasion, and available drug.

3. The misuse of prescription-type and over-the-counter drugs by adults is seen in many countries. The sleeping pills, the minor tranquilizers and the amphetamine-like compounds are being taken without supervision or particular knowledge about the hazards involved.

4. Heroin addiction, at one time seen only in the cosmopolitan centers of the Western World, has spread to small communities and to countries where it has previously been unknown.

5. Tobacco consumption continues to increase each year around the world despite the well-documented risks involved.

SPECIFIC COUNTRIES AND THEIR PROBLEMS

A brief description of the drug problem in various countries follows. Omission from the list does not mean that the nation has no drug abuse concerns. Rather, it signifies that either no information is at hand, or that the situation is not unlike neighboring countries mentioned.

North America

Canada. Canada's drug problem is similar to that of its neighbor to the south, but in miniature. For example, in 1971 Canadians had an estimated 1.5 million people who had ever used marihuana. At the same time the estimate in the United States was over 20 million. About 15,000 opiate dependent people are believed to live in Canada, many of them concentrated in Vancouver. LSD, MDA, and PCP are in use. Volatile solvent sniffing is reported from various parts of the country, particularly Manitoba. Of course, the major public health problems are excessive drinking and smoking.

The LeDain Commission (roughly equivalent to our Shafer Commission) report recommended the legalization of marihuana under a system similar to their regulation of alcohol.(1) It is unlikely that the recommendation will be acted upon by the government, but one or more of the provincial governments may move in that direction.

Mexico. The unusual number of hallucinogenic drugs indigenous to Mexico makes their native use fairly predictable. The peyote cactus, the psilocybe mushroom, and the psychedelic morning glory seeds (ololiuqui) are consumed by some. In addition, marihuana was introduced in 1910 and has been widely cultivated and used by the peasants. Opium has been an illicit cash crop for the export trade. It is now estimated that 50 percent of the heroin consumed in the U.S. comes in from Mexico. During the past few years some Mexicans in the large cities have become involved with heroin.(2) Students and other young, middle and upper class members have become interested in marihuana and stimulants. At least one working class community outside Mexico City is deeply involved in solvent sniffing.

Jamaica. An. N.I.M.H. funded project has been completed by the Research Institute for the Study of Man.(3) The Jamaican situation is of particular interest because about 40-50% of all working class males smoke ganja (a potent form of cannabis) from adolescence on. They use it to achieve the energy to labor, and as a relaxant at the end of the day. They do not describe mind-altering experiences or fantasies. This is in sharp contrast to the folk experience in the United States. In fact, here we are concerned that our youth will suffer from the amotivational syndrome if they become over-involved in marihuana. The study showed little difference between the ganja users and a matched, control group on a wide variety of physical and psychological examinations. Note should be made of a diffusion of ganja use into middle and upper socioeconomic groups in Kingston.

South America

Aside from a special problem with coca chewing in Bolivia, Ecuador, and Columbia, the drug problems in the South American countries are similar to other developed nations. Marihuana, sedatives, and stimulants are of first concern. Heroin is a minor, but growing, issue.

Africa

Egypt. Hashish has been forbidden for almost a century in Egypt, yet 20 percent of males 20-40 years old smoke it. The penalties for smuggling it in from Syria and Lebanon are harsh, but there is no shortage.(4) In the large cities alcohol and opium are becoming more widely used despite the religious taboos.

South Africa. Dagga (cannabis) is widely used among the Bantu. It has been used as an energizer among South African mine workers who had dagga breaks long before coffee breaks were known. Other groups are increasingly adopting the custom. Government officials express strong concern and have instituted severe penalties.

Nigeria. The death penalty is on the statute books for transporting cannabis for sale. It is not known whether the sentence has ever been carried out.

Australia

In Australia and New Zealand excessive drinking is the major drug problem. Sedative and tranquilizer misuse would rank next. Chronic bromide intoxication persists in some places due to the availability of patent medicines containing bromides. There are also a number of people who use excessive amounts of aspirin and phenacetin for chronic pain. Cannabis, amphetamines, opiates, and LSD are lesser issues.

Europe

England. The "British system" of heroin maintenance for the treatment of heroin addiction is a well-known and an interesting aspect of the problem in the United Kingdom. It is, perhaps, too soon to make a final judgment about its effectiveness in England.

In addition to opiate dependence, England has other chemical dependency problems. Cocaine and amphetamines are being abused, the latter often in the form of amphetamine-barbiturate combinations. Sedative-tranquilizer overuse plagues the socialized medicine system. Marihuana and hashish are widely used, and penalties approximate those in the United States. The per capita consumption of alcohol and tobacco seems to increase each year as everywhere else.

France. All the drugs of abuse are encounterd in Paris, the port cities, and a few others. The problem of alcohol intoxication is particularly serious in France. The Marseilles area has traditionally been the major area for conversion of morphine base to heroin. Until a few years ago little of the product was disposed of within France. Recently, this pattern has changed, and heroin has appeared on the street. The increasing number of addicts had produced a more vigorous control effort, and heroin factories have recently been raided in southern France.

Netherlands. With the most liberal enforcement policies in Europe, hashish smoking is acceptable in certain youth entertainment centers in Amsterdam. In 1971 some 20 percent of school age children reported having used hashish, 6 percent more than 20 times.

Sweden. Sweden, and, to a much lesser extent, other Scandinavian countries have a stimulant problem that extends back to the early 1960s. Preludin was easily available after its introduction, and intravenous use became a popular activity. Over 10,000 abusers of amphetamines and Preludin were estimated for Sweden, but that number may have decreased since more vigorous controls and additional treatment facilities became available. At every international meeting Sweden asks that amphetamines be more vigorously controlled. All the other common drugs of abuse are available and used. Scandinavia shares a large alcoholism problem with every other European nation.

U.S.S.R. The problem is alcoholism. It preoccupies the authorities in the U.S.S.R. and other Communist countries. Despite the fact that it is considered a crime against the State to be a chronic inebriate, the numbers are not diminishing markedly despite stringent laws and severe penalties. Poland, Czechoslovakia, and other Iron Curtain countries share in this dilemma.

It is not possible to obtain information on the extent of the drug problem in Soviet Russia. Officially, drug abuse does not exist. Nevertheless, periodically increasingly severe laws are publicized, which would be superfluous if non-existence were a fact.

Asia

Japan. Japan's methamphetamine epidemic started at the end of World War II and peaked in 1954 when 550,000 persons were involved. With the introduction of compulsory hospitalization and stricter law enforcement, the number rapidly subsided only to start increasing again during the last decade.

Japan was also the first country to experience a methaqualone epidemic during the early 1960s. Young people swallowed large quantities of Quualude until supplies were decreased by stronger controls. Analgesics and solvents have become popular more recently. Heroin is a lesser problem, and marihuana is only now beginning to be used in increasing amounts.

India. India has made the use of strong cannabis preparation illegal although the weaker bhang is a popular tea. Nevertheless, the stronger forms, charas (hashish) and ganja, are traditionally used, especially by low income groups. Potent cannabis is now being employed by upper and middle class youth, and they are also using alcohol in increasing amounts. It is not uncommon to observe at a family gathering in some Indian city, the old folks drinking bhang and the younger people sipping the taboo Scotch, precisely the opposite drugs which might be consumed by the two age groups in this country.

Opium is a traditional substance among peasants in some parts of the country. Heroin use is sporadic. Medicinal opiates like Demerol are abused by well-to-do older people.

Nepal. State charas shops are visible in Katmandu. Nepal may be the only country where the sale of cannabis is legal. A large smuggling trade into India also exists.

China. Little is known about the drug abuse situation in China, although it is doubtful that it is more than modest. Control over individual behavior is greater than in Russia, and intoxication and addiction are political offenses. An alcohol problem of unknown extent exists. In Yunan province opium is still grown and smoked in the remote areas.

Iran. Iran has a long history of opium cultivation and use. In 1955 the cultivation of the poppy was banned. This led to a vast flow of opium into the country from neighboring lands, particularly Afganistan. By 1969 it became economically necessary to reinstitute limited opium production. Addicts older than 60 were registered and permitted to buy 2-5 Gm of opium daily.(5) About 100,000 such individuals are maintained on opium in this fashion. Over 200,000 other people are believed to be addicted to opium. Heroin addiction is estimated to exist among 10,000 upper and middle class youth, principally in Tehran.

Iran has a death penalty for smugglers and traffickers of opium and heroin. Firing squads and hangings are mentioned in the newspaper with regularity. Nevertheless, the traffic continues without substantial decrease in opiate availability.

Turkey. Turkey, where a large proportion of America's illegal heroin came from, banned the cultivation of the Oriental poppy in 1971 and subsidized alternate crops. A limited planting of opium was planned during the 1975 growing season, and we don't know how much of it was diverted into the production of illegal heroin.

What is interesting is that Turkey has only a small opium and practically no heroin problem.(5) The farmers customarily have a ball of gum opium in the house and use it for dysentery, to put cranky children to sleep, and for other medical purposes. The abuse seems to be minimal.

The concern of the authorities is with the growing hashish problem in the large cities, but even that is not large when compared to other countries. The laws are harsh, including life imprsonment for transportation of heroin, cocaine, and cannabis. The Turkish jails have nothing to recommend them, and your author has visited a number of Americans now incarcerated there who can only look forward to lengthy stays in a miserable setting.

Pakistan. Among the Pakistani the smoking of charas is considered an illegal, socially unacceptable act.(5) Charas is often laced with opium. The smoking practice is restricted to men. What is striking in conversations with officials in Pakistan and neighboring countries is that a hardening of the restrictions on cannabis is evident. On the other hand, in the West the trend is toward a more lenient legislative approach.

Hong Kong. The highest rates of opium and heroin addiction in the world are to be found in this crowded, crown colony. Good quality heroin is available at reasonable prices. "Chasing the dragon" is more popular than injecting heroin. It consists of mixing it with a barbiturate, heating the mixture, and inhaling the smoke in a tube. Hong Kong is also a major transhipment point for heroin destined for the Pacific coast ports.

NOTES

1. Final Report of the Commission of Inquiry Into the Non-Medical use of Drugs. Information Canada, 171 Slater Street, Ottawa, 1973.
2. Bueno, D. V. The Problem of Drug Addiction in Mexico. In R. T. Harris, et al., Eds. Drug Dependence, Austin, Texas: University of Texas Press, 1970.
3. Marihuana and Health. Third report to the U.S. Congress from the Secretary of DHEW Publication No. (ADM) 74-50, 1974, U.S. Gov't, Printing Office, Washington, D. C. 20402.
4. Soueif, M. I. The Social Psychology of Cannabis Consumption: Myth, Mystery and Fact. Bull. Narcotics 24:1-10, 1972.
5. CENTO Seminar on Public Health and Medical Problems Involved in Narcotics Drug Addiction, 1972.

2. Trends in Substance Abuse

What is the national picture in drug abuse trends—both of the culturally acceptable and the nonacceptable drugs?

In recent years all sorts of shifts have been noted for each abused chemical agent, some sloping down, some essentially flat, and some slanting upward. A recent report provides us with some good estimates of the current substance abuse situation.(*)

ALCOHOL

As might be expected, beverages containing alcohol are the most widely used and abused of the psychoactive substances. More than nine million people are believed to have definite problems in connection with their drinking. Alcoholic women are becoming more visible in American society, and the preponderance of male alcoholics over females seems to be diminishing.

Younger people are drinking more, with 6 percent of high school seniors consuming alcohol-containing beverages daily. Drinking patterns established during adolescence are believed to carry over to adulthood with some regularity. More than 200,000 deaths are reported yearly as alcohol-related. This constitutes 8 percent of all the deaths in this country. The past 15 years have shown a 30 percent increase in alcohol consumption.

TOBACCO

Tobacco is second to alcohol in its widespread use. Fifty-five million Americans smoke cigarettes daily. It is estimated that more than 300,000 citizens die prematurely each year from illnesses related to smoking. Currently about 22 percent of youths and 40 percent of adults are regular smokers, and these figures are essentially unchanged since 1974. What has changed drastically has been smoking by high school females. Their rate now approximates that of high school males. By age 12, one out of five youngsters smokes. The hope of a few years ago that the younger generation would not indulge as much in establishment drugs has not come to pass.

MARIHUANA

Cannabis is the most commonly used illegal drug. The rates are highest among 18 to 25-year-olds, but its use is spreading to those younger and older. About 16 million Americans have used marihuana during the past month. Of these, four million are between 12 and 17 and 8.5 million are in the 18 to 25-year-old age group. Ten percent of high school seniors are daily users. Very few deaths due to marihuana use are recorded.

HEROIN

The number of those addicted to heroin has stabilized during the past few years at about a half-million people. It should be recalled there was a ten-fold increase in heroinism between 1960 and 1969—from about 60,000 to more than 600,000. This was followed by a slow decline and then a levelling off during the mid-1970s.

Heroin potency in street material is now down to 5 percent, and the cost per pure milligram of heroin has risen to about $2. The increased price and decreased potency are believed to reflect a diminished availability. These factors make heroin less attractive to novices and tend to move addicts into treatment. Heroin-related deaths and the number of emergency room visits involving this drug are down, another sign that the numbers involved are either stabilized or decreasing.

METHADONE

Methadone as a drug of abuse derives from its use as a maintenance treatment for about 80,000 clients. Since it is effective for about 24 to 36 hours during maintenance therapy, take-home supplies are given to those patients who are given the privilege of visiting the clinic only two or three times weekly.

Some of these supplies may be sold off; less frequently clinic robberies or sales by staff are sources of street methadone. More than 200 methadone-related deaths were reported in 1977, half of which were in New York City. This represents a decrease over previous years due to a tightening-up of take-home regulations. When LAAM, the longer acting methadone analogue becomes available, this problem should be further reduced or eliminated entirely.

BARBITURATES

The source of black market barbiturates and other hypnotics is usually from prescribed materials, but they are supplemented with illegitmately manufactured products. Barbiturate deaths have been decreasing gradually since 1970 when physicians started prescribing the safer benzodiazepines more often for sleep. For example, in 1970 there were 1,873 barbiturate deaths due to suicide. In 1975 the number decreased to 1,036, despite a slight rise for all suicides from 23,488 to 1970 to 27,063 in 1975. Additional federal efforts are underway to curb the abuse of the barbituric acid derivatives and related drugs.

MINOR TRANQUILIZERS

Ninety million prescriptions for minor tranquilizers were filled in 1977, a slight decrease from the previous year. Although the majority of these drugs was used for proper indications, a number of patients and nonpatients misused and abused the anxiolytics by taking large quantities to achieve a state of intoxication or unconsciousness. A quarter of all drug-related emergency room visits is connected with tranquilizer use. The number of deaths due to anxiolytics alone is relatively small, but when used in combination with alcohol or other sedatives anxiolytics' depressant effects are enhanced.

AMPHETAMINES

Amphetamines and other appetite suppresent prescription drugs accounted for almost 17 million prescriptions in 1977. Most of these were properly used for narcolepsy, minimal brain dysfunction, and, in short courses, for weight control. Four million of the prescriptions were for amphetamines of which 85 percent were for long-term weight control, a practice that has been demonstrated not to be effective. In addition, an unknown amount of illicit amphetamines is available. Their level of abuse is holding steady, and the intravenous injection of large amounts, the speedfreak phenomenon noted during the late 1960s, almost has disappeared. Nevertheless, the amphetamines remain a potential item of increased abuse.

COCAINE

Cocaine use continues to increase, with most of those who indulge doing so sporadically. This pattern may be due to high cost and relative unavailability. The average purity has dropped to 30 percent cocaine, whereas a few years ago 90 to 100 percent cocaine was the product most often available on the illicit market. The number of occasional recreational cocaine users and also of "cokeheads" will predictably increase during the next few years.

LSD AND OTHER HALLUCINOGENS

LSD, DMT, and other hallucinogenic drugs have declined in use since the mid-1960s although they have, by no means, disappeared from the drug scene. Emergency room visits in connection with hallucinogens also have become much less frequent. However, there is one exception. Phencyclidine (PCP, Angel Dust) not only is increasing in usage, but the results of its ingestion are a matter of considerable concern to health care and law enforcement officials. The person under the influence of phencyclidine is more apt to engage in unpredictable, violent behaviors than have been encountered with other hallucinogens. The individual may present a variety of neurologic and psychiatric toxic reactions that are neither easily diagnosed nor treated.

INHALANTS

The sniffing of commercial products containing volatile solvents or the contents of aerosol sprays is a juvenile practice that does not always terminate when one becomes an adult. The practice is not decreasing; indeed, among high school seniors it has been gradually increasing during the last few years. Acute lethality (sudden sniffing death) and chronic organ damage have been documented. At present the following products are popular in various regions of the country: gold and bronze spray paints, Texas shoeshine aerosols, lacquer thinner, the volatile nitrites, gasoline, clear plastic spray, Transgo transmissioin fluid, and PAM, an aerosol spray.

SPECIAL POPULATIONS AT RISK

Certain groups vulnerable to overinvolvement with drugs have been identified. The ratio of female to male drug abusers is rising, particularly with regards to alcohol, sedatives, tranquilizers, and certain other psychochemicals. Youths have shown dramatic increases in the abuse of all drugs during the past decade. In recent years, the increase continues for cocaine, marihuana, and phencyclidine. The elderly is a group at risk in the misuse of sedative prescription drugs singly and in combination. Geriatric patients in some long-term care facilities may be exposed to poor or improper prescribing practices to their detriment.

Ethnic minorities usually are over-represented in drug abuse survey data, and special prevention and treatment measures must be devised to deal with this serious issue. All of these populations at risk will require careful, thoughtful planning to reduce the prevalence of their dysfunctional drug use.

DISCUSSION

As we reflect on the implications of the current trends in the abuse of various psychochemicals, no clear pattern can be discerned. If we use the analogy of a few years ago, the "war on drugs" has resulted in neither victory nor defeat. We seem to be engaged in a sort of trench warfare where hard-earned gains on one salient are cancelled out by losses in another sector. Barring some unforseen breakthrough, the tough, obstinate battling will continue, with the final issue remaining in doubt for years to come.

It may be, as some believe, that a significant degree of the drug problem will remain with us—and that it will never recede to the lower levels of the good old days. They claim that the quality of life, especially for the young, will have to change markedly before the abuse of drugs will revert to more acceptable levels.

The changes will have to be in the direction of enhanced aspirations, goals that are not compatible with the overuse of drugs, and hopes for the future that include emotional and physical growth, not impairment. Such a shift in the value system of youth is not impossible. It has happened before, and it is happening now to an all-too-small number of young people.

But what about the great majority?

Will it take a modern Children's Crusade—a spiritual renaissance dominated by some charismatic leader? Or can we work our way to a more sober, less stoned society through research and development? The final solution is evidently in prevention, but the large-scale prevention of substance abuse is a remote prospect at this time.

NOTE

*Drug Use, Patterns, Consequences and the Federal Response: A Policy Review, Office of Drug Abuse Policy, Executive Office of the President, March, 1978.

ADDITIONAL READING

1. Cohen, S. Narcotism: *Dimensions of the Problem.* N.Y. Acad. Sci. 311:4-9, 1978.

2. DAWN Quarterly Report: *A Report from the Drug Abuse Warning Network,* January-March, 1977, IMS America, Ltd. Contract No. DEA-77-11. Heroin Indicators Trend Report, DHEW Publication No. (ADM) 76-378, 1976.
3. National Survey on Drug Abuse: 1977, Eds.; H. I. Abelson and I. Cisin.
4. Project DAWN V: *Phase Five Report of the Drug Abuse Warning Network,* May, 1976-April, 1977, IMS America, Ltd. DEA Contract No. 76-25, DHEW Publication No. (ADM) 78-618, 1977.

3. The Epidemiology of Heroin Addiction

The major variables in the spread of heroin addiction are:

1. the availability of the drug,

2. the number of current users,

3. the number of non-using people in distress.

Other variables are of some importance, but their impact is of lesser significance. They include:

4. the legal and moral deterrence,

5. the availability of successful treatment facilities,

6. the quality and pharmacology of the drug,

7. the manner of its usage.

THE AVAILABILITY OF THE DRUG

Sufficient quantities of heroin exist within the national boundaries to provide all current addicts' needs for the next two to three years. Estimates that no more than 10-15 percent of all contraband heroin is confiscated, are probably correct. Therefore, it cannot be expected that supply curtailment will, in itself, solve this problem in the near future. Local shortages may occur from time to time, but these will have an insignificant effect upon addict numbers. While awaiting new supplies, the addict population goes over to codeine cough syrups, barbiturates and other sedatives, or enters a methadone detoxification program for a short period of abstinence to reduce the size of the daily requirement. Now that methadone detoxification capabilities have markedly expanded, this has become a popular means of dealing with a drug "panic."

One undesirable aspect of methadone maintenance programs (and of other successful narcotic treatment programs) is that it expands the quantity of opiates available to other consumers and potential consumers. We can assume that 15 percent of all heroin addicts (about 75,000) are under treatment in methadone maintenance programs. It is proper to inquire into the fate of the heroin that these people are not using. Does it go into new consumer markets? Does some of it go into a higher quality "bag" that the user buys? Or does it somehow go away? There is no evidence to believe that the latter possibility is the major rechanneling mode.

Leakage of methadone onto the street results in a direct expansion of total illicit opiate supplies. In some cities like New York methadone from licit sources has constituted a black marketed commodity which satisfies the primary needs of fair numbers of addicts, and tides others over until their heroin connection is re-established. Therefore, methadone diversion in substantial amounts is a serious matter in the epidemiology of narcotic addiction.

If *heroin* maintenance clinics were ever established in communities where illicit supplies are also plentiful, a catastrophic expansion of available opiates would result. The increase in the numbers of new addicts would be staggering. It is not only that a majority of heroin addicts would enter treatment freeing their unused supplies of clandestine heroin for other persons. At that point we would be confronted with the fact that heroin has to be injected three to five times daily, and therefore "take home" heroin supplies must be issued to the user from the first day of treatment. In contrast, to maintain an individual on methadone, swallowing the material only once a day is required. Thus, a better control over supplies can be retained.

Heroin maintenance is only rational at the end of an epidemic to treat the last few recidivistic addicts, thereby eliminating the remaining foci of reinfection. Even then, it might have to be done in a closed environment to prevent leakage.

Heroin maintenance in a closed situation, for example, a "rehabilitation camp," might be a successful venture for certain kinds of addicts. Used in an open situation it will tend to destroy other treatment efforts such as methadone maintenance and therepeutic communities. Most addicts will certainly prefer heroin maintenance to more difficult or less pleasureable alternatives.

It cannot be argued that the "British System" has proven the success of heroin maintenance. The lack of a large illicit source of supply in England makes comparison with the problem in the United States improper. The "British System" was radically changed in 1968, and a definitive evaluation of the new program is yet to be made. It is interesting to note that more methadone is being prescribed to British addicts than heroin. We will deal later with the issues involved in the approach to treatment of opiate addiction in Great Britain.

Along with treatment and rehabilitative measures it will be necessary to try to limit supplies as much as possible. It is difficult to visualize how any national treatment strategy could succeed in the presence of a plentiful heroin supply situation.

For those who still retain the notion that heroin supplies are still controlled by a single syndicate, an unhappy development must be reported. At present, multiple, parallel supply channels exist so that destroying some single major operation will not produce more than a minor impact on the market.

The destruction of opium plantings amply reported in the press may not have its hoped for resolution of the problem. Only a relatively small planting area will meet the needs of the nation's addicts and this can occur in remote, well-camouflaged terrain. Less than 100 tons of opium are needed to produce the 6-9 tons of heroin needed yearly for the American black marketplace.

The eradication of opium poppy plantings is no simple matter. The oriental poppy can grow in many climates. It is ordinarily cultivated where labor is cheap and detection is difficult. Those who produce the crop are generally unaware of and unaffected by the moral issue of helping provide a highly addicting substance to a user in some city thousands of miles away. To interdict opium cultivation would be ruinous to the peasant-farmers for whom it represents the only possible cash crop. The attractive profits involved at every stage of marketing invite new production areas and new heroin entrepreneurs.

The easy assumption that mandatory capital punishment for the large scale dealer will deter these people ought to be carefully studied. The rewards of dealing are enormous, and it seems that risk-taking people will always be attracted under such conditions. In Iran hundreds of smugglers of opium and heroin have been publicly executed, still the smuggling situation remains.

THE NUMBER OF CURRENT USERS

Every addict is a potential focus of spread of his addiction. The analogy with the dissemination of contagious diseases is very suitable except that the vector is not a pathogenic virus or bacteria, but a chemical which will make one feel better or keeps one from withdrawal sickness. In a small group situation in which some are using, it is inevitable that others in the group eventually will. When a woman becomes closely involved with a male addict, the statistics predict a strong likelihood that she will become addicted. When a husband and wife are addicted, treating only one is useless because of inevitable reinfection.

Communities have been studied where one or a small number of addicts moved in and produced a centrifugal spread that resembled the pattern of a typhoid outbreak from an infected food handler.

It is not difficult to understand why addiction spreads. During the early phase of the addiction the rewards of the "high" make the addicts proselytizers. What can one give a friend or a loved one which is better than instant joy? As the addiction matures, and the euphoria becomes less apparent, the drive to avoid the withdrawal sickness becomes dominant. At this point other motives for transmission of the addiction state become more apparent. One is the "turning on" of friends and relatives so that they can become the source of support for one's own habit. Another reason is to bring others down to one's own level of misery.

If all the "junkies" could somehow be removed from a community the infection would naturally disappear. The addict must be seen, not only as a consumer and casualty, but also as a transmitter of his disorder. It is this obvious fact which causes the heads of governments to advocate mandatory treatment or mandatory incarceration of addicts. At a certain point we are told, civil rights of addicted individuals become meaningless. That point occurs when the social order is in danger of collapsing if severely punitive action is not taken. "Has that point been reached here?" is a question asked by some of our government enforcement officials.

A LARGE NUMBER OF NON-USING PEOPLE IN DISTRESS

Dysphoric people constitute the susceptible reservoir of potential addicts. At one time it was thought that only addictive personality types could become addicted. Although immature, psychologically unstable people may be over-represented among the addicted, it seems that almost anyone can become an addict under certain conditions. The stable person who becomes addicted in the course of a painful illness is an example. Therefore we should think of vulnerability to addiction as a continuum from those highly susceptible to those who are very resistant, depending on their character structure and their level of distress.

"Distress" requires some definition. It includes all sorts of conditions in which psychological pain is experienced. It may be due to a low toler-ance to frustrating experiences or a pervasive feeling of hopelessness about one's situation. High anxiety levels, an existence without goals, ex-cessively high, unrealistic expectations, a real or imagined dismal life situation, these and other factors can cause psychic distress. The drug is used to relieve that distress.

To change a person's misperception of himself and his life situation is no easy task. Such attitudes are usually non-rational and the derived feel-ings and opinions are a complex admixture of reality and fantasy. Atti-tude change is best approached on a revivalistic, exhortative basis. As times become more desperate, it is the preachers and prophets with sim-ple, emotional messages who gain listeners and converts.

We know that improving an individual's social situation is no guaran-tee of freedom from the distress that can lead to destructive drug usage. In fact, affluence is as difficult a milieu for human development and maturation as poverty. However, we also know something of the tech-niques that seem to diminish a group's distress. Feelings of communion, strong beliefs in a religious, social, or political cause, feelings of mean-ingfulness and gratification in one's activities—these and other qualities are protection against compulsive drug taking.

SUMMARY

The choices, then, in attempting to contain the dissemination of heroinism are these: reduce the quantity of drug available, reduce the number of active users, or improve the quality of life so that relief from psychic unease will not be needed. Since these are difficult long-term solutions to the problem, a rapid resolution must not be expected.

4. The Latin American Connection

HEROIN: SHIFTING SUPPLY LINES

Those who think of the narcotic traffic still operating as shown in "The French Connection" are about 75 percent wrong these days.

Five years ago opium and morphine base flowed from Turkey and other Middle Eastern countries into southern France where they were processed into heroin, later to be transhipped to the United States at the rate of about 10 tons a year. Ten tons of heroin will supply about 100-200 million person/days of heroin. The street material averaged about 15 percent heroin. The Mediterranean route was a major source of heroin for the eastern half of the United States and Canada. The southwestern cities were supplied with brown (Mexican) heroin. Smaller amounts came in from the Golden Triangle (Burma, Thailand, Laos) via Hong Kong, Macao and Saigon to Vancouver, Seattle and San Francisco.

It was during 1972 that the French-Corsican traffickers sustained a number of setbacks. Narcotic agents at the North American ingress points for heroin shipments were able to confiscate large shipments, including one seizure of almost half a ton. Meanwhile, back in France the authorities finally felt the pressure to search out heroin laboratories, arrest the entrepreneurs, and seize the raw and processed materials. In addition, Turkey's 1972 decision to prohibit poppy cultivation was a blow to the syndicates since they had not yet prepared new poppy production areas. As if these reverses were not enough, the route of entry of a third of the French heroin into North America had been through Latin America. This supply network was successfully disrupted when the major French-Corsican traffickers were arrested in South and Central America during 1972.

Apparently, a decision was made by the large operators to restrict transatlantic supplies to the northeastern United States market. But the harassed French heroin suppliers could not even provide for this shrunken territory. By 1973 the bag on the street averaged as little as 2 percent heroin, and sometimes less. Two percent heroin means less than 5 mg of heroin, an amount which may hardly be noticed by an addict with a fair degree of tolerance. This sort of situation leads to a "panic"—addicts cleaning themselves up on their own or going into detoxification programs. Others bought methadone on the street. Still others went over to sleeping pills and booze.

Unfortunately, the story does not have a happy ending because of recent events. During the past two years Mexico has replaced France as the main supplier of heroin in this country. According to a series of articles in the *New York Times* (April 21-24, 1975), which are well worth reading, 60 percent of the heroin consumed today is of Mexican origin. Brown heroin, which assayed at about 17 percent heroin, was seen for the first time in New York in 1975. Entirely new criminal syndicates have sprung up to manage the new distribution chain, and they are dominated by Latin Americans. The Mexican heroin story goes back to World War II when, with overseas supplies cut off, some New York Mafiosi financed Mexican poppy production in the hinterland. When the French monopoly weakened a few years ago, Mexican poppy production bloomed, and efforts by Mexican authorities have interdicted only a fraction of the opium fields and heroin supplies.

Meanwhile, with enormous profits at stake, the French suppliers have been busy reorganizing. Some of their shipments now go to midwestern cities where the narcotic officials have been somewhat less vigilant compared with those in New York, Miami and, Baltimore. Turkey has announced that 100,000 farmers will be allowed to raise opium poppies this year. Although the government promises no diversion of gum opium into illegitimate channels, it is difficult to believe that the farmers will not hold out some fraction of their crop for the much better prices paid by the dealers. The amount of French heroin in the New York bag has increased to 7 percent during the past year—a sure sign that supplies are more plentiful. New York, it should be recalled, contains about half of the country's heroin addicts.

HEROIN: ADULTERATION IS THE NORM

If the heroin has not been adulterated by the time it arrives in this country, it will be cut many times over here. A bag of pure heroin would be lethal if it happened to be sold on the street. It has been mentioned that heroin constitutes only a fraction of the contents of the bag. What are the other contents?

Diluents

Lactose, mannitol, and inositol are the common sugars used to make up the bulk of the white powder that is purchased. They are inert and are added to make the material bulkier. Unfortunately, sometimes insoluble substances like flour, cornstarch, or talc are used for the same purpose. These lodge in the lungs and other organs causing infarctions by blocking the blood vessels in which they are carried.

Other Drugs

Quinine is commonly found in eastern heroin. It is added to provide a bitter taste in case it should be tasted. Cutting with large amounts of sugar will mask the bitterness of the small amount of heroin present, therefore, it is reconstituted with quinine. It is said that the lightheadedness and ringing in the ears, which a full dose of quinine provides, will add to the "rush' of the injected material. As a fringe benefit, it may cure the malaria that is sometimes transmitted from contaminated syringes. Disadvantages, however, also exist. Many cases of overdose are not due to narcotics. Quinine is suspected of causing some of them in those people sensitive to intravenous quinine. Procaine and other local anesthetic agents are being found in confiscated or purchased street heroin these days. It is not clear what function these synthetic local anesthetics serve in heroin. It may be the dizziness that is noted when they are injected intravenously enhances the narcotic effect.

COCAINE GROWTH INDUSTRY

Cocaine and heroin have nothing in common pharmacologically, but they have a few elements of similarity. They are the "hard" drugs, whatever "hard" may signifiy. They are sometimes used together: the "speedball" of the old days. And now they both come to us from the lands to the south.

Coca leaves grown in South America have always been the source of cocaine. During the past few years the demand has grown so rapidly that both prices and acreage have increased enormously.

Peru and Bolivia are the only South American countries where the coca bush is legally cultivated. Last year Peru produced 20 million kilograms of coca leaf, only a quarter of which was used for legitimate purposes: chewing by the local Indians and export for chemical use. Since it takes 150 kilos of leaf to make a kilo of cocaine, Peru alone produced about 100,000 kilos of illicit cocaine last year. We hear of a Silver Triangle of coca paste distribution in Bolivia, Paraguay, and western Brazil.

One hundred and fifty kilos of coca leaves become a few kilos of coca paste by a simple extraction with potassium carbonate in an oil drum. This is reduced to a kilogram of cocaine in any of one of hundreds of cocaine factories that exist all over South America. In Colombia alone about 70 major criminal organizations are into the cocaine traffic. American authorities have indicted more than a hundred drug traffickers in Colombia, but because of existing restrictive extradition treaties, they remain safely in Colombia actively plying their trade.

Police action has been less than effective in the South American countries involved, with the exception of a recent cleanup in Chile. The Drug Enforcement Administration estimates that cocaine exports from Chile to the United States have been reduced from 200 kilos a month to less than 10. The Chilean Junta also sent 17 major traffickers to this country despite the fact they were Chilean nationals.

Imagine any way to smuggle cocaine across the national boundary and you can be assured that it has been tried. One of the most dangerous ways is to put the cocaine in rubber sheaths and swallow them. Fatalities have occurred when gastric juices and movements broke the sheaths. After arrival in a city like New York the cocaine will sell for $2,000 an ounce, or if fairly pure, up to $4,000. When broken down into gram packages and cut, an ounce will bring in $4,000 to $6,000. This means that the cocaine bought in Colombia, Ecuador or Peru for $5,000 a kilo will bring in about $200,000 in Los Angeles, New York, or Miami.

COCAINE: IT USED TO BE THE REAL THING

Only a few years ago pure cocaine was available to the few who were into "snow." Now, even the best cocaine has been cut 25 percent, and 5 and 10 percent cocaine is easy to find. There is little relationship between its strength and its price. A batch of 13 percent cocaine sold for $1,250 an ounce in Austin recently, while 86 percent cocaine brought only $1,000 an ounce in Petaluma. The diluent is one of the sugars, but caffeine, amphetamine, or phencyclidine also are picked up on analysis. The principle adulterants are the local anesthetics: procaine, xylocaine, lidocaine, pontocaine, and benzocaine. Like cocaine, these substances will produce numbness of the tongue or nose if the material is sniffed or tasted. They might also contribute a slight giddiness which some may interpret as a "high."

SUMMARY

Federal enforcement authorities believe that no more than 10 to 15 percent of illicit drugs can be seized. With the vast expansion of poppy and coca plantings in Latin America, the revival of Turkish production, and the potential of Southeast Asian production, it is evident that heroin and cocaine will be with us for a long time. We will have to learn how to live in cities where these drugs are plentiful. The major barrier to a bedrugged society will depend upon the resilience of each person, not on the hope that these drugs will go away. They will go away only when the demand for them no longer exists.

REFERENCES

1. Gage, N. New York Times, Series of four articles on drug trafficking. 4/21/75-4/24/75.
2. Perry, D. C. *Heroin and Cocaine Adulteration.* PharmChem Newsletter, Vol. III, No. 2, April, 1974.

5. West Berlin: A Drug Abuse Microcosm

The heroin epidemic of the 1960s, which involved only a few countries including the United States, has given way to a worldwide pandemic.

All the countries of Western Europe, Iran, Thailand, Burma, and many other nations are reporting an upsurge in problems with heroin dependency. If other drugs and alcohol are included it can be said that no country is spared the impact of large numbers of its citizens made ineffective or impaired by chronic chemical intoxification.

A recent visit to West Berlin has provided some current information on that democratic outpost surrounded by communist East Germany. The West Berlin situation is unique in that it is a compact community of two million people. Furthermore, except for about 100,000 guest workers, mostly Turkish, Pakistani, and Indian, it is culturally homogenous. It is relatively isolated, with access available via plane, motor vehicle, and barge.

Although West Berlin's known heroin situation is more extensive than that found in other West German cities, it is described here because it provides us with a problem in miniature, and one that is recent and circumscribed. Perhaps, something can be learned from it.

BACKGROUND

Something must be said about the political events of the last 60 years in order to understand the present state of affairs. Germany has lost two great wars, experienced a ruinous inflation, has barely contained anarchistic and communistic uprisings, lived through a decade of Nazism, and was split in two after the World War II. Berlin was 60 percent destroyed by war's end. Despite these disasters, Germany is a revitalized and prosperous country today. Some individual and national psychological uncertainty and confusion remains. What once was the paradigm of strict and disciplined child-rearing, for example, now seems to be transformed into indulgent or even uncaring parenting. Neither the family, nor the church, nor the state have the strong influence over the minds of young people that they once had.

These changes led to two distinct and divergent trends. One was the search through drugs for relief from lack of direction and meaninglessness. The other was terriorism, a mindless destruction, not easily understood. Although the Baader-Meinhof terrorists—a small band that originated in Berlin—may have been involved in hashish or LSD earlier, they stopped the use of drugs when they became activists. These few intellectuals without a cause chose one deviant path, many of the psychologically impaired slipped into a junkie life-style.

Like most cosmopolitan centers, Berlin had experienced some traditional abuse of cocaine, hashish, opium, and prescribed psychotropic drugs. During the chaotic period after World War I, the misuse of these agents increased, but eventually it subsided to minimal levels. Alcoholism had always been a problem, but was in no way an unusual situation for a city of its size.

CURRENT SITUATION

An increase in the use and confiscation of illicit gum opium was noted in 1966. Shortly after, something called "Berliner Tinte" (Berlin Ink) appeared. This was a concoction that resulted when morphine base was treated with vinegar instead of acetic anhydride, the usual compound used in the manufacture of heroin. About 1970, high quality heroin began appearing, ranging in potency from 16 percent to as high as 60 percent purity. By comparison, these street materials are about 10 times stronger than present United States supplies.

A gram of such heroin costs about 200 to 400 marks ($100 to $200). It is believed that 2,500 to 4,500 persons are addicted to heroin in West Berlin. It would take only about a kilogram of pure heroin a day to keep all users supplied, and, when the volume of traffic entering Berlin is considered, it is difficult to believe that such an amount can be stopped.

During the early 1970s heroin arrived from Turkey, where it was manufactured from opium brought in from neighboring states. It was then shipped to Dutch ports and arrived in Berlin by air or surface transportation. In 1974 the Dutch hardened their attitudes about the heroin traffic, deported a number of the Chinese traffickers, and were able to cut off most of these supplies. Since then it is believed that most of the heroin arrives in one to five kilogram packages carried in by the guest workers as they enter or return to West Berlin from a holiday. Another source of opiates was apothecary thefts, but these have been controlled by improving security and reducing opiate stocks.

A strange political situation makes the apprehension of these illicit supplies difficult. The guest workers take charter flights to Shoenfeld airport in East Berlin. Although they go through a customs inspection, the East German authorities are not too concerned about searching out the heroin since it does not stay in that country. From East Berlin, the workers can go to West Berlin by subway or elevated trains without going through customs again. This open border is a reflection of West Germany's political position that all Berlin is a single city despite the 15-foot wall that splits it.

It is believed that a kilo of heroin costs dealers 80,000 to 110,000 marks ($40,000 to $55,000) in West Berlin. This brings an enormous profit to the transporter and to the dealer who may cut it once or twice.

The presence of occupation forces does not make the problem easier. It is believed that about 3 percent of the American brigade might be on hard drugs. Random, unannounced urine screens are not permitted so that precise figures are not available. The American authorities are well aware of the situation and have instituted preventional, educational and rehabilitational measures.

Some 84 overdose deaths were reported in West Berlin during 1977. This figure is high in relation to the presumed number of addicts, at least when compared with the United States experience. It may be that the stronger heroin explains the high ratio of overdose deaths. Another possibility is that the number of addicts is underestimated.

Of course, West Berlin has other drug concerns. Hashish is said to be used on a regular basis by 10,000 Berliners. Sleeping pills and tranquilizers are misused there as elsewhere. Cocaine has not arrived in any quantity. A thinner called Pattex, containing toluene and other solvents, is used by children in some poor neighborhoods. Pattex and gasoline sniffing are said to involve about 1,000 youngsters, and two Pattex youth centers have been established in West Berlin. LSD use has diminished, and PCP has not yet appeared.

TREATMENT

The major treatment modalities are therapeutic communities and the so-called "therapeutic chain." The therapeutic communities are similar to the North American versions, in fact, they seem to have been inspired by our groups. They tend to have smaller numbers of members. Part of their funds comes from the government. In one Synanon house, for example, 100,000 marks was provided by the city and 400,000 marks was raised by members' work or donations.

At the Synanon visited, about 400 addicts had been accepted since 1971. Of these, 45 remain and 15 others live on the outside but are believed to be clean. Three hundred and forty have left. Withdrawal is "cold turkey," and, despite the good quality heroin, serious symptoms have never been encountered. It is preferred to retain the member rather than graduate him. About 250 people live in all West Berlin therapeutic communities.

The therapeutic chain consists of some outreach activities by social workers. Counseling and motivation centers usually are manned by professionals. They are available for interview and evaluation of the addict. From here the addict might go to an inpatient detoxification unit for three to six weeks when Valeron, an opiate not available in the United States, may be used. Some detoxification centers only provide sedatives and tranquilizers. Methadone is rarely used for detoxification and never for maintenance. After detoxification a therapeutic community or outpatient treatment may be recommended for stabilizing the new, abstinent state. Finally, a period of months is spent in vocational or educational rehabilitation after which a job is obtained at the regular employment centers.

The authorities are almost universally against a maintenance philosophy having obtained their information about maintenance from what seems to have been "methadone mills." Perhaps also, the lesser addict-crime problem in Germany makes maintenance therapies less urgent. In Germany every indigent person is entitled to financial assistance that almost covers his food and rent. This arrangement may decrease criminal activity, but it may also reduce the pressure to enter treatment. Narcotic antagonists, drugs that prevent the effects of heroin and other opiates, do not appear to have been tried. The long-acting antagonists might have some contribution to make toward dealing with their problem one day, but they are not used now.

The ex-addict paraprofessional is employed in the treatment system, but far less so than in this country. Socialized medicine and the third party payment system tends to exclude paraprofessionals to some extent.

Followup data on treatment efficacy hardly exists at present. A survey of the number of heroin addicts in West Berlin known to the police and treatment establishments is about to begin.

It appears that only 10 to 15 percent of all addicts are in treatment at any one time. This means that the bulk of addicts are either in jail or on the street. The large proportion of untreated addicts may be a serious factor in the spread of addiction. In the United States a third to a half are in some kind of treatment situation at any point in time.

PREVENTION

The budget for prevention for 1978 is 900,000 marks. TV spots, films, and a theater-in-the-round with audience participation are some of the Berlin efforts in this area. Information about where to seek help, the risks and dangers of addiction, and similar subjects are made available.

DISCUSSION

West Berlin's drug situation is at a relatively early stage of maturation—perhaps where North American countries were 10 years ago. Nevertheless, there is a possibility that things will get worse. The unfavorable factors are:

(1) The ease of supplying the city with large amounts of heroin under present conditions.

(2) The high quality heroin on the street.

(3) The fact that a large majority of addicts are not engaged in a treatment program.

(4) Although the authorities are concerned, it is unlikely that a major effort will be mounted to reverse the present trend. At the early phase of a drug epidemic, a major effort to suppress its spread ought to be made in the hope that the full-blown consequences will be avoided. Vigorous efforts to interdict supplies and to treat as many users as possible could abort the spread of addiction.

(5) The absence of treatment programs that will be attractive to the addict with low levels of motivation.

(6) As in this country social changes, particularly in child-rearing practices, do not seem to be underway.

WHAT CAN WE LEARN FROM WEST BERLIN

A number of points merit reflection and experimentation on our part. The reported minimal symptoms from relatively strong heroin even under conditions of unassisted withdrawal requires that we re-evaluate our approach to the withdrawal process. Perhaps we have assumed that these symptoms are worse than they are. It may be that in healthy young people, the abstinence syndrome is uncomfortable, but needs less treatment than we have been giving it. This may explain the innumerable "cures" and remedies for detoxification that keep coming forth here. The common denominator may be a placebo effect.

The importance of a balanced approach between supply and demand reduction is re-emphasized. By this time the heroin distribution networks have formed in West Berlin. The only approach that seems to offer promise is to put a number of enforcement people underground for extended periods of time to identify the important links in the distribution system. Naturally, if the opium plants can be eliminted where they grow, it will be so much the better.

Further research in searching for practical therapeutic measures is still needed. The ones we have are unappealing to the addict or only partly effective. A narcotic antagonist imbedded in a plastic polymer and requiring an injection only a few times a year is under development. The longacting antagonist combined with an effective behavioral maturation program could attract those who would not enter therapeutic communities, or who would fail when they did.

6. The Many Causes of Alcoholism

Why is that of two rather similar-appearing social drinkers, one will continue his modest consumption indefinitely, while the other will come to use increasing amounts and wind up with his drinking out of control, and his health, family situation, or his career seriously impaired?

Since there is rarely a single cause for a person becoming alcoholic, the answer is usually complicated. It seems worthwhile to review the various theories that attempt to explain why nearly 10 percent of the drinking class drink in destructive ways, while 90 percent appear to handle their intake satisfactorily.

Causes of alcholism are usually sorted into three groups: biological, physiological, and sociocultural. This classification will be followed here, recognizing that alcoholism is normally the interplay of all these factors.

BIOLOGICAL

Genetic

There are a number of points at which genetic differences can impinge on the drinking pattern.

A person might inherit a susceptibility to the acute, intoxicating effects of alcohol, so that small quantities produce loss of control over one's subsequent intake.

Ethanol is broken down in a series of metabolic reactions. People, perhaps even races, differ in the rate of enzymatic degradation. A genetically determined, impaired ability to catabolize ingested alcohol would be associated with a poor ability to "hold" one's liquor.

The brain cells of different people may have an inherited, variable ability to adapt to high or chronic levels of alcohol.

Certain personality features may be genetically determined. In the case of the potential alcoholic, it may be an inherited difficulty in dealing with anxiety, frustration, and depression.

An organ vulnerability, genetically determined, may make one person more likely than others to develop certain of the complications of chronic alcohol consumption.

A considerable interest in the inherited aspects of destructive drinking is now occupying the attention of certain investigators, especially in Scandanavia. The issue of the inheritance of alcoholic traits becomes a practical matter when counseling children who have one or more alcoholic parents. The well known fact that excessive drinking runs in families is obviously no grounds for attributing noxious drinking behavior to one's chromosomes. Environmental factors would also play a significant role in such instances. Studies of families of alcoholics always show higher rates among relatives than in the general population, commonly quoted as about 4 percent for men and a half to 1 percent in women. Sons of alcoholic parents have rates as high as 25 to 50 percent, while the rate for daughters is 3 to 7 percent. The environmental factor could be sorted out if the children of alcoholic parents who were adopted by non-alcoholic foster parents soon after birth were studied. This has been done by Shuckit[1] and Goodwin.[2] They believe that genetic factors do play a role in the transmission of an alcoholism potential to the children. In a Danish twin study 25 percent of non-identical twins and 65 percent of identical twins who had at least one alcoholic parent became alcoholics whether they were reared by alcoholic parents or by non-alcoholic foster parents.

This evidence is far from conclusive for a predetermined dipsomania. At most it would speak for an inherited vulnerability to become an excessive drinker, perhaps on the basis of a diminished capacity to tolerate stress. It is therefore not inevitable that a son will follow his father's drinking patterns, especially if he is aware of the predisposition.

Biochemical

Defects in carbohydrate metabolism, for example, a sensitivity to insulin, or episodes of spontaneous hypoglycemia are apparently associated with heavy drinking. Instances of adrenal insufficiency under such conditions have also been reported. However, these endocrine abnormalities are more likely to be the results of unphysiologic drinking practices than their cause.

Alcoholics Anonymous considers the alcoholic to be a sick person whose chemistry is different from others in that alcohol affects him idiosyncratically. It is true that people vary in their metabolism of alcohol with identical twins having very similar metabolic curves. One study has found that the metabolic pathway in certain drinkers tends to be pushed into anaerobic metabolism. When the anaerobic metabolites combine with acetalehyle, a product of alcohol breakdown, a compound with a morphine-like structure is formed. This work is far from confirmed, but it has been used to attempt to explain the addictive quality of alcohol.

Endocrine

It is a rather common clinical observation that alcoholic cirrhosis is found in an unusual number of men with scanty body hair. Upon questioning, these people will say that the hair on their chest and extremities has always been sparse. Perhaps, consistently low levels of androgenic hormones predispose to cirrhosis. This finding may indicate that an endrocrine basis for some of the complications of heavy drinking exists. In turn, cirrhosis of the liver interferes with the metabolic breakdown of sex hormones, particularly estrogens.

PSYCHOLOGICAL

Tension Relief and Anxiety Control

When people are asked why they drink, a common response is: "Because I feel better, I feel relaxed." In those who are tense under ordinary conditions, or those who are tense because of constant situational pressures, such feelings of relaxation are sought very much. One can visualize that the definite relief from frustration and anxiety, which is often noted from modest amounts of alcoholic beverages, could lead to its excessive use in chronically distraught people. Feelings of guilt, shame, poor self-esteem, depression, and loneliness are soluble in ethanol.

It is interesting that studies done by Mendelson have demonstrated that while small amounts decrease, large amounts of alcohol increase tension states.(3) The heavy chronic drinker, while still conscious, is even more nervous and upset than he was while sober. Therefore, having previously treated one's anxiety with liquor successfully, the search for tension relief can lead to increased drinking. Under these conditions one is driven to drink to the point of unconsciousness.

Personality Disorders

The possibility that some predisposed people have an "alcoholic personality" was once invoked to explain their aberrant drinking. There seems to be no one personality structure involved. Instead, a variety of personality configurations may predispose to a career of alcoholism. The immature, dependent person who does not tolerate life stress well is one sort of individual who may find that drink temporarily solves his perpetual problems. Depressed people, schizophrenics and sociopathic persons are overrepresented in alcoholism statistics. It is more what alcohol does for a person who has difficulty coping than any particular character structure which makes alcoholism a career.

Psychodynamic Formulations

The psychoanalytic literature suggests that alcoholics (among others) are oral dependent types. The orality developed because of deprivation during early life. Some analysts have suggested that alcohol is a symbolic substitute for mother's milk. Their oral dependency is assuaged by drinking, and when they become incapacitated their dependency needs come to have a real, physical basis.

Learning Theory

According to learning theory the tension reduction that results from drinking provides a positive reinforcement to continue to imbibe. The rewards of feeling better, the social approval, one's group endorsement of drinking or of getting drunk all tend to perpetuate the intake of alcohol. When someone abstains after a period of drinking, the shakiness, the hangover or the impending DTs constitute a negative reinforcement and tend to push the person trying to remain sober, right back to drinking. Whether or not one subscribes to conditioning theory, it is important in treatment to know what positive rewards the person is obtaining from drink, and to know what factors keep him from remaining abstinent.

Role Modeling

When some significant person in one's life relies upon alcohol to deal with the vicissitudes of existence, then the adolescent whose coping patterns are being formed, may adopt similar unhealthy practices by identification. The opposite can also occur: the young person may be so repelled by the parent's drunken behavior that he develops opposite and negative attitudes toward the use of alcohol.

Traditionally, the family setting was the place where drinking habits were formed. Today, this is somewhat less true. Peer groups make a significant contribution to the formation of drinking practices. Adolescent drinking habits often reflect what the "rest of the kids" are doing. Adolescent alcoholism tends to be an activity clustering among friends. If the gang is involved in heavy drinking or in drugs, it is difficult for any one member to abstain. It is also evident that the adult in certain kinds of work (public relations, for example) is exposed to considerable pressure to drink too much. Some people succumb to alcoholism as a sort of occupational disease.

SOCIOCULTURAL

Culture Specific

Certain cultures (French, American, Irish) have traditionally had high levels of alcoholism, and others (Italian, Chinese) apparently have a low prevalence of alcoholism. A number of reasons for the varying frequency have been offered: The meaning of alcohol in the society, early child rearing pactices, or acceptance or rejection of intoxication as a social practice. People living within a culture with considerable pressure to drink and with a high rate of destructive drinking are at great risk. For certain groups in that culture (young, urban males, for example) very heavy drinking is almost the cultural norm. In such a society drinking is equated with manliness; it becomes the way to show group identification and solidarity, and it is the institutionalized way to release inhibitions.

Subcultures under Stress

A subgroup, which finds itself overwhelmed with severe conflict, in a non-win situation, or one living in considerable turmoil, will find that large numbers of its members resort to drinking themselves into oblivion as the only way out. Subcultures have been obliterated, in part at least, by alcoholic overindulgence of a major segment of its key people.

ALCOHOLISM: A SYNTHESIS

It seems reasonable to think of alcoholism as the end product of a combination of the various factors mentioned. The McCords described a chain of events as a result of their studies that often lead to destructive drinking.(4) The following model draws upon their work.

A person with a genetic vulnerability (manifested psychologically or biochemically) had an early childhood of exposure to considerable family stress. This led to an inadequate, erratic satisfaction of his dependency needs, and an inability to form a clear self-image, including a definition of his male role. As a result, he developed intensified dependency needs and was conflicted about the means to satisfy them. As an adolescent he became aware of the cultural pressures as expressed both in the mass media and in daily life to "be a man," and not to be dependent. He, therefore, adopted an "independent facade" of self-reliance and toughness while still searching to satisfy his underlying dependency.

As he grew up, the pressures for him to accept the independent male role continued. Other alternatives for him to satisfy his dependency needs were not at hand. He found in alcohol a transient release from the underlying struggle between what he was, and what he ought to be. Furthermore, drinking was not only culturally acceptable, it was equated with manliness and self-sufficiency, the very qualities in which he felt inadequate. His drinking did not solve the problem, rather it aggravated it. Finally, his tenuous self-image collapsed, his dependency traits broke forth, and his drinking went completely out of control.

Such a chain of events seems to have occurred in some of the children the McCords follow. Other sequences applicable to other men and women, and terminating in alcoholism, also exist. Although one specific event might at times seem to precipitate someone into a life of drink, antecedent factors would surely be required for such a dramatic change in life style.

NOTES

1. Shuckit, M. A., et al. A study of alcoholism in half siblings. *Amer. J. Psychiat.* 128:1132, 1972.
2. Goodwin, D. W. et al. Alcohol problems in adoptees raised apart from alcoholic biological parents. *Arch. Gen. Psychiat.* 28:238, 1973.
3. Mendelson, J. H., et al. Experimentally induced chronic intoxication and withdrawal in alcoholics. *Quart. J. Stud. Alc. Suppl. No. 2,* 1964.
4. McCord, W. and McCord, J. *Origins of Alcoholism,* Stanford University Press, Stanford, 1960.

7. How Social Drinkers Become Alcoholics

The transition from being an abstainer to suddenly becoming an alcoholic is not the usual course. What is much more frequent is that someone who had been drinking moderately for years will shift the pattern of imbibing to one of problem drinking or alcoholism.

Many students of the phenomenon separate alcoholism from problem drinking. Alcoholism is considered to be a physical addiction to alcohol: the build-up of tolerance over time, and an alcohol withdrawal syndrome varying from shakiness to DTs on sudden reduction or discontinuance of alcohol. A strong desire to continue to drink heavily is an associated effect. Problem drinking consists of difficulties in living directly related to overdrinking. Marital, job, social, or health problems are some of the areas affected. Addiction may or may not coexist. In this essay alcoholism refers to both problem drinking and alcohol addiction.

It is most unlikely that an alcoholic person deliberately makes a decision to become one. Instead, he or she slips imperceptibly, without conscious intent, into excessive drinking styles that culminate in alcoholism. This transformation period is important to identify by the individual and by the clinician.

People in a pre-alcoholic phase may be able to correct their drinking behavior more readily if they become aware of their progression toward destructive alcohol usage patterns. This incremental drinking mode probably accounts for the majority of alcoholics, and the question is: Can an early warning system be designed that will alert the drinker when he or she approaches a hazardous consumption level?

The problem is not a simple one. It consists of more than a quantitative change in consumption. Some people can be impaired by daily amounts of alcohol that others seem to consume without apparent difficulties. A fatty liver or alcoholic hepatitis may develop in a person whose intake is "no more than the others in my group." In this country many occupational and social groups imbibe rather heavily and consistently. Some of their members will get into difficulties early. Others may go on indefinitely without encountering alcohol-related adverse effects.

Usually, an escalation of drinking practices occurs during periods of increased stress. A few extra drinks are taken to unwind, to forget or to sleep. (A drink is equivalent to one and one-half ounces of 100 proof whiskey, six ounces of wine, or 16 ounces of beer. They each contain about three-quarters of an ounce of ethanol.) When the stressful period is past, the newly established drinking routine continues. Under conditions of further stressful episodes, alcohol consumption increases again. Eventually, a point is reached when attempts to cut down or stop fail because of early withdrawal symptoms like the shakes or insomnia; these require alcohol for relief.

The pleasures of drinking can have an entrapping quality. The mild euphoria and social relaxation provided by a few drinks produce feelings of amiable fellowship and good cheer. This is an attractive state, very attractive to some, but some people make the error of assuming that the additional ingestion of potable beverages will serve to increase the fun. The memory of the immediate pleasure is of greater importance than the memory of distant bad effects.

With additional amounts, because of the biphasic action of alcohol, the mild and pleasant stimulation changes to an increasing depression and then to a substantial loss of control over behavior. This up-then-down effect of ethanol on the central nervous system also is well known when alcohol is used as an anti-anxiety agent. Initially, alcohol reduces tension and anxiety. As heavy drinking becomes chronic, anxiety levels are elevated. It may be that this increase in anxiety perpetuates drinking in a vain search for relief. Using alcohol to evade an unpleasant reality, to forget one's worries, or to achieve mastery over life's stresses usually turns out to be a poor effort at self-treatment that is compounded by the period of intoxication, the post-intoxication ineffectivenesss and debility, and the pre-intoxication drive to escape from the consequences.

The dilemma is that the socially drinking individual has few guidelines to indicate that he may be at risk when his drinking pattern gradually changes. If one stays below two drinks a day, and does not save up the drinks to go on a binge, impairment over the years will not occur (Anstie's Rule). But many people in this culture drink more than that and appear to do well. At what point do we approach our personal danger zone? The answer is not entirely in the amount of ethanol ingested over time, but in how and why one drinks and what the effects are.

We must also remember that even two drinks a day are too much for some people. There are those who are hypersensitive to very small amounts of ethanol, reacting with a flush, hypotension, tachycardia, and chest constriction. Then there are the pathologic drinkers who become violent under the influence of one or two glasses. In addition, a long list of drugs interact adversely when combined with alcohol. These range from antibiotics, antihypertensives, and anticonvulsants to anticoagulants, diuretics, sleeping pills, and many other groups. Of course people with peptic ulcer, pancreatitis, or liver ailments may increase the severity of their disorder by exposing themselves to alcohol. Diabetics and epileptics would be unwise to use alcohol if only because of the risk of smelling like a drunk during a period of unconsciousness, let alone the deleterious effects of alcohol in such conditions.

As a rule the shift to dysfunctional drinking is a gradual one. In large doses alcohol is a protoplasmic poison, but the dangerous level varies for each individual. Furthermore, to tell a person who has been regularly taking four drinks a day, and who has crept up to eight a day that he is at risk will predictably accomplish little. In fact, anger at being unjustly accused, or a complete denial that a problem exists, are the usual responses. The advice is interpreted as nagging and may, in itself, lead to additional drinking. It would seem more desirable for each person who drinks to regularly examine his own drinking practices and be willing to change them if the suspicion of overdrinking is uncovered.

Self-examination should be a part of the drinking person's routine, and every effort should be made to be as candid with oneself as possible. Examples of questions that could be indicative of a pre-alcoholic or an early alcoholic situation include the following.

DO I GET DRUNK WHEN I INTENDED TO STAY SOBER?

This question speaks to early loss of control over one's drinking. The inability to stop, once drinking has commenced, is an ominous sign. Even an occasional loss of control may be a warning signal. Some confirmed alcoholics are unable to stop drinking after a single drink has been consumed.

WHEN THINGS GET ROUGH DO I NEED A DRINK OR TWO TO QUIET MY NERVES?

Using alcohol as a tranquilizer can be precarious because the dose is difficult to adjust, and no other person is supervising the medication.

DO OTHER PEOPLE SAY I'M DRINKING TOO MUCH?

If the negative effects of drinking are evident to more than one person, or to a single person on a number of occasions, this means that one's behavior is exceeding the social limits. It would be well to listen to such comments, remembering that most people are usually reluctant to talk about the drinking troubles of their friends and relatives.

HAVE I GOTTEN INTO TROUBLE WITH THE LAW, MY FAMILY OR MY BUSINESS ASSOCIATES IN CONNECTION WITH DRINKING?

Being arrested for drunk driving or drunk and disorderly conduct are not reliable early signs of excessive drinking. Only a minority of these acts are apprehended, so it is unlikely that this was the first such offense. Being confronted with difficulties at home or at work also tend to be the cumulative effect of a long series of objectionable behaviors.

IS IT NOT POSSIBLE FOR ME TO STOP DRINKING FOR A WEEK OR MORE?

Resolving to stop and not being able to carry it off would indicate a definite psychological or physical dependence and reflect a serious future outlook. Being able to stop is encouraging, but it does not eliminate the possibility of binge or other types of destructive drinking. Many alcoholics remain dry for long intervals. It is not being able to stop that is indicative of a dangerous situation.

DO I SOMETIMES NOT REMEMBER WHAT HAPPENED DURING A DRINKING EPISODE?

Blackouts due to alcohol consist of variable periods of amnesia for what happened during the drinking bout. They are to be differentiated from passing out into unconsciousness, which is the end state of intoxication. Blackouts, which are complete and cover periods of hours or more, are definite evidences of alcoholism. Passing out is an unfavorable sign.

HAS A DOCTOR EVER SAID THAT MY DRINKING WAS IMPAIRING MY HEALTH?

Although it is now possible to pick up early evidences of harmful drinking, by the time a medical examination reveals abnormalities attributable to alcohol it is clear that continuing to drink as previously will further damage one's health. Abnormalities of amino acid ratios, plasma lipoproteins, or hepatic enzymes are signals that too much ethanol is being ingested for the liver to cope with.

DO I TAKE A FEW DRINKS BEFORE GOING TO A SOCIAL GATHERING JUST IN CASE THERE WON'T BE MUCH TO DRINK?

Assuring oneself of a sufficient supply of alcohol just in case is evidence of an unhealthy preoccupation with such beverages and speaks for a need to feel "loaded" on social occasions.

AM I IMPATIENT WHILE AWAITING MY DRINK TO BE SERVED?

The urgency to obtain a drink reflects a craving. Gulping drinks is another sign of overinvolvement with alcohol.

HAVE I TRIED TO CUT DOWN BUT FAILED?

As with the inability to stop drinking for periods of time, the inability to cut down is a warning that dependence is present or impending. Cutting down successfully, but eventually slipping back up is another sign of possible future trouble.

DO I HAVE TO HAVE A DRINK IN THE MORNING BECAUSE I FEEL QUEASY OR HAVE THE SHAKES?

The relief obtained from a drink after arising is apparently due to the relief of early, mild withdrawal symptoms. Therefore, a degree of physical dependence is present, and this means future trouble.

CAN I HOLD MY LIQUOR BETTER THAN OTHER PEOPLE?

Being able to hold one's liquor is not necessarily an evidence of manliness or freedom from complications of drinking. It may indicate the development of tolerance due to the persistent consumption of large quantities. Although social disabilities may be avoided by holding one's liquor, physical impairment due to the amount consumed is inevitable.

HAVE MANY MEMBERS OF MY FAMILY BEEN ALCOHOLICS?

There seems to be a genetic component to some instances of alcoholism. People whose parents or siblings had serious problems with alcohol have reason to be extra careful of their drinking habits. Not only may there be an inherited vulnerability, but the early life experience of a child of alcoholic parents may predispose to seeking out consciousness changing drugs or alcohol in later life.

The indicators mentioned above are early or somewhat advanced signs of alcoholism. They should be assessed seriously by the individual concerned or by the health professional who is evaluating him. The recognition that a threat to one's future exists is a first step. The second step is taking realistic action on the basis of the threat. The third step is sustaining the new behavior. These steps are the critical blocks in altering the course of destructive drinking: refusal to accept the information, refusal to do anything about it, and refusal to maintain a corrective course of action once it is initiated.

SUMMARY

We have about 10 million alcoholics in this country. The human burden of these people to themselves, their families, and the rest of the population is immense. Primary prevention, the education of those not involved in the disorder, will be the eventual solution, but it is a distant goal. It is in secondary prevention, the redirection of those threatened with alcoholism, that will lead to more immediate results. Meanwhile, tertiary prevention, the rehabilitation of the 10 million who can be considered alcoholics, must also be carried out as effectively as possible. Alcoholism is the most important drug problem of all from a public health, or any other, point of view.

8. The Volitional Disorders

It may be worthwhile to consider the disorders of volition—the conditions we bring upon ourselves. This eassy will deal only with those involving the intake of some substance, the consumatory volitional disorders.

It is a bit old fashioned to speak of volition, of free will, at a time when enormous forces seem to dominate our existence. But no matter how compelling these are, a measure of choice still seems to remain.

As these disorders are examined, they do not seem to arise from some defect of the will. No one decides: "I will become an alcoholic—or an addict—or obese." Ordinarily, these maladies emerge after a long series of minimal decisions such as "I'll have another drink," or "I'll get stoned," or "I'll have a piece of pie a la mode." No conscious choice was ever made. Instead, the person slipped unknowingly into a pattern of behavior that culminated in a disturbance of some consequence.

Rather, will power could be operational after the condition has become manifest, and it is evident that a life-threatening disorder exists. We must be aware, however, of the overriding difficulties that the over-indulger will experience in trying to eliminate the habits of a lifetime.

To stop doing something that allayed psychic distress for decades, either pharmacologically or symbolically, is extremely difficult. The usual rewards of tension reduction, relaxation, or unconsciousness are no longer available. Aversive life experiences can no longer be dealt with by the usual means, however harmful they may have been. Even the psychomotor satisfactions of the habit—whether it be fixing, gorging, guzzling, or smoking—are gone.

Six consumatory volitional disorders will be discussed. Others exist but they are less frequently seen than the half dozen to be mentioned.

EXCESSIVE SMOKING OF TOBACCO

Smoking is one of the more difficult of the disorders of volition to understand. The substance is widely available, legal, and socially acceptable. Most adults are or have been smokers.

When cigarette users are asked why they persist despite the hazards involved, they are hard-pressed to describe the rewards of smoking. Some will mention feelings of relaxation, others mild stimulation, but many notice little or no mood alteration. It is a trivial reward when compared to the exaltation of cocaine, the vast alterations of consciousness that is LSD, the orgasmic pleasure of a good bag of heroin, or even the oblivion that sleeping pills or booze can bring. The joys of smoking can hardly be a significant reason for its perpetuation.

Instead, we should look at the ritual of smoking as being rewarding, and the reinforcement of repetitive oral-manual routines many thousands of times a year as the element that serves to fix and perpetuate the behavior. In addition, nicotine has been shown to produce a withdrawal syndrome in laboratory animals when its administration has been suddenly discontinued. This has been confirmed in humans whose pitiful tales of the abstinence effects are rather commonplace.

A few years ago the Synanon administration decided that a noxious practice like smoking should be abolished in Synanon houses. Most of the residents were people who successfully had kicked their heroin addictions cold turkey. But a number of these residents had to leave Synanon because they were unable to kick cigarettes. Some of the others felt that coming off heroin was less stressing. What does this mean? Apparently, the cigarette habit is so dependency-producing because of the social mimicking displays, cultural persuasion, personal gratifications, and some physiologic reinforcers that relapse is more frequent than remission.

One of the memorable moments of my medical career took place almost 40 years ago when, as an intern, I was doing a history and physical on a newly admitted patient with Buerger's disease. He had had amputations of both upper arms, and a mid-thigh and a tarsal amputation of the legs. I asked, as is usual, what had brought him into the hospital. "Doc," he said, with a certain urgency in his voice, "Could I have a flap fixed on my stump so that I will be able to hold a cigarette?"

Of all the volitional disorders, smoking is as dangerous as any. In fact, although there are those who rationalize the data and say that the final proof is not yet in, the statistical and experimental evidence is better than we will ever have for any of the other drugs called dangerous. Next to excessive drinking, it probably causes more morbidity and mortality than any other drug, including one named heroin. It is a major factor in development of lung and other cancers and chronic pulmonary disease like bronchitis and emphysema, and it contributes to a variety of cardiovascular and gastrointestinal problems.

Unfortunately, the earlier hopes of a reduction in smokers and smoking that arose during the late 1960s have been frustrated. More people are smoking more now than ever. In the United States more than 4,000 cigarettes a year are consumed for every adult person over 15.

OVEREATING

Obesity is common in affluent societies. A quarter of the population in this country are obese; that is, more than 20 percent over their ideal weight. With increasing age, overweight conditions increase. Interestingly, even in non-affluent countries obesity is also present. This is probably a reflection of the high symbolic value placed on food and the high carbohydrate diet available, usually consisting of potatoes, bread, and other starches.

Juvenile obesity is usually due to genetic-metabolic factors, familial-cultural patterns that encourage overeating, evidences of emotional deprivation (such as separation from mother), and combinations of these. Eating habits learned early tend to continue into adult life. Adult obesity increases the severity and mortality from diseases like hypertension, arteriosclerosis, diabetes, gout, and cholecystitis.

Eating is a gratifying sensory experience. People who have little to enjoy in other aspects of daily living may overeat to achieve a measure of satisfaction with their existence.

The ingestion of food can also be anxiety-reducing, the feeling of "being full" is relaxing to child and adult alike. Depression is generally accompanied by anorexia and weight loss, but compulsive overeating is also seen, and the extreme hyperphagias are either depressive or psychotic equivalents.

In such studies done to examine the psychological characteristics of very adipose people, a rather common finding consisted of a lowered self-esteem. There was an expectation of personal failure and rejection. Their anger was turned inward upon themselves with depressive equivalents and self-inflicted injuries occurring at a higher rate than among the non-obese control groups.

Like many other volitional conditions, overeating is an exaggeration of a normal process. It might be assumed, therefore, that obesity should readily respond to treatment. This is not so. When evaluated over long periods of time, the conventional therapies are unsuccessful. What is needed, of course, is a thorough reeducation and a reduction in the emotional problems of the patient.

EXCESSIVE USE OF SUGAR

Every child knows that sweets are reward foods. The taste of sweetness is sought by members of all societies and even by other species, including the dog and the monkey. This almost universal craving has led to a vast production and refining of sugar, which is one of the few foods we eat that is virtually 100 percent pure. In fact, it is too pure, stripped of valuable nutrients in order to be snow white.

The association between sugar intake and childhood dental caries is well established, but we prefer to fluorinate our water rather than reduce sucrose consumption. The stress of high loads of sugar over many years is presumed to contribute to adult-type diabetes by exhaustion of the islet cells of the pancreas.

A number of primitive cultures have been studied following the introduction of refined sugar into their diet. It has been found that when the per capita consumption per year rises to about 70 pounds, the incidence of diabetes approaches that of civilized societies such as England and the United States, whose use is more than 100 pounds per person each year. The sweet tooth also gives rise to obesity over time. Using the above statistic, about 600 to 700 calories a day are derived from sugars.

No one is going to take our refined sugar away. But those who use large quantities should be aware of some possible undesirable consequences, especially if they are overweight or have an abnormal glucose tolerance test.

EXCESSIVE DRINKING OF CAFFEINATED BEVERAGES

Coffee and tea have long been inveighed against, more so in bygone times when it was the drink of extremists who wanted to overthrow the establishments of the day. Coffee houses were seditious places where plots were brewed along with the coffee. Today it is the most innocent of beverages, and the 100 mg of caffeine a cup it contains is harmless—except for certain people. A collaborative heart study that looked into the effects of various drugs, alcohol, and beverages suggested that drinking more than six cups of coffee daily increased the risk of myocardial infarction. Tea drinking was less damaging because it contains half as much caffeine and also has some theophylline, which is a mild coronary vasodilator.

Probably more common than coronary artery effects are the psychic disturbances that consistent coffee drinking evokes in some people. Disturbed sleep is a well-known occurrence, but daytime irritability, nervousness, restlessness, and headache are not so uncommon. Some people describe withdrawal effects from caffeine, including impaired alertness, headache, and shakiness.

The drinking of caffeinated beverages is one of the more benign of the volitional disorders. It would be regrettable if that pleasure were eliminated. However, with the advent, at last, of potable decaffeinated coffees, those sensitive to the effects of the alkaloid can switch. Perhaps those who are double-digit coffee drinkers should do likewise.

VOLITIONAL DISORDERS ASSOCIATED WITH ABUSABLE DRUGS

The inordinate use of mind-altering drugs can be life-impairing and life-endangering. Almost all of these drugs, used in large amounts over prolonged periods, are hazardous to health by producing physical damage or some mental disorganization. What must be remembered is that drug abusers do not consciously want to shorten or terminate their lives. Some of them are self-treating their depression or their schizophrenic symptoms. Some are using drugs as a means of coping, however maladaptively, with stress. Some have little or no future orientation, no concept of tomorrow, and thus no need to be concerned about survival. Therefore, what we called risk-taking may not be that to the risk taker. When we see a heroin addict looking for the "pusher" whose junk has just killed someone, he is merely looking for extra good stuff, not death.

The chronic lethal states will not be considered at this time. Instead, the focus will be on the acute disasters that can befall a chemically intoxicated individual.

Narcotics

The junkie is engaged in a high risk occupation. He is apt to incur accidental or deliberate injury or death from many sources: muggers, his friends, his pusher, the police, and others. His suicide rate is 20 to 50 times that of the population at large. It is believed that each year 1 to 2 percent of the heroin addicts die from overdose, or other acute reactions to the injected material. The numbers of street addicts over 60 are remarkably few. Some mature out, it is true, but most will die before achieving that age.

Sedatives

Like the narcotic addict and the alcoholic, the habitual user of sleeping pills is accident prone and suicide prone. Barbiturates are now the second most popular means of suiciding, and they are first among the methods used by women. The "accidental suicide" has been well described by Kubie and others. This is the person who uses combinations of depressants in sufficient quantities to knock out the respiratory center. The most popular combination at the moment seems to be alcohol, a minor tranquilizer, and a barbiturate. The additive or potentiating effects of such polydrug use can result in death without any overt intent to do one's self in.

Stimulants

The heavy amphetamine user, as epitomized by the "speedfreak," is indeed a "death tempter" and "death defier" as described by Shneidman. Injecting gram quantities of amphetamines into one's vein can be devastating pharmacologically and behaviorally. The resulting combination of impulsivity, hyperactivity, and paranoid thinking can lead to all kinds of trouble. A half-dozen years ago something called "speed roulette" was still around. It consisted of two "freaks," each attempting to outdo the other in the amounts of "speed" they injected. The one who could not walk away lost.

Hallucinogens

Sudden death in connection with taking a drug like LSD is infrequent. When it occurs, it is usually due to a grandiose overestimate of one's powers. This results in attempts to fly or walk on water, all unsuccessful to date. Suicide is rare, and homicides even more so.

ALCOHOLISM AND ALCOHOL ABUSE

Alcoholism abounds with paradoxes. It is the most common and serious problem of all the drug dependencies, yet it is the most socially acceptable. While 95 percent of the adult drinkers apparently can drink without harming themselves, 5 percent are drinking destructively. It is not easy to predict who will become one of the 5 percenters. It is a malady in which the etiologic agent is obvious, but the prevention and cure elude us. One man's heavy social drinking is another's pathological dependence on alcohol.

Booze is ordinarily consumed to reduce anxiety, except that its chronic use increases anxiety levels. It is employed as a social lubricant to increase friendliness and good cheer, yet it is clearly the most violence producing of all drugs. And then, of course, the paradox of volition: why do millions impair their health, shorten their lives, disorganize their families and destroy themselves socially and financially by drinking excessively?

Information needs no retelling here about physical and mental damage, about the social and economic costs, about accidents, and the other prices paid by the 10 million alcohol abusers and 190 million nonabusers.

What we are interested in is: Why? Is it genetic predisposition, maladaptive response to environmental stress, permissive cultural attitudes, personality susceptibility, metabolic deficiency or some malignant, learned behavior? The answer is: It's all of these in varying degrees in different individuals. And what of the will? Volition could overcome all of these factors, but extreme loading makes willful correction much more difficult.

Since the abuse of alcohol is so widespread and disastrous in its effects, perhaps a solution might be to replace the personal will with a political will. When a substance is so intermeshed into the social structure as alcohol, no government interdiction or prohibition can work. The only point to be made is that if alcohol were a newly discovered drug, and if it were submitted to the F.D.A. for marketing, it could hardly be approved for sale. The adverse effects and complications of extensive use are simply too many.

III
DIAGNOSIS

1. Symptoms and Signs of Drug Abuse

In this essay the following definitions are used:
Depressants: *All narcotics, sedatives, tranquilizers, volatile solvents, alcohol.*
Narcotics or opiates: *Opium, heroin, morphine, Demerol, methadone, Dilaudid, codeine.*
Sedatives: *Barbiturate and non-barbiturate sedatives and hypnotics.*
Tranquilizers: *The minor tranquilizers such as meprobamate and chlordiazepoxide.*
Stimulants: *Amphetamines, cocaine, Ritalin, Preludin.*
Hallucinogens: *LSD, mescaline, DMT, MDA Sernyl, psylocybin.*

The widespread misuse of drugs makes it necessary to consider this condition in the differential diagnosis of a wide variety of medical, surgical, and psychiatric illnesses. This is particularly true in adolescent medicine, but adults are by no means excluded from the untoward effects of mind-altering drugs. The more common symptoms and signs that are encountered will be reviewed by system.

ASSOCIATED CONDITIONS

A number of ailments that occur more frequently in heavy drug users than in the population at large are mentioned here. They are not the result of drug ingestion; they are due to the life style of the "head" particularly when he congregates in urban ghettos or in unsanitary communes.

Poor hygiene and a lowered resistance to infection produce an increased incidence of upper respiratory infections, trench mouth, scabies, pediculosis, and impetigo. Poorly healing sores are frequently seen. Dietary faddism may induce mineral, vitamin, or protein deficiencies. Dental caries is one of the frequent reasons for visits to free clinics and other emergency health facilities. Lacerations of the soles of the feet are occupational hazards for the unshod. Streptococcal sore throat, viral hepatitis, mononucleosis, tuberculosis, and leptospirosis, along with other infections including the childhood contagious diseases, are present in greater than average community levels because of malnutrition, crowding, dirt, or neglect. Food poisoning epidemics from poorly prepared or improperly stored food or contaminated water have occurred during a few rock festivals.

Ringworm, seborrhea, and jock itch are well known. The incidence of acne is high even for this age group. Whether this is the result of poor skin care is uncertain. Some investigators believe that marihuana can exacerbate acne.

Because of casual attitudes toward the variety of sexual activities, syphilis, gonorrhea, and other venereal diseases are increasing in this population. The chancre may sometimes be found in extragenital sites such as the lip, tonsil, finger, or nipple. Nonspecific urethritis and cervicitis, trichomoniasis, and moniliasis are also prevalent. Hemorrhoids and anal fissures in male or female youngsters may be a complication of unusual sex practices.

With the increased violence that has come to the scene, the results of beatings, shootings, and stabbings have required treatment. Only a minority of these assaults have been due to drug-induced aggressiveness. Usually they are the result of the intervention of criminal or psychopathic elements into a colony of innocents who are unable to cope with them.

GENERAL SYMPTOMS

Weight loss or malnutrition can accompany chronic, heavy use of most drugs. Amphetamines and cocaine have a direct effect upon the satiety centers producing anorexia. The heroin addict, in addition to a reduced appetite, tends to use money for drugs, not food. Exhaustion is the end state of "speed" runs and other extended drug binges. Impotence and amenorrhea are reflections of a general drug-induced debility, with depressant drugs further dampening libido and hormonal function.

Fever is found when stimulants or hallucinogens increase sympathetic tone and the metabolic rate. It is also present during the depressant withdrawal period. Needle-borne infections, of course, will also produce elevated temperatures.

SKIN

Color Changes

Jaundice is often noted when the patient has serum or viral hepatitis. Cyanosis is maximal in opiate overdose, but can also be present in sedative overdoses and during convulsive episodes. LSD produces a flush during its period of action. The discoloration of the fingers in heavy cannabis smokers differs in location from tobacco stain. In the "pothead" it is on the thumb and forefinger, in the tobacco smoker it is on the fore and middle finger.

The "tracks" of long standing opiate (and less frequently long term barbiturate and amphetamine "mainliners") are pigmented, linear markings along the course of superficial viens of the arms, legs, and penis. They are caused by injected foreign particles or low grade infections. Since they last indefinitely, efforts are sometimes made to cover them with a tatoo. Long sleeved clothing is worn during warm weather for similar reasons. The puncture needle marks can be detected for only a few days or a week unless an inflammatory reaction has occurred. Thrombophlebitis of the veins is occasionally seen and is the result of injecting irritating or infectious material. Abscesses or depressed, scarred areas are present in "skin poppers" particularly when the opiate injection has been made into the fatty tissue of the upper arm or thigh.

Other Skin Changes

Ankle edema can be found in an occasional patient on methadone maintenance. Gooseflesh is a reliable, objective sign of withdrawal from opiates. Sweating is prominent during the withdrawal states and during high dose amphetamine use. Patients on methadone maintenance may complain of it. Almost any drug can cause a rash. Barbiturate and tranquilizer rashes are quite common. The pustular rash of chronic bromidism should be recalled. Acne rosacea and dilated facial venules accompany heavy alcohol intake. Solvent inhalers may present with a rash around the mouth and nose.

EYE, NOSE AND THROAT

Eye

The conjunctivitis (red eye) of the cannabis user and the alcoholic is well known. Dilated pupils are encountered during hallucinogenic, volatile solvent or stimulant exposure. Anticholinergic drugs like belladonna, henbane or Jimson weed will also dilate the pupils. Constricted pupils are the hallmark of opiate activity. During withdrawal or following Nalline injection they will dilate. Solvents will cause tearing, and lacrimation is also a part of the opiate withdrawal state.

Nose

Runny nose occurs during the opiate abstinence syndrome. Septal ulceration in connection with cocaine and amphetamine "snorting" is documented. The intense vasoconstriction from cocaine can cause a septal perforation.

The odor of some misused items can be detected during and after use. Volatile solvents and alcohol are partially excreted via the respiratory tract, therefore they can be smelled for an hour or more after intake. The odor of marihuana smoke resembles burnt rope and is perceptible in the exhaled breath, the clothing, or the room for a while. Incense may be used to disguise the odor.

Throat

Uvular edema is described following heavy bouts of hashish smoking. Users of marihuana, anticholinergic compounds, amphetamines, and opiates may complain of dryness of the mouth. Sernyl (phencyclidine) is said to cause salivation. Laryngeal spasm and freezing occur when aerosol sprays are inhaled rapidly for purposes of intoxication.

RESPIRATORY

Bronchitis is a symptom in those who persistenly smoke such irritating substances as tobacco, marihuana, and hashish. Bronchial carcinoma and emphysema have not yet been demonstrated to be related to cannabis use as they have to tobacco. Asthmatic attacks have been precipitated by LSD and cannabis in predisposed individuals. Aspiration pneumonia can take place during a coma due to depressant drugs. Pneumonia, pulmonary abscesses, embolism, and fibrosis all may develop in connection with injection of insoluble or septic materials into a vein. Talc emboli occur after Ritalin, Pyribenzamine or other talc base tablets are dissolved and injected.

Apnea is a manifestation of depressant poisoning. Acute pulmonary edema is the common cause of death in opiate overdose. It is associated with right ventricular dilation, hypotension, hyperpnea, and cyanosis. Hyperpnea is a possible sequel to high amphetamine doses. Chest pain is also a component of the amphetamine overdose picture.

Instances of suffocation are known in which glue sniffers fell unconscious on the rag containing the material. Other cases have occurred when volatile solvents were sniffed in closed spaces, for example, a plastic garment bag.

CARDIOVASCULAR

Endocarditis of bacterial or fungal origin is a recognized complication of unsterile intravenous injections. Cardiac arrhythmias are associated with amphetamine overdose. This condition, also called "overamped," is manifested by tachycardia and hypertension. Other reasons for a rapid pulse are cannabis, hallucinogen, or cocaine use. During opiate withdrawal the pulse rate is often rapid. Sino-atrial or A-V arrest is precipitated by the Freon sprays in the presence of hypoxia.

Cerebral hemorrhages in young people may be caused by dramatic elevations of blood pressure due to amphetamine injections. Bradycardia and hypotension are concomitants of opiate overdose. Shock is a development in serious poisoning due to narcotics or sedatives. An angiitis of small and medium calibre arteries has been reported after prolonged amphetamine use, particularly in high doses.

GASTROINTESTINAL

Nausea and vomiting accompany the ingestion of many drugs. This is particularly true of peyote. The first few injections of opiates may produce vomiting, but tolerance to this effect is rapidly acquired. Loss of appetite is noteworthy when stimulants are used. It is also routinely present during the LSD state. On the other hand, hyperphagia is remarked upon by about half of cannabis users. A ravenous appetite is also present during amphetamine withdrawal. Opiate users are usually constipated, with diarrhea and abdominal cramps occurring during withdrawal. Diarrhea is experienced by some cannabis users. In folk medicine it has been used in the treatment of constipation. Complaints of abdominal pain have been heard from an occasional amphetamine abuser and during opiate withdrawal. Sometimes the pain is severe enough to cause one to consider a surgical emergency.

Hepatitis as a disease of the unsterile needle or of the life style of the "head" needs no additional comment. Large amounts of amphetamines and alcohol have a hepatotoxic capability. The role of malnutrition and hypovitaminosis in liver damage due to these two drugs is acknowledged. Liver damage due to volatile solvents, particularly carbon tetrachloride is known.

HEMATOPOIETIC

Case reports of aplastic anemia due to benzene inhalation are in the literature. Nutritional anemias are found whenever intense preoccupation with mind-altering drugs occurs. Malaria is not encountered as frequently as in the past in connection with the use of group syringes and needles. Blood stream infections are always a possibility under such circumstances. Bleeding tendencies are a real possibility in heavy drinkers due to their varicosities and prothrombin deficiency.

MUSCULOSKELETAL

Serious musculoskeletal disorders do not play a noteworthy role in drug abuse problems. Muscle wasting as a part of the severe weight loss in "speedfreaks" is seen. Tremors are a common symptom during hallucinogen and stimulant use. In chronic alcohol, sedative, and opiate users the tremor may persist after the drugs are no longer used. During opiate withdrawal muscle cramps and spasms can cause considerable discomfort. The muscle jerks may involve an entire extremity (kicking the habit). The aches and pains of all withdrawal states are referred to the muscles and bones.

NEUROLOGICAL

The hallucinogens and stimulants increase and quicken the deep tendon reflexes. The opposite is true of the sedatives and narcotics. Headache is complained of during amyl nitrite inhalation. Occasional marihuana users will speak of a hangover headache. The prototypical symptom of the hung-over drinker or solvent sniffer is headache.

The stimulants and hallucinogens produce insomnia. Sedatives, cannabis, tranquilizers, and narcotics induce drowsiness. The depressant drugs can result in stupor or in coma. This includes the anesthetics such as nitrous oxide, the aerosols and volatile solvents. Convulsions are infrequently observed during LSD and amphetamine use. They constitute a part of the abstinence syndrome for all depressant drugs. Hyperactivity is associated with the amphetamines and cocaine. Stereotyped activity is also characteristic of these drugs. Repetitive, useless activities of a simple nature such as picking the skin, pacing, or stringing and unstringing beads might be continued for hours. A cerebellar syndrome consisting of ataxia, nystagmus, diplopia, clumsiness, and slurred speech is associated with depressant intoxication.

Some of the disease entities seen in connection with drug abuse include peripheral neuritis, Korsakoff's and Wernicke's syndromes, (alcohol) tetanus, and encephalitis (needle borne infection). A case of lead encephalopathy due to gasoline sniffing has been reported. A single report of cerebral atrophy in chronic cannabis users must await confirmation.

PSYCHIATRIC

Some of the signs of involvement in the drug life include behavioral toxicity; that is, behavior becomes destructive to the individual or those around him. Changes from previous behavior patterns occur: changes in the sleep-wake cycle, changes in choice of friends and associates, changes in mood including unpredictability and impulsivity, changes in the direction of decreased school or work performance, and changes in truthfulness and honesty. Other changes observed are in goal-directedness, drives, and attitudes. This is the amotivational syndrome. These alterations are not diagnostic of drug abuse, but that condition ought to be considered when they become obvious.

During cannabis, stimulant, and hallucinogen trips panic and anxiety states can prevail. An acute psychotic or paranoid reaction may intervene. A toxic delirium is possible with every drug that has been used for its mind altering properties. Deliria are also characteristics of the depressant abstinence syndromes, with confusion, hallucinations, and delusions regularly seen. It is said that certain drugs have specific hallucinatory qualities. For example, cocaine is supposed to provide tactile hallucinations usually of insects in or on the skin. Folk beliefs allege that alcoholic deliria consists of seeing strange animals such as pink elephants. These tales are often mistaken. Alcohol can induce an acute auditory hallucinosis during which the individual is quite well oriented except that he hears voices, music, or other sounds that are not present. Depressions may develop during LSD experiences, but are seen more often following that event. Particularly during the withdrawal phase following a binge of high dose amphetamines can the depression be profound. The suicide rate among all drug dependent persons is high both during the intoxication and during the drug-free interval. Homicides may be more frequent with amphetamine in large doses than any other drug. Accidental death due to miscalculation of the environment is a possibility with every agent. Prolonged psychotic breaks are well known with the hallucinogens, the stimulants, alcohol, and the sedatives. Clinicians have diagnosed chronic brain syndromes in people who have taken LSD, amphetamines, and depressants over a long period of time.

CONCLUSION

Almost any organ system may be involved in the side effects of drug misuse. The possibility that presenting symptoms might be caused by drug exposure is worth entertaining. Occasionally, a perplexing diagnostic problem will be clarified when a detailed licit and illicit drug history is taken.

RECENT REFERENCES

General

1. Cherubin, C. E. Acute addictive states. N.Y. State J. Med. 71: 2391-2394 (Oct 14) 1971.
2. Louria, D. B. Medical complications of drug abuse. Drug Therapy. (Aug) 1972, pp. 35-44.
3. Lundberg, G. D. Complications of drug abuse. Calif. Med. 114: 77-78, 1971.

Amphetamines

4. Kramer, J. C., Fischman, V. S. and Littlefield, D. C. Amphetamine abuse. JAMA 201:305-309 (July 31) 1967.
5. Lynn, E. J. Amphetamine abuse. A "speed" trap. Psychiat. Quarterly 45:92-101, 1974.
6. Margolis, M. T. and Newton, T. H. Methamphetamine (speed) arteritis. Neuroradiology 2:179-182, 1971.
7. Tinklenberg, J. R. A clinical view of the amphetamines. Family Physician 4:81-86 (Nov) 1971.

Barbiturates

8. Deveniji, P. and Wilson, M. Abuse of barbiturates in an alcoholic population. Canad. Med. J. Assn. 104:219-221, 1971.
9. Norton, P. R. E. Some endocrinological aspects of barbiturate dependence. Brit. J. Pharmacol. 41:317-330, 1971.
10. Shubin, H. and Weil, M. H. Shock associated with barbiturate intoxication. JAMA 215:263-268, 1971.
11. Smith, D. E. and Wesson, D. R. A new method of treatment of barbiturate dependence. JAMA 213:294 (July 13) 1970.

Hallucinogens

12. Bakker, C. B. The clinical picture in hallucinogen intoxication. Hospital Medicine. (Nov) 1969, pp. 102-114.
13. Cohen, S. A classification of LSD reactions. Psychosomatics 12, 182-186, 1966.
14. Frosch, W. A. The abuse of psychotomimetic drugs. Int. J. Addictions. 6:299-308 (June) 1971.
15. Malleson, N. Acute adverse reactions to LSD in clinical and ex-

perimental use in the United Kingdom. Brit. J. Psychiat. 118: 229-230, 1971.

16. Schwartz, C. J. The complications of LSD: A review of the literature. J. Nerv. Ment. Dis. 146:174, 1968.

17. Stern, M. and Robbins, E. S. Clinical diagnosis and treatment of psychiatric disorders subsequent to use of psychedelic drugs. In, *Psychedelic Drugs,* Grune & Stratton, New York, 1969.

18. Taylor, R. L. Maurer, J. I. and Tinklenberg, J. R. Management of "bad trips" in an evolving, drug scene. JAMA 213:422 (July 20) 1970.

Marihuana

19. Campbell, AMG, Evans, M., Thomson, J. L. G. and Williams, M. J. Cerebral atrophy in young cannabis smokers. Lancet 2(7736) 1219-1224 (Dec 4) 1971.

20. Clark, L. D., Hughes, R. and Nakashima, E. N. Behavioral effects of marihuana. Arch. Gen. Psychiat. 23:193 (Sept) 1970.

21. Keup, W. Psychotic symptoms due to cannabis abuse. Dis. Nerv. Syst. 31:119 (Feb) 1970.

22. Kolansky, H. and Moore, W. T. Effects of marihuana on adolescents and young adults. JAMA 216, 486 (Apr 19) 1971.

23. Talbott, J. A. Marihuana psychosis. JAMA 210:299, 1969.

24. Tennant, F. S., Preble, M., Pendergast, T. S. and Ventry, P. Medical manifestations associated with hashish. JAMA 216:1965 (June 21) 1971.

25. Weil, A. T. Adverse reactions to marihuana. N. E. J. Med. 282: 907 (Apr 30) 1970.

Narcotics

26. Cherubin, C. E. Infectious disease problem of narcotic addicts. Arch. Int. Med. 128:309-314 (Aug) 1971.

27. Dole, V. P., Foldes, F. F., Trigg, H., Robinson, J. W. and Blatman, S. Methadone poisoning. N. Y. State J. Med. 71:541-543, 1971.

28. Saylor, L. F. Induced vivax malaria among users of intravenous heroin. Calif. Med. 114:73-75, 1971.

29. Stone, M. L., Salerno, L. J., Green, M. and Zelson, C. Narcotic addiction in pregnancy. Amer. J. Obstet. & Gynec. 109:716-723, 1971.

30. Tartakow, I. J. Narcotic induced hepatitis. Amer. J. Med. 50: 313-316, 1971.

Volatile Solvents

31. Bass, M. Sudden sniffing death. JAMA 212:2075, 1970.

32. Chapel, J. L. and Thomas, G. Aerosol inhalation for kicks. Missouri Med. 67:378, 1970.

33. Press, E. and Done, A. K. Physiologic effects and community

control measures for intoxication from the intentional inhalation of organic solvents I. Pediatrics 39:451, 1967. II. Pediatrics 39: 611, 1967.
34. Taylor, G. J. and Harris, W. S. Cardiac toxicity of aerosol propellants. JAMA. 214:81, 1970.

2. Skin Signs of Substance Abuse

The skin is almost all that we see of a person and it can be very revealing.

A glance at the skin may be rewarding for a clinician seeking diagnostic support in an obscure instance of some chemical dependency, or for an emergency room physician trying to understand why the patient is comatose, hardly breathing, and without a perceptible pulse.

ACUTE ALCOHOLIC INTOXICATION

Direct Signs of Drinking

The vasodilating effect of alcohol often produces a *flush*. Certain hypersensitive Asians and Eastern Europeans will flush strongly about the head and neck after ingesting very small quantities of alcoholic beverages. Drinkers who are receiving one of the antidiabetic sulfonamides tend to flush readily.

Naturally, anyone who takes a drink after swallowing Antabuse would show an intense red skin color in addition to the other symptoms of the alcohol-Antabuse reaction. The severe erythemas are thought to be caused by a sensitization to acetaldehyde. Since Antabuse inhibits the breakdown of acetaldehyde by interfering with the action of aldehyde dehydrogenase, the flush in that instance is almost certainly due to a high acetaldehyde blood level. *Red eye* is a suffusion of the conjunctiva associated with a prolonged bout of drinking.

Indirect Signs of Drinking

The clumsiness and the stuporous condition of the intoxicated person results in a number of cutaneous stigmata. *Cigarette burns* between the fingers and over the upper body are well known. Falls may result in *bruises* or *bleeding*. *Pressure ulcers* over the bony prominences reflect long periods of immobility due to unconsciousness. In the south, drinkers who fall asleep out-of-doors may awaken with disseminated *fire ant stings,* while those who do the same in northern states in winter will develop *frostbite,* to say the least.

CHRONIC ALCOHOLISM

Direct effects

Jaundice may be seen in patients with either alcoholic hepatitis or cirrhosis. *Spider angiomata and telangiectasis* are distributed over the upper thorax, neck, and head in steady drinkers.

The *caput Medusae* is a dilated, tortuous collection of veins surrounding the umbilicus in some cases in portal vein obstruction. It represents an attempt to form collateral pathways for the return of blood from the abdominal organs bypassing the scarred and occluded portal system in the liver. The phrase refers back to the head of Medusa, a mythological woman whose hair was turned into a mass of writhing snakes by Athena. Whoever looked at her was turned into stone.

Palmar erythema is a common sequel to heavy drinking. The syndrome of male *gynecomastia,* and sparse *chest, pubic,* and *axillary hair* is due to a toxic effect of alcohol on testicular hormone production.

Bleeding tendencies due to prothrombin deficiencies result in *purpura, nose* and *gum bleeds,* and other hermorrhagic displays. The *melanosis* seen in some cirrhotics might be caused by an associated pellagra. Alcoholic beri beri presents with a *scaly dermatitis* and *glossitis.* Cirrhosis is associated with *flat, opaque nails* with white transverse bands and tendency to develop *Dupuytren's contracture.* The nail fold is thinned and the cuticle is widened. About 10 percent of cirrhotics show *clubbing* of the fingers. *Erythematous skin nodules,* particularly on the legs, sometimes can be found. These are necrotic fat clumps secondary to the high lipase levels assocated with pancreatitis.

Some skin diseases are caused by consistent heavy drinking, others are made worse by such indulgence. The nasal area can be involved with *acne rosacea* and *rhinophyma. Seborrhea* is common, and *nummular eczema* and *psoriasis* may be exacerbated. *Leukoplakias* are detectable on the oral mucous membranes, and a *black hairy tongue* or a green, *chlorophyl-stained tongue* are sometimes visible.

Indirect Signs

The life style of the Skid Row type of chronic drinker makes him liable to develop a number of cutaneous changes. Personal hygiene is neglected, and the dermatoses of improper diet and infection become apparent. *Sores* and *ulcerations* of the extremities, *scabies, pediculi* of the hair parts, and folliculitis of the bearded areas are seen. *Abcesses,* even *carbuncles,* are more frequent in this group than in the general population. *Tooth decay* and *gum boils* are common.

NON-MEDICAL NEEDLE USE AND SKIN SIGNS

Opiates, and in particular, heroin, are the most commonly injected drugs for non-medical purposes. However, amphetamines, cocaine, sedative-hypnotics, and an array of other substances are also injected subcutaneously, intramuscularly, or intravenously. The possible intravenous injection sites are numerous. After the veins of the arm are "buggered," those of hands, fingers, legs, neck, penis, and sublingual veins have been used.

Needle puncture marks may be identified for up to a week. They can be found over any accessible skin area, usually over the superficial veins. They should be looked for before punctures for medical purposes are begun. *"Pop" abcesses, ulcers, and scars,* the results of skin "popping," are visible over the upper arm, back, abdomen and thigh.

The toxic effect of quinine, often used as an adulterant for heroin, causes a necrotic breakdown of fat and skin. *Tracks* are linear, discolored, brownish streaks found along the course of subcutaneous veins. They are the result of unsterile injections along with deposition of particulate materials. They can last for years and become lighter as they age. Attempts to obliterate tracks by *bleaching* or *tattooing* have been made. *Thrombophlebitis* is a common finding that is associated with less-than-sterile punctures of the veins.

Two other cutaneous infections occur much less frequently: *camptodactylia* (edema and fibrosis of the fingers preventing their flexion) and *sphaceloderma* (necrosis of the skin).

"Shooting tattoos" are black spots caused by the carbon from a flamed needle being repeatedly injected under the skin. *Tourniquet discolorations* are circular markings where belts or ropes were repeatedly applied to occlude veins prior to injection. They represent cutaneous bleedings and pressure pigmentations of poorly fitting tourniquets applied over years. A mistaken intra-arterial injection can lead to *pain, swelling, cyanosis,* and *gangrene* of the extremity. Injecting barbiturates and related substances outside the vein can give rise to a woody cellulitis that is painful and inflamed. *Jaundice,* as one symptom of hepatitis, is often transmitted by the group use of infected needles.

SKIN MANIFESTATIONS OF THE ADDICTED LIFE STYLE

When existence centers around a chemical, many common health-sustaining practices are neglected. Skin and oral care are seldom practiced, and *trench mouth, skin infestations,* and *caries* are likely. *Linear, transverse scars* across the wrists are occasionally seen, the residuals of some unsuccessful suicide attempt in a person whose character structure and life-style contribute to a depressive state. Dirt and infestations also result in *scratch excoriations.* Cigarette and match *burns* result from "nodding" while under the influence of heroin or sleeping pills. *Tattoos* indicating adherence to some deviant group or a deviant life style might be encountered. These are sometimes homemade. *Acanthosis nigcicans* is sometimes seen in the armpits and may be related to inadequate hygiene or poor nutrition. The dermal consequences of avitaminosis, including *peleche,* have been observed. *Scabies* and *pediculosis* are found under conditions of inattention to cleanliness.

SKIN MANIFESTATIONS OF NARCOTIC USE

Opiate overdose is characterized by *pinpoint pupils, cyanosis, apnea,* and *coma.* As an exception, the pupils may be *dilated* when meperidine (Demerol) has been used. Terminally, extreme anoxia may cause constricted pupils, due to opiate overdose, to become dilated. During withdrawal from heroin and related drugs and pupils are usually dilated.

The potpourri of materials that go into the bag of heroin make allergic reactions a good possibility. A *fixed drug eruption* at the injection site, *urticaria,* and *purpura* have been recorded. The hives are the result of a histamine reaction and are supposed to be common when morphine is injected intravenously. These lesions may be *pruritic,* and *scratch marks* may be seen. *Piloerection* represents a valuable objective sign of narcotic withdrawal. An occasional patient on methadone maintenance will have *ankle edema. Sweating* is also a complaint of methadone maintenance patients.

COCAINE SKIN REACTIONS

The sniffing of cocaine can lead to *redness, ulceration,* and more rarely, *perforation* of the nasal septum. Cocaine has a vasoconstricting effect that impairs nutrition to the mucous membranes and, over time, causes necrosis. The paresthesias reported by cocaine users may account for the hallucinated "coke bugs." These imaginery insects, crawling under or on the skin, producing itching and can result in considerable *scratch marks,* sometimes with secondary infections.

SKIN CHANGES WITH OTHER DRUGS

During the period of LSD activity, the face is *flushed. Sweating* accompanies high dose amphetamine use. Allergic rashes to barbiturates and other sedative-tranquilizer drugs occur from time to time. They may be *erythematous, purpuric,* or *urticarial.* Barbiturate or other sedative-hypnotic overdose is accompanied by either *contracted* or *unchanged pupil* size.

On the other hand, in glutethimide (Doriden) overdose, the *pupils* are *dilated* or *anisocoric. Bullae* on the dependent and pressure-bearing surfaces of the skin might be encountered in any deeply comatose patient. It is believed, however, that barbiturates adversely affect epidermal metabolism, and the sweat glands excrete a certain amount of barbiturates. Therefore, blisters may form more readily in the person unconscious from barbiturates.

Solvent inhalers may present with a *dermatitis* around the nose and mouth. Those who inhale spray paints may appear in an emergency room with the metallic silver or gold pigment on their face.

Gynecomastia in males who use marihuana chronically has been described, but it is a rarity. *Discolorations* of the fingers due to the marihuana tars might be seen between the thumb and index finger in heavy smokers who do not use a holder. A *conjunctivitis* is regularly seen during the period of marihuana use. An association between cannabis use and *acne* has been suggested. Chronic bromide use is associated with an *acneiform* or a *pustular eruption.*

SUMMARY

The skin is a revealing organ, and it can be helpful in clarifying some puzzling clinical problems. Most illicit drugs or their mode of use will produce cutaneous signs that can assist in the diagnostic process.

ADDITIONAL READING

1. Committee on Alcoholism and Drug Dependence, A.M.A. *Medical Complications of Alcohol Abuse,* 1973.

2. Young, A. W. et al. Skin stigmata of adolescent drug addiction. *Modern Treatment.* 9:117, 1972.
3. Korn, L. and Weidman, A. I. Pathogenesis and age of skin stigmata of narcotic addiction. *J.A.M.A.* 224:1433, 1973.
4. National Drug Abuse Training Center, Medical Monograph Series, Vol. 1, No. 1, *Diagnosis and Evaluation of the Drug Abusing Patient,* Nov., 1976.
5. Richter, R. W. *Medical Aspects of Drug Abuse.* Harper & Row, Hagerstown, MD, 1975.

3. Urine Testing for Abusable Drugs

The need to determine the drug or drugs recently ingested by a user may be required for a variety of reasons. The emergency room physician would like to explain the life-threatening symptoms by learning what substances had been consumed. The clinic staff is interested in whether the methadone used for maintenance purposes was actually swallowed, and whether street drugs were also consumed. Personnel physicians in industry are interested in the current drug-using practises of their job applicants. The psychiatrist seeks help in explaining bizarre behaviors that do not fit the usual psychiatric syndromes. The Armed Forces commanders want information on the prevalence and kinds of drugs used in their troops. Every practising physician will, at one time or other, request a urine screen for various reasons.

WHAT CAN BE DETECTED IN A DRUG SCREEN?

Most drugs of abuse are excreted in the urine in amounts sufficient to show as positive within 24 to 48 hours after their consumption.

All Opiates, Natural and Synthetic
Heroin. This drug is the most frequently tested for and found. Depending on the quantity injected, it may be found up to 72 hours after last use. Since it is completely deacetylated in the body, it is excreted and reported as morphine.

Codeine. Codeine is excreted as codeine, however, 10 to 15 percent may be found in the urine as morphine. Therefore, a small amount of morphine in a urine sample that contains considerable codeine does not mean that morphine or heroin was used. If the urine shows a large amount of morphine and codeine, then heroin or morphine was taken along with codeine.

Propoxyphene (Darvon). Darvon and its metabolite norpropoxyphene are usually detected together in the urine.

Methadone. Methadone is also excreted along with its metabolite. It is frequently found, especially when methadone maintenance patients are among those whose urines are being tested. The absence of methadone in a patient maintained on it requires explanation.

Pentazocine (Talwin) and meperidine (Demerol). These synthetic narcotics can be successfully differentiated from others in this class.

Sedative Hypnotics

Barbiturates. All the common barbiturates, including phenobarbital can be identified.

Non-barbiturates. The benzodiazepines are readily detectable. Many of the other non-barbiturate sedatives, including methaqualone (Quaalude), are identifiable.

Psychostimulants

Amphetamines. All amphetamines are detectable, but the test is less sensitive than for the opiates. Twenty mg may produce a positive up to 24 hours; large amounts give positive results for 48 to 72 hours. Some methamphetamine is excreted as amphetamine.

Cocaine. Cocaine itself is to be found in the urine, but its metabolite, benzoylecgonine, is invariably present with it. Benzoylecgonine may be present alone.

Hallucinogens

LSD and THC. Commercial laboratories do not perform tests for these substances at present; however, research laboratories can find these substances in the urine.

Phencyclidine (PCP). PCP can be detected in blood and urine. It is frequently found in many urban centers.

Quinine. Quinine is a common adulterant of heroin in some areas. It is used to impart a bitter taste to the highly diluted heroin should the buyer wish to pre-taste his purchase. Quinine in small quantities is readily detectable. The urine will remain positive for quinine after morphine can no longer be identified. A positive quinine test in an addict is suspicious of prior intake of heroin. However, the ingestion of quinine water or of proprietary cold tablets will give a positive reaction for quinine.

Nicotine

At times the nicotine spot may be confused with opiate spots.

Multiple Drugs

It is not uncommon to find more than one drug. In one series of 10,000 urine samples done on probationers: 72.8 percent were negative, 18.4 percent contained one drug, 6.4 percent contained two drugs, and the remaining 2.4 percent had three or more drugs.

WHAT ARE THE LIMITS OF DETECTABILITY FOR VARIOUS DRUGS?

The detection limits are about: 0.5 ug/ml for amphetamine, methamphetamine, for the rapid acting barbiturates, codeine, and morphine; 0.7 ug/ml for phenobarbital and phencyclidine; 1.0 ug/ml for methadone, propoxyphene, cocaine, and methaqualone.

WHAT TECHNIQUES ARE USED FOR URINE TESTING FOR DRUGS?

A number of advanced technologies are used. Ordinarily, if a positive urine is found, it is tested again utilizing a second method to reduce the possibility of false positives. The most common techniques include:

RIA = radioimmunoassay,

EMIT = enzyme multiplied immunoassay technique,

FRAT = free radical assay technique,

GLC = gas-liquid chromatography,

TLC = thin layer chromatography.

WHEN SHOULD THE TEST BE DONE?

1. The screening of large numbers of individuals within an organization to determine the prevalence of drug abuse. Such organizations may be military units, hospitals, prisons, schools, business firms, etc. The ex-

tent of the problem must be ascertained in order to plan proper preventative, educational, and rehabilitative programs. If it is known that urine testing is done, this will have some deterrent effect upon drug misuse.

2. Treatment, detention, and rehabilitation centers for drug abusers may be checked periodically for contraband drugs. Spot checks, including urine examinations, will help determine how serious the problem is. Drug smuggling into such installations is usually greater than the authorities assume.

3. In the differential diagnosis of coma and psychosis, urine testing has an important role to play. Some examples: Acute PCP and amphetamine psychoses may be indistinguishable from acute paranoid schizophrenia. Comatose patients who have an alcoholic odor on their breath may also have swallowed significant amounts of barbiturates. Patients in a coma with constricted pupils should be screened for opiate overdose by means of the urine test, but given an immediate therapeutic trial of 0.4 mg of Narcan (naloxone) i.v.

4. The response of the opiate addicted patient to long-term treatment can be objectively evaluated by periodic urine testing. It has been calculated that testing a patient's urine every five days at random intervals is an efficient time period for determining abstinence from dangerous drugs.

5. One method of evaluating narcotic treatment programs is by determining the frequency of "dirty" urines among the patients. A gross discrepancy often exists between the staff's estimate of the success of their program and the abstinence of their patients as determined by sequential urine tests.

6. Before placing a narcotic user on a program like methadone maintenance, which may extend as long as the patient lives, it would be well to be sure that the patient is addicted. He may be a "needle freak," or he may be using so little heroin that tolerance has not developed, and his "withdrawal" symptoms are due to anxiety or are bids to obtain drugs from the doctor. A series of urine tests will determine if he is taking sufficient heroin for it to appear in the urine.

7. Methadone maintenance programs are required to test urines periodically. The staff can ascertain from the testing whether the methadone is being taken and whether heroin or other drugs are being used regularly or sporadically. Most failures in methadone maintenance programs are

not due to a relapse back to heroin usage. More often the patient will turn to excessive use of barbiturates, amphetamines, or alcohol. The latter drug cannot be found on TLC but can be readily identified on examination or by breath analysis.

8. Medicolegal requirements make urine screening mandatory under certain conditions, for example, crimes committed under bizarre circumstances, criminal and civil cases in which drug use is suspected or alleged, certain motor vehicle or plant accidents, and when destructive behavior occurs which may have been drug induced.

9. The identity of illicit materials obtained from a patient or his family can sometimes be clarified by TLC.

10. An employer may require spot checks for abusable drugs if an addict in treatment is to be hired.

WHAT ARE THE PROBLEMS OF COLLECTING A URINE SAMPLE?

The results of testing for dangerous drugs are worthless or misleading if the collection of the urine specimen is not carried out carefully.

Certified Urines

As a matter of policy, or whenever valid test results are desired, certified urine examinations should be carried out. Certified urines are those collected under the direct observation of an experienced technician or aides. The observer should be of the same sex as the observed. The observer should be cognizant of the various techniques addicts can employ to deceive the staff. Such ingenious efforts are too well known to require repeating here, except to note that the standard purchase price for a drug-free specimen is $2.00 on the street.

Occasionally, the question of the staff not trusting the patient is mentioned as an argument for either not performing urine tests or not requiring certified urines. Such an attitude does not take into account the addict's previous way of life. He has survived as a "junkie" by skillful deceit and subterfuge. He tends to be contemptuous of those he can "con," and respects those who are not taken in by him. To freely trust an addict or a recently addicted person does him a disservice. He needs the external control imposed until the time when responsible control over his own behavior is achieved. Urine testing is an important, impartial control measure.

The Stall

A common evasion by a person who has recently taken one of the drugs of abuse is to claim that he cannot void. He will claim that he forgot instructions and urinated just before arriving at the place where the urine is collected and is now unable to provide a specimen. Coffee or fruit juice can be offered. If he is working or going to school and cannot wait at the clinic, he should be asked to report later or the next day. The incident should be recorded. A series of stalls is suspicious of continuing drug abuse. Such a person may attempt to clean up for a few days prior to submitting a sample of urine. If he is physically dependent on opiates or barbiturates he might show some early withdrawal signs after arriving at the office.

Pale Urine

It is common knowledge among "junkies" that the chances of a positive urine are diminished if considerable beer or water are drunk prior to the test. In urine with a very low specific gravity, the dilution of morphine may be so great that a negative test is reported. Pale urines should be recorded. They have the same significance as stalls. Instructions to those who will supply urine specimens ought to mention that only small amounts of fluid be taken for a few hours prior to the test.

Actual Inability to Void

Some people find it difficult to void upon request, especially if they are being observed by a stranger. This is not to be considered a stall. Such a person given fluids and encouragement will eventually supply a sample. A specimen brought into the clinic has little value. Various laboratories request from 10 to 50 cc of urine for drug testing.

WHEN ARE URINE TEST RESULTS CONFUSING?

Interfering Substances

Certain drugs may make the reading of a test plate difficult because the spot may be masked. Sometimes a spot not due to dangerous drugs is found in the region where such metabolite spots will ordinarily migrate. The phenothiazines exemplify a class of drugs that could cause interference. Heavy smokers may absorb and excrete sufficient nicotine to make a morphine test difficult to interpret. Experienced laboratory technicians should be able to distinguish the two substances.

False Positives

A laboratory test that is always accurate hardly exists. A well run laboratory will have reduced the incidence of false drug positives and negatives to a minimum by maximizing specificity while preserving sensitivity. In addition to the interfering substances mentioned, certain of the antihistamines and anti-tuberculosis drugs have caused a rare false positive reaction.

Labeling or other administrative errors are a possible source of incorrect reports. A single positive test found on an individual is not conclusive proof that he has used heroin recently. It is certainly no proof that he is heroin dependent. Only repeated random tests that are positive are good evidence for regular heroin use. To confront a patient accusingly on the basis of a single positive is poor policy. It may be unfair and demoralizing to the patient. A series of "dirty" urines should be discussed with the person concerned. Decisions about changing the therapeutic approach or discontinuing his treatment ought to be made on the basis of the total response to treatment, not simply from urine analysis.

False Negatives

Occasional urine tests on a person using street heroin may be reported as negative. There are a number of reasons for false negatives and their causes are listed below. A false negative will allow the patient to cheat on the program for awhile. When urine test results are used to help evaluate the effectiveness of some treatment program, a large number of false negatives will provide the staff with an incorrect feeling of optimism about their achievements. Actually, they may be using a testing technique that is relatively insensitive.

(1) The heroin used was too poor to appear in the urine. On the east coast a "bag" may contain 0 to 10 percent heroin. On the west coast and along the Mexican border it may have 0 to 20 percent heroin. When urine is tested after "bum" heroin was used, the report will be negative. Some heroin users are pseudoaddicts; they have a "needle habit" and derive some psychologic gratification from injecting water containing minimal quantities of heroin. The pseudoaddict displays only purposive signs (behavior directed at getting more drugs from the observer) on sudden discontinuance of heroin for he has not developed tolerance and will not experience true withdrawal. Naturally, he will have a urine negative for heroin, but this is not a false negative.

(2) The problem of pale urine has been mentioned. Some clinics will routinely not test pale urine; others have the test performed, but record the sample as pale urine.

(3) The last dose is taken too long before the test. The dose-time relationship will determine whether sufficient material is available to give a positive result. When less than 5 mg of heroin is injected, a false negative

may be obtained even when tested within a few hours. Fifteen mg of heroin may be detectable for 36 to 48 hours after which a negative will be reported. When large amounts of heroin have been taken three days prior to testing, the drug is generally still detectable.

(4) The test procedure is not sensitive enough. Certain testing methods give a high percentage of false negatives that are positive when more sensitive procedures are utilized. Cation exchange paper collection of urine is less sensitive than when the urine specimen is submitted to the laboratory. A third to three-quarters of the morphine and codeine appears in the urine as conjugated glycuronides. Therefore hydrolysis will increase sensitivity.

(5) Administrative errors are made. Mistakes in properly identifying urines, incorrect recording of results, and other clerical errors can produce false positives. In a properly run laboratory this source of error can be virtually eliminated.

SUMMARY

Well-performed, double-checked urine examinations can provide results with almost 100 percent accuracy these days. In order to be meaningful, the tests should be quickly reported. Because of its expense, the urinanalysis of drug abusers in treatment is being reevaluated at this time.

ADDITIONAL READINGS

1. DeAngelis, G. G. Testing for drugs—Techniques and issues. Int. J. Addict. 8:997, 1973.
2. Goldstein, A. Is on-site urine testing of therapeutic value in a methadone treatment program? Int. J. Addict. 12:717, 1977.
3. Jain, N. C. A survey of drug use among probationers in the Los Angeles area in 1976. Int. J. Addict. 13:1319, 1978.

4. Flashbacks

A relatively unique mental phenomenon has emerged since the recent widespread use of the hallucinogens. This is the flashback, the spontaneous reappearance of certain effects that were experienced while under the influence of a drug like lysergic acid diethylamide (LSD).

I was apparently the first in this country to mention the emergence of an altered state of awareness following recovery from a psychedelic experience in an article written many years ago (J. Nerv. Ment. Dis. 130: 30-39, 1960). The subject remains one of clinical and mediocolegal importance since the use of psychedelic drugs continues, although with much less news media coverage.

The term "flashback" appears to have originated with those who underwent the state. It was, doubtlessly, derived from motion picture industry jargon signifying a short cutback in a film story to an earlier point in time. To "flash" is the verb form, the act of being in a flashback. This essay will deal with frequent inquiries about flashbacks in a question and answer format.

WHAT ARE FLASHBACKS LIKE?

Most often they are visual phenomena that suddenly appear days, weeks, or months after the last ingestion of an hallucinogen and without apparent cause. The intensification of a color that is perceived, the increased dimensionality of an object or vibrancy of its form are visual effects that may be noted. Illusions, the ostensible movement of a fixed object, or the misinterpretation of an image for something else are frequent. Pseudohallucinations and actual hallucinations can be perceived.

Other flashback experiences include a slowing of the perception of time just as it slowed under the influence of the hallucinogen. Likewise, the rearousal of a strong emotion felt during the drug experience is a possibility. Ego boundaries can become diffuse, and the differences between "Me" and "Not-Me" seem less sharply defined.

It is one's interpretation of these novel events that is critical in determining whether or not psychological impairment ensues. Since they appear suddenly and unexpectedly, often at inappropriate times, they are usually associated with foreboding or dread. The person may interpret the strange events as a sign of "cracking up." Or the content of the flash itself may be horrifying. In other instances the response to a flashback may be one of enjoyment and pleasure, a surprising but welcome "free trip." It is the dysphoric responses that the mental health professional will encounter.

The precipitation of an anxiety or depressive reaction following exposure to an hallucinogen is not considered to be a flashback, although some writers have included such cases in reports of reemergence of hallucinogenic manifestations. These are longer lasting conditions. They do not make their appearance as abruptly, and have none of the associated sensory and self-concept changes.

WHAT CAUSES FLASHBACKS?

The answer to this question is unknown, but it certainly is not due to a retention of LSD in the body. LSD is almost completely eliminated within the first 24 hours after its intake. Nor are flashbacks due to some structural change in the brain. A good possibility is that they represent a behavior learned during a state of psychophysiologic arousal that later can be precipitated under conditions of nervous system arousal. They can be conceptualized as a form of state dependent learning.

What has been experienced under the effects of LSD is laid down in the memory banks. When a level of nervous system excitation similar to the LSD state occurs subsequently, state bound recall occurs. This means that the flashback is a partial reentry into the memory of some aspect of the hallucinogenic experience at a time when the brain is at an equivalent level of arousal. It is quite likely that another factor contributes to the emergence of flashbacks, and that is a relative reduction in one's control over the sorting and integration of information. For example, some people report that their flashbacks are most likely to appear during entry into and return from sleep.

Drugs associated with the later appearance of flashback phenomena include all hallucinogenic agents. LSD, mescaline, psilocybin, PCP, and others in this class have this capability. In addition, marihuana has been considered to be the causative factor for some flashback incidents. Other related drugs with the potential include Ketamine (an hallucinatory anesthetic resembling PCP), morning glory seeds, and large amounts of amphetamines.

WHAT PRECIPITATES FLASHBACKS?

A common precipitant is stress. Flashbacks emerge most frequently during periods of intense psychological or physical pressures. It is known that extremely severe stress, in itself, can provoke a dissociative state, and flashbacks can be thought of as acute, brief, recurrent dissociative phenomena. Stress is, obviously, a period of heightened arousal. Fatigue and a condition of diminished sensory input are sometimes associated with the unfolding of a flashback.

Certain drugs are considered precipitants of flashbacks. Marihuana is one, and since some of the symptoms of marihuana are reminiscent of flashbacks, marihuana-precipitated flashbacks are said to occur when marihuana use produces a greater response than would be expected from marihuana alone. Antihistamines and cold remedies, nitrous oxide and even caffeine have been accused of provoking flashes.

Returning to the scene of a psychedelic trip is supposed to induce flashbacks. This observation is probably valid when the person is quite suggestible and has a strong expectation that he might flash.

HOW OFTEN DO THEY OCCUR?

It is estimated that less than 5 percent of hallucinogen users will undergo some sort of subsequent altered state of consciousness that could be called a flashback. When a sample of frequent hallucinogen users is studied, then the figure increases to as high as 80 percent. This number includes, however, those with very transitory and fragmentary episodes and those whose altered states of consciousness were elicited by direct questioning.

WHAT OTHER FACTORS FACILITATE THEIR APPEARANCE?

In addition to frequent, high dose exposures, "bad trips" are more likely to be followed by a flashback than good ones. It is claimed that personality factors play a role in their induction. Individuals with an immature, unstable character structure and those with looser ego controls are more liable to be susceptible to flashbacks.

WHEN CAN ONE BE CONFIDENT THAT FLASHBACKS WILL NOT OCCUR OR RECUR?

If a year has elapsed since the last use of hallucinogens or since the last flashback, then it is unlikely that such an incident will break through thereafter.

WHAT WILL BE THE COURSE OF SOMEONE WHO REPORTS MULTIPLE FLASHBACKS?

Most people who flash will do so once or a few times, and then the condition will disappear. The phenomenon will diminish in frequency and intensity over time, assuming that causative drugs are not used.

There are rare instances on record where individuals have had very distressing recurrences for many years.

HOW IS THE DIAGNOSIS MADE?

Ordinarily, people bring their diagnosis with them. Flashing is rather generally known among those who use exotic substances. In fact, they tend to overdiagnose their condition, calling post-hallucinogenic anxiety or psychotic reactions flashbacks. Establishment of a proper diagnosis would include, (1) the prior ingestion of an hallucinogen or related drug within a year or so, and (2) the brief recurrence of feelings, sensations or body image changes that are reminiscent of the hallucinogenic state.

WHAT IS THE DIFFERENTIAL DIAGNOSIS?

Not all prolonged adverse reactions to an hallucinogen are flashbacks. The paranoid or anxiety reactions should be separated out because their management is different. Certain temporal lobe epilepsies may present as momentary altered states during which colorful visual displays are seen. Flashbacks resemble paramnesias in which feelings of estrangement and detachment from existence occur. These culminate in uncomfortable feelings of depersonalization and derealization. Certain *deja vu* and fugue experiences are reminiscent of flashbacks. Hypnagogic and hypnopompic imagery experienced while falling asleep or waking up are similar to flashback hallucinatory episodes.

There are other momentary states of altered awareness that may be confused with flashbacks. Maslow called them peak experiences and believed that many people have undergone such events during their lifetimes. They range from brief intense feelings of "all rightness," a fleeting vision or some other ephemeral perceptual moment, to very profound experiences variously called mystical, religious, or transcendental. These can be confused with those flashbacks that are experienced as insightful, pleasant, or awesome.

WHAT ARE THE ADVERSE CONSEQUENCES OF FLASHBACKS?

The immediate reaction to the appearance of a flashback may be panic with its consequences. As they recur, the person can become alarmed that they will result in serious mental disorganization. Suicide has been reported, apparently because the individual was upset about the peculiar and uncontrollable experiences that were taking place. Accidents are possible since judgment and psychomotor skills are impaired. When the recurrent flashes persist, a chronic anxiety or depressive reaction can set in.

ARE LEGAL IMPLICATIONS INVOLVED?

Since the individual is in a partially dissociated state, the plea of diminished capacity has been made if a defendant committed a crime in connection with a flashback. Such pleas generally have not been successful except to reduce the severity of a sentence.

Certain sensitive and highly responsible jobs have been denied to people with a history of hallucinogenic drug use on the basis that they might later develop flashbacks. Such precautions seem overly restrictive when one considers the remote possibility that flashbacks will develop, and the even more remote possibility that they may occur on the job. This is particularly true if an interval of a year or so has elapsed since the intake of an hallucinogen or of the onset of the last flashback.

WHAT IS PROPER TREATMENT FOR
RECURRING FLASHBACKS?

The most important aspect of treatment consists of reassurance that the condition will pass, that the brain is not damaged, and that the strange occurrence is not a precursor of a psychotic break. Support should be provided until the condition wanes. The precipitating factors for that particular patient should be studied and eliminated. The patient should be counselled to reduce arousal-elevating activities as much as possible.

Some people will smoke marihuana for the reactive anxiety in connection with the undesired flashbacks. This is not recommended. The flashbacks may represent a weakening of ego integrity as a result of the hallucinogenic event. Marihuana would tend to attenuate ego function and reality testing even more. It is obvious that the stronger hallucinogens never should be used while flashbacks are occurring.

If sedation is needed, a minor tranquilizer like diazepam (Valium) in just effective doses is preferred. A lighted room at bedtime may be helpful for those whose flashbacks come during the presleep period. Exhaustion and tension should be avoided. Anything that will improve the physical and mental state (balanced diet, necessary dental care, psychotherapy, etc.) ought to be undertaken. There is a remote possibility of suicide, and this must be considered.

SUMMARY

The hallucinogenic experience is one of extremely high arousal levels and of diminished ego controls over the processing of information. It is therefore not surprising that during the subsequent non-drug state, a fragment of the experience may break through. An especially favorable time for the emergence of such reexperience would be during high levels of central nervous system arousal or during times of diminished ego functioning.

RECOMMENDED READINGS

1. Brown, A. and Stickgold, A. Marihuana flashback phenomena. J. Psychedelic Drugs 8:275-283, 1976.
2. Heaton, R. Subject expectancy and environmental factors as determinants of psychedelic flashback experience. J. Nerv. Ment. Dis. 161:156-165, 1975.
3. Horowitz, M. J. Flashbacks: Recurrent intrusive images after the use of LSD. Am. J. Psychiatry. 126:565-569, 1969.
4. Keeler, M. H. Adverse reactions to marihuana. Am. J. Psychiat. 124:674-677, 1967.
5. Siegel, R. K. and West, L. J. *Hallucinations: Behavior, Experience and Theory.* Wiley, New York, 1975.
6. Stanton, M., Mintz, J. and Franklin, R. M. Drug Flashbacks. Int. J. Addictions, 11:53-59, 1976.

5. Alcohol Withdrawal Syndromes

When heavy and consistent drinkers suddenly stop or markedly reduce their intake, an array of symptoms and signs sometimes emerges. Full-blown alcohol withdrawal syndromes rarely occur in those who have been drinking excessively less than five years.

A well-known precipitant of withdrawal symptoms is severe physical stress such as pneunonitis or a major surgical intervention. However, users would tend to stop or be unable to continue drinking in connection with such stressful events.

WITHDRAWAL MECHANISMS

The alcohol abstinence syndromes can be conceptualized as release phenomena from the depressant effects of alcohol. Excitatory activity of the central nervous system dominates over CNS depressant activity. Therefore, symptoms such as tremulousness, hallucinations, convulsions, insomnia, delirium, hyper-reflexia, and autonomic stimulation become evident. Convulsive thresholds, for example, which were elevated due to the depressant effects of alcohol, are lowered during the withdrawal phase. Similarly, psychomotor hyperactivity is released when the depressant effects of ethanol are terminated.

Other findings are consistently associated with specific withdrawal effects. Stimulation of the respiratory centers as a rebound from the depressant effect of alcohol can cause hyperventilation and respiratory alkalosis during the 48 hours after abstaining. As a result of alkalosis, hypomagnesemia occurs due to a shift of magnesium ions from intravascular to intracellular.

Low magnesium intake due to poor nutrition while overdrinking adds to the low plasma magnesium level during withdrawal. Respiratory alkalosis and hypomagnesemia correlate quite well with withdrawal seizures, tremors and hyper-reflexia.

CLASSIFICATION

A completely satisfactory classification of the alcohol withdrawal states is not yet available. Many atypical and incomplete clinical pictures are seen. Some do not readily fit into current nomenclature. The following categorization does not reflect the highly diverse pathways that withdrawal states can take.

Relative (or Early) Withdrawal

A condition called relative (or early) withdrawal has been described recently. It consists of tremulousness and shakiness upon awakening after a night of abstinence from alcohol. Thus, the morning after sickness in binge or persistent alcohol abusers can be understood as an early, partial withdrawal syndrome. It is also believed by some investigators that certain withdrawal symptoms build up during chronic heavy drinking and become even more manifest during the post-alcoholic state. These include the sleep disturbances (to be described), agitation, muscle aches, tremors, nausea, tinnitus, anxiety, and depression.

Impending Delirium Tremens

This category includes manifestations such as shakiness, sweating, and low-grade fever. Agitation is not uncommon and a mild degree of mental confusion may exist. However, when a full-blown delirium, hallucinations, or convulsions develop, they constitute a progression to other abstinence syndromes. Impending DTs is the most common of the withdrawal syndromes. It can begin as early as 12 hours or as late as 72 hours after the last drink. For some people this condition will constitute the entire withdrawal experience. A fewer number will go on from there to the more advanced syndromes.

Alcoholic Hallucinosis

Within a day after drinking has stopped an acute onset of auditory hallucinosis can evolve. It may follow the impending DTs, or it may appear without prodromal symptoms. The sensorium is usually clear and orientation remains intact. The sounds that are heard may be musical, or they may be voices. Frequently the voices make derogatory, accusatory, or persecutory remarks about the listener. The observation that the hallucinated material is auditory, and the content is paranoid has prompted some psychiatrists to assume that the hallucinosis is evidence of an underlying schizophrenic process.

Alcoholic Convulsions

Grand mal convulsions without aura may occur 12 to 24 hours after cessation of drinking ordinally associated with the impending DTs. Both epileptics and non-epileptics may convulse, and a workup for epilepsy is indicated in a person who has his first seizure during withdrawal. Having convulsed once, subsequent withdrawal episodes are likely to be accompanied by convulsions. A third of those who have seizures will go on to develop the full-brown delirium tremens. Status epilepticus is another possible complication in the patient who starts convulsing.

Delirium Tremens

This is a late manifestation of alcohol withdrawal. It peaks three to four days after cessation of drinking. The delirium is a fluctuating type, worse during periods of reduced sensory input. Visual hallucinations are the homey or occupational type. A truck driver, for example, may vividly describe long journeys along the highway while lying in his hospital bed.

The hallucinations can be distinguished from the abstruse, paralogical hallucinatory activity of the schizophrenic. Stereotyped ideas of alcoholic hallucinations, such as seeing pink elephants, have had little clinical confirmation. The misperceptions are generally frightening, but pleasant ones also have been described. For instance, a drunk tank occupant was enter-tained over a long holiday weekend by the visions on his private television screen. Marked confusion and variable disorientation are accom-paniments to the DTs. The tremors are gross and irregular and become worse when the patient is asked to perform an act. High fever, tachycard-ia, and elevated blood pressure are associated signs.

The DTs can be life endangering to elderly or seriously ill individuals. With improved treatments hospitals are reporting a less than 1 percent mortality except where large numbers of very ill delirium tremens patients are being treated. Hyperthermia or peripheral vascular collapse are the usual causes of death.

Wernicke-Korsakoff Syndrome

Although not strictly a withdrawal phenomenon, the Wernicke-Korsa-koff complex often appears after one of the before mentioned postalco-holic states. The syndrome is marked by impaired eye muscle control, lid paralysis, deficient recent memory often resulting in confabulation, delu-sional thinking processes, peripheral neuritis, and ataxia. The condition is sometimes reversible with thiamin and other B complex vitamins. It seems to represent a severe B avitaminosis and, in fact beri-beri and pellagra may coexist.

SLEEP DISTURBANCES DURING WITHDRAWAL

Considerable research has been done in recent years concerning changes in sleep patterns during heavy drinking and withdrawal. During a binge, REM (dreaming) sleep may diminish and some intoxicated people might have 0 percent REM time during sleep. During withdrawal, REM sleep rebounds and may occupy as much as 100 percent of sleep time. Some workers believe that the high REM levels relate to the awake hallucinatory activity with postalcoholic hallucinations being a sort of waking dream. Exactly the opposite effect is seen on delta wave (slow wave, or Stages III and IV) sleep. It is increased during the intoxication period and decreased during withdrawal.

Total sleep time may be increased during the intoxication period al-though sleep fragmentation is regularly reported. Insomnia is a common concommitant of withdrawal. Sleep onset is delayed and multiple awaken-ings occur. Some patients are afraid to close their eyes because of the hor-rors (frightening hallucinations). Nightmares waken them from sleep.

A number of clinicians speak of a terminal sleep in which a patient gets a night of deep, refreshing sleep during his DTs. He then awakens essentially recovered from this postalcoholic withdrawal state.

TREATMENT OF WITHDRAWAL

General

Correction of pre-existing malnutrition, avitaminosis, and anemia should begin as soon as oral feeding is possible. A fluid and electrolyte imbalance may exist but intravenous rehydration must be accomplished cautiously, and the oral route used when possible. Hypokalemia and hypomagnesemia are the most frequent electrolyte abnormalities. Potassium and magnesium sulfate are worth supplying when these deficits exist. A search for infections and injuries should be routinely made.

These patients have a reduced pain sensitivity and poor thermal regulatory capability. Therefore, a serious infection or surgical emergency may be smoldering without being clinically apparent. Those diseases associated with chronic alcoholism must be looked for, otherwise disasters can occur. For example, the patient may seem to recover from his withdrawal syndrome only to become increasingly confused and drowsy. This might be considered a relapse by his physician. There is a possibility that a decompensated liver, unable to handle the protein provided during refeeding, has resulted in aminoacidemia and impending hepatic coma. Other general supportive measures include regulation of urinary and bowel function, correction of hyperacidity, skin care, and oral hygiene.

Preventive

Some physicians routinely prescribe broad spectrum antibiotics when temperatures exceed 101 degrees. Others wait for more definite proof of infection. For very high fevers cooling measures become mandatory.

It is common practice to use Dilantin and phenobarbital or Valium as a prophylactic during detoxification from alcohol. Ordinary amounts of Dilantin orally may not act quickly enough to prevent convulsions. Oral Dilantin in 300 mg doses or intramuscular Dilantin in full doses are preferable.

Large quantities of thiamin and the remainder of the B complex are routinely given to correct a massive deficiency that most alcoholics have and to prevent such conditions as Wernicke-Korsakoff's syndrome.

Soon after mental functioning recovers, the patient should be engaged in conversations leading to a long-term treatment program for the drinking problem.

Sedation

Librium is the preferred drug but other agents such as paraldehyde, the phenothiazines like Mellaril, and the antihistamines like Vistaril also are widely used. The principle is to quiet the patient so that he does not exhaust. There are hazards with these sedatives but the benefits outweigh them.

Sleep is important and chloral or Dalmane are indicated for withdrawal insomnia. They do not produce the same REM disturbances alcohol does.

After recovery, sedatives should gradually be reduced and eliminated if possible. For long-term use, noneuphoria producing sedatives may be preferable in patients prone to abuse substances. Placebos are satisfactory support for a few recovered patients.

Outpatient Management

Hospitalization is necessary for the severe alcohol withdrawal syndromes—particularly convulsions and delirium tremens. If impending DTs exist and the symptoms are mild, and if no significant medical or surgical complications are present, outpatient management can be considered. It is important to see the patient daily and to provide only a day's supply of sedatives. A reliable caretaker in the home is also a necessity.

SUMMARY

The various alcohol withdrawal syndromes described appear as multiple, variegated symptom complexes. If the concept of an early withdrawal syndrome is accepted, then they are frequent. Alcohol withdrawal syndromes are serious medical-psychiatric problems, especially when intercurrent illness coexists. With existing medical capabilities, survival is to be expected in most instances.

REFERENCES

1. Gross, M. M., *et al.* Acute alcohol withdrawal syndrome. In *The Biology of Alcoholism,* Eds.: B. Kissin and H. Begleiter, Vol. III, pp. 191-263, Plenum, New York, 1973.
2. Gross, M. M., *et al.* Sleep disturbances in alcoholic intoxication and withdrawal. In: *Recent Advances in Studies of Alcoholism,* pp. 317-397, Pub. No. (HSM) 71-9045, Washington, D.C., 1971.
3. Mello, N. K. and Mendelson, J. H. Alcoholism: A Biobehavioral Disorder. In: *American Handbook of Psychiatry.* M. F. Reiser, Ed., Vol. IV, 1974.
4. Wolfe, S. and Victor, M. The physiological basis of the alcohol withdrawal syndrome. In: *Recent Advances in Studies of Alcoholism.* Pub. No. (HSM) 71-9045, 1971, Washington, D.C.

6. Alcohol and the Liver

New information is being generated concerning the metabolism of alcohol. This substance is a most important public health drug, and anything that is learned of its transformation in the body might be a help in treatment of acute and chronic alcohol toxicity.

Alcohol (also ethyl alcohol or ethanol) is quickly absorbed from the stomach and upper intestinal tract. Less than 10 percent is excreted unchanged from the lungs and skin and only a trace from the kidneys, so that the liver must deal with the bulk of ingested ethanol. Other organs do not have the necessary enzymes to metabolize it. So the liver cell is crucial in detoxifying alcohol and, as will be seen, impaired hepatic ability to metabolize alcohol causes further damage to the liver.

ALCOHOL, NUTRITION, AND LIVER DISEASE

At one time it was thought that a disease like cirrhosis was due to malnutrition rather than from the direct toxic effect of ethanol on the liver. After all, heavy drinkers spend little money for food and less time eating. Balanced diets are rarely consumed by alcoholics. Alcoholic gastritis causes a loss of appetite and vomiting if food is taken in. Alcoholic pancreatitis produces steatorrhea with its loss of nutriments.

Alcohol and its metabolites interfere with the release of water soluble vitamins from the liver. The metabolism of alcohol utilizes thiamine (vitamin B1), and alcoholic beverages contain hardly any vitamins. It is quite likely that a chronic heavy drinker will be malnourished in the essential vitamins and minerals.

This does not mean that he or she will be cachectic, although in the end stages of alcohol abuse that can certainly occur. Alcohol does have a caloric value of about 7 calories per gram, or about 1375 calories per pint of distilled spirits. This is more than half the daily caloric requirements for an average-sized person. A heavy imbiber of beer, wine, or whiskey may be obese but still could be malnourished in specific nutritional components such as vitamins, minerals, and proteins.

It is now well established that when chronic alcoholics do eat a balanced diet, they still may develop cirrhosis. Leiber and his associates fed a group of healthy volunteer subjects a very adequate diet plus vitamin and mineral supplements. They also received six drinks a day, or a total of 10 ounces of 86 proof alcohol daily for an 18-day period.

The investigators found a progressive rise in liver fat (by serial needle biopsies). At the end of the experiment there was eight times as much fat in the liver cells as at the start. The liver cells were distorted with striking changes in the mitochondria, the organelles, and the endoplasmic reticulum. During the 18-day period the blood alcohol concentration never rose above 90 mg/100 ml, which is below the level that is considered legally intoxicating.

These findings signify that consistent, spaced drinking, even without producing drunkenness, might still induce liver impairment over time. Cessation of drinking brought about a reversal of the fatty deposition in the liver.

These results were replicated in rats fed an adequate diet with 50 percent of their calories supplied as alcohol. The rats did not go on to develop alcoholic hepatitis or cirrhosis. Alcoholic cirrhosis is a later manifestation of liver toxicity (cirrhosis takes about 10 years to develop), and the rat's life span is only about 2 years. Lieber's group repeated their study on 16 longer-lived baboons, providing half the caloric requirement as alcohol and otherwise giving the animals an adequate diet. A control group received an alcohol-free diet of the same caloric content. The control group all had normal livers at the end of the study. The experimental group all turned out to have fatty livers, five baboons developed alcoholic hepatitis, and six others eventually showed cirrhosis of the liver. No doubt the combination of large amounts of alcohol plus associated malnutrition induces cirrhosis more easily than either factor alone, but the experiments described above indicate that alcohol, by itself, is capable of causing cirrhosis.

THE METABOLISM OF ALCOHOL

The breakdown of alcohol in the liver proceeds over acetaldehyde to acetate, which eventually becomes water and carbon dioxide. This simple statement actually describes a complicated process involving a number of liver enzymes and coenzymes. The first step, the formation of acetaldehyde and hydrogen ions, is a significant one.

Ethyl alcohol	alcohol dehydrogenase	Acetaldehyde + Hydrogen
$CH_3 \bullet CH_2OH$	$\longrightarrow$	$CH_3 \bullet CHO + H_2$

The enzyme, alcohol dehydrogenase, is available to deal with the modest amount of alcohol produced by intestinal microorganisms acting on sugars. Alcohol manufactured in the intestine is almost entirely cleared in the liver before it can reach the systemic circulation.

The alcohol dehydrogenase pathway is rate limited. Other metabolic systems (catalase) can be brought into play when large amounts of alcohol are introduced into the organism. The auxiliary systems may account for the partial tolerance acquired by chronic drinkers.

The first breakdown product of alcohol metabolism, acetaldehyde, has a toxicity of its own. It impairs certain functions of the liver cell, which causes higher acetaldehyde levels in heavy drinkers than in non-alcoholics drinking similar amounts. High acetaldehyde levels disturb the synthesis of heart and skeletal muscle protein. In the brain acetaldehyde interferes with the metabolism of some of the neurotransmitters.

Hydrogen ions convert pyruvate, a step in the gluconeogenesis of protein to glucose, into lactate. If this happens when little or no carbohydrate is eaten, and when glycogen stores in the liver are depleted, hypoglycemia can result. A low blood sugar is a possible cause of the anxiety, shakiness, and mental confusion in some alcoholics. Prolonged, severe hypoglycemia could cause brain damage.

The excessive amounts of lactate diffuse into the blood stream and produce lactic acidosis. The kidneys cannot excrete uric acid well in the presence of lactic acidosis. Uric acid accumulates in the blood and other tissues producing hyperuricemia and gouty attacks. This explains the well-known association of gout with drinking bouts in predisposed individuals.

The excessive hydrogen ions derived from alcohol catabolism displace the hydrogen that would have been generated from the breakdown of fat. This means that lipids will accumulate and cause fatty infiltration of the liver. Even when no fat is ingested, a fatty liver can result from stored fat that is mobilized from body fat cells by alcohol-induced hormonal discharges from the liver, fat which the liver is incapable of handling.

The inability of the liver to metabolize fat produces a number of consequences. Some of the excess fat is combined into lipoproteins in the liver. The enzymes responsible for the reaction continue to be secreted even after alcohol has been eliminated, producing elevated lipoprotein levels in the blood. In predisposed people, alcohol acts to elevate their blood lipid levels with its danger of coronary atherosclerosis. Some of the excessive accumulation of fat is broken down to ketones. These are acid-reacting substances and, in combination with the lactic acidosis, can produce a ketoacidosis manifested by drowsiness, stupor, or coma.

The long-noted clinical observation that chronic alcoholics being detoxified are resistant to the effects of drugs like sedatives, tranquilizers, and anesthetic agents has been confirmed in the laboratory. The reason for the lack of effect of these drugs in ordinary doses is that alcohol induces excessive quantities of the enzymes that are also effective in metabolizing these other drugs. When actively drinking, however, the alcohol interferes with the liver's ability to detoxify drugs and causes a prolongation of the drugs' effects and, perhaps, potentiation of the sedative effect of alcohol.

As liver cells become damaged from exposure to alcohol, their ability to degrade ethanol also fails. Serious hepatic insufficiency is one reason why heavy drinkers may lose their capacity to consume more than small amounts, because whatever alcohol is consumed continues to recycle. The well-known susceptibility of excessive drinkers to carbon tetrachloride poisoning might be explained on the basis of the competition of both drugs for certain hepatic enzymes.

Consistent drinking will cause fatty liver cells to become inflamed, with some cells becoming necrotic—alcoholic hepatitis. Still later, the inflammatory process causes scarification of the liver parenchyma—cirrhosis. The blood supply to many liver cells becomes impaired because of the scarring. The results of the partial or complete obstruction of the portal veins are many: esophageal and rectal varices with bleeding, ascites with worsening of the hypoproteinemia, uremia due to an inability to clear ammonia from the blood, and hepatic coma. In large urban areas cirrhosis is now the fourth leading cause of death in males between ages 25 and 45. Sudden deaths have occurred in people who had been drinking heavily enough to develop a very fatty liver. Fat emboli were found in the pulmonary vessels, and it is believed that the emboli came from the liver.

The systhesis of protein is impaired when the liver is damaged. This causes hypoalbuminemia with reversal of the albumin:globulin ratio. Prothrombin is not manufactured in sufficient quantities. Combined with a deficient intake or malabsorption of vitamin K, coagulation is defective, and hemmorrhagic tendencies compound the danger when thin-walled varices rupture.

ALCOHOL AND SEXUAL DYSFUNCTIONS

The combination of impotence, gynecomastia, and testicular atrophy in male alcoholics was long assumed to be an effect of underlying liver damage. More recently it was found that the gynecomastia and atrophy of the testicles were seen in drinkers who had no evidence of substantial liver impairment.

Acute alcohol intake was shown to decrease the testicular synthesis and increase the metabolic disposition of testosterone. The decreased plasma testosterone levels lead to an increased leutinizing hormone production by a hypothalamic-pituitary feedback mechanism. These endocrine changes may explain the paradox noted by Shakespeare and many others that alcohol "provokes the desire but takes away the performance.'' Leutinizing hormone appears to increase sexual drive, but the low testosterone level does not permit sustained penile erection.

CIRRHOSIS AND CANCER OF THE LIVER

Primary cancer of the liver is not common in North America. Its substrate, in most cases, is cirrhosis. In Lee's series, only 11 percent of such malignancies occurred in nonalcoholic cirrhotics. In other parts of the world, cancer of the liver is often secondary to parasitic or viral liver disease. In this country, primary hepatic cancers develop at the site of hyperplastic liver nodules, which are regenerative attempts by the alcoholic's cirrhotic liver.

SUMMARY

In the absence of malnutrition large amounts of alcohol taken over extended periods of time can cause fatty liver, hepatitis, and, with continued drinking, progression to cirrhosis. It is difficult for a chronic alcoholic not to be malnourished in essential food elements so that these deficiencies contribute to the liver damage.

Excessive amounts of alcohol increase the synthesis of fat, prevent its breakdown, and mobilize peripheral fat. This results in fatty infiltration of the liver and elevated plasma lipoprotein levels with its consequences.

Heavy drinking can produce hypoglycemia by converting pyruvate, a precursor of glucose, to lactate. Contributory factors are a poor carbohydrate intake and a depleted glycogen reserve in the liver.

Hyperuricemia and gout can develop in predisposed individuals because of the lactic acidosis and its effect upon the renal tubule's ability to excrete uric acid.

Alcoholic ketoacidosis is due to a combination of increased ketones formed from the hyperlipemia and the shift in the Krebs cycle from pyruvate to lactate.

Large quantities of alcohol have dual effects on the metabolism of other drugs. Alcohol accelerates the metabolic breakdown of certain drugs, making the alcoholic being detoxified less sensitive to anesthetics, sedatives, and tranquilizers. The actively drinking alcoholic, however, may be more sensitive to such drugs because the metabolic pathways are preempted by alcohol.

The impotence of alcoholics is not necessarily caused by liver dysfunction, although it may be contributory. Rather, it may be a direct toxic effect upon gonadal steroid secretion.

Hyperplastic nodular cirrhosis is a favorable site for hepatoma development.

Acetaldehyde rather than alcohol may be the toxin involved in muscle, neuronal, and possibly hepatocyte dysfunction.

Hypoproteinemia, hypoprothrombinemia, hypovitaminosis, and their sequellae are a consequence of alcoholic liver disease.

ADDITIONAL READING

1. Leiber, C. S. The metabolism of alcohol. *Scientific American,* 234:25-33, 1976.
2. Leiber, C. S., et al. Sequential production of fatty liver, hepatitis and cirrhosis in subhuman primates fed with adequate diets. *Proc. Nat. Acad. Sci.,* 72:437-441, 1975.
3. Kissen, B. and Bigleiter, H. *The Biology of Alcoholism.* Plenum, New York, 1971-1973.
4. Lucia, S. P. Alcohol and the liver. *JAMA,* 229:391, 1974.
5. *Alcohol and Health: New Knowledge.* Second Special Report to the Congress. Supt. of Documents, U.S. Govt. Printing Office, Washington, D.C., 20402, 1974.

7. The Fetal Alcohol Syndrome: Alcohol as a Teratogen

"BEHOLD THOU SHALT CONCEIVE AND BEAR A SON: AND NOW DRINK NO WINE OR STRONG DRINK." JUDGES 13:7

In medicine, as in life, until the mind has been prepared to see something it will pass unnoticed, as invisible as though it did not exist.

Only five years ago the fetal alcohol syndrome (FAS) was rediscovered by Jones and Smith, and since then thousands of cases have been found. It was a rediscovery, not a discovery, because the ancients knew of a connection between alcohol intake during pregnancy and birth defects. It was also common folk knowledge that alcoholic women tended to have "small, shriveled children with an imperfect look."

It was known that pregnant alcoholics miscarried more often than non-drinking women. As recently as 1968, Lemoine and his French colleagues (Quest. Med. 25:477, 1968) described 127 infants of chronic alcoholic females with "very peculiar facies, considerable retardation of growth in height and weight, and an increased frequency of malformations and psychomotor disturbances." Little attention was paid to this report.

THE SYNDROME

The FAS consists of a variable number of the following developmental defects.

1. Low birth weight and small size due to prenatal growth deficiencies. After birth growth is also retarded. These children never catch up in size or weight.

2. Mental retardation with an average I.Q. in the 60s. It is now believed that the FAS is the third most common known cause of mental deficiency.

3. A variety of birth defects including, but not restricted to, microencephaly, short palpebral fissures, ptosis, epicanthal folds, maxillary hypoplasia, cleft palate, joint anomalies, anomalous genitalia, capillary hemangiomas, and altered palmar creases. As many as 50 percent of the children have some cardiac abnormality. The major heart defects include the Tetralogy of Fallot, septal defects, and patent ductus arteriosus.

ETIOLOGY

The cause of the FAS is unknown, but many of the defects can be explained on the basis of a profound effect of alcohol or its metabolite, acetaldehyde, on the fetal central nervous system during its earliest development. An abnormality of neuronal migration may be the pathological basis for much of the clinical picture.

Malnutrition secondary to chronic alcoholism does not seem to be the underlying mechanism since well-nourished pregnant women who drink also have produced FAS offspring. Furthermore, offspring of malnourished mothers tend to catch up in growth and weight after birth; FAS children do not.

The condition appears to be related to blood alcohol levels and the ability of alcohol to diffuse freely across the placental barrier. Therefore, intermittent binge drinking might produce such problems even if the total intake during pregnancy was modest. The entire period of gestation may be at risk, with the first trimester producing the malformations and the second and third trimesters inducing growth impairments.

The fetuses are very quiet *in utero*. This lack of movement may account for the undeveloped palmar creases the frequency of breech presentations, and the joint anomalies. The decreased fetal activity might be due to the sedative effect of alcohol.

Since heavy drinkers also tend to be heavy smokers, the interaction with tobacco has made the question of causation difficult. The animal studies have demonstrated, however, that alcohol alone can be a teratogen to the fetus.

In one study 43 percent more alcoholic pregnant women produced FAS infants than a matched control group. Twelve percent of nonalcoholic women who drank moderately had children with anomalies consistent with the FAS. It is estimated that about 4,000 to 5,000 children a year are born with varying degrees of the syndrome.

HOW MUCH ALCOHOL?

A safe level of alcohol consumption has not yet been determined. The National Institute for Alcohol Abuse and Alcoholism has suggested that no more than two mixed drinks or their equivalent in beer or wine be consumed daily during pregnancy. Other authorities recommend complete abstinence.

The risk factor appears to be great when more than six drinks are consumed daily. It is with lesser amounts—two to six drinks—that the risks remain imprecisely established at this time. Animal models of the FAS are being developed. They may assist in the determination of how much and when the drinking of alcoholic beverages is harmful to the fetus. Mice, rats, rabbits, and other species produce litters that show features of the FAS when on a diet that includes sufficient alcohol. Some of the embryos are so defective that resorption or spontaneous abortions occur.

ATYPICAL FAS VARIANTS

Milder variants of the FAS are probably common but are less often diagnosed. Children of heavily drinking parents may show borderline intelligence, behavioral problems, including minimal brain dysfunction (MBD), and poor learning ability. MBD is a significant clinical problem and a certain number of these children could have derived their poor attention span and hyperkinetic behavior from a mother's alcoholism.

In a study at Washington University, 20 percent of the fathers and 5 percent of the mothers of MBD children were alcoholics. In the control group of nonhyperactive children only 10 percent of the fathers and none of the mothers were alcoholics. These findings have been confirmed in a subsequent UCLA study.

Another possible variant of the FAS is the child who is "slow in everything," "fails to thrive," or just looks "funny." Despite the dangers of overdiagnosing this condition, it is likely that the range of damage must extend from the fetus that is so disabled by alcohol that it is stillborn, through the readily diagnosed FAS infant, to the child with only minimal evidence of psychophysical impairment.

THE PROSPECTIVE STUDIES

Three major studies funded by the NIAAA are now exploring the relationship of alcohol to teratogenesis. In the Boston City Hospital survey, 74 percent of the infants born to women who imbibed more than 10 drinks a day demonstrated the FAS. In the Seattle (University of Washington) study 12 percent of women who used two ounces of ethanol (about 4 to 5 drinks) a day delivered FAS children. Of 90 women who used less than two ounces of ethanol, two cases of FAS were found (2.2 percent).

From Loma Linda University and four cooperating Southern California hospitals, some preliminary results are available. Heavy alcohol users had more spontaneous abortions than moderate, low, or non-users. In fact, they had 10 times as many spontaneous abortions as non-users of alcohol. Other points emerging from this study are that heavy drinking is ordinarily associated with heavy smoking, greater coffee use, a tendency to use more drugs, and to eat junk foods.

In addition to these investigations, many other studies in animals and humans are underway. The newborn of a variety of animal species showed hyperactivity and poor learning ability when the mothers had received an adequate diet nutritionally plus alcohol that produced a blood level of 200-300 mg/dl.

PREVENTION

It seems clear that the FAS is a major cause of congenital mental and physical disorders. It is probably the most important preventable cause of birth defects. What is needed is an educational program aimed at the public, especially heavy drinking women, and all physicians that will change our attitudes about drinking during pregnancy.

It was not uncommon in the past to recommend that expectant mothers take some wine or an alcohol-containing tonic before meals. Even this amount of ethanol may be undesirable, especially when combined with certain kinds of social drinking.

A bill has been introduced into the Congress that will require warning labels addressed to pregnant women on all alcoholic beverage containers (whiskey, wine, and beer) including alcohol-containing proprietary medicines.

Alcoholics should not conceive, and for those who do, termination of pregnancy should be available. If such women want to have a child, they should stop drinking before conception and throughout the pregnancy.

The developing information about the FAS combined with the increased prevalence of drinking by women, especially young women, requires that a special effect be made to make all of them aware of the potential for serious adverse effects upon the fetus.

SUMMARY

The FAS has an overall pattern of defects that is so similar that it probably is due to a single cause. The likelihood that the cause is alcohol's effect upon the maternal and fetal metabolism is great. The number of involved offspring increases as the amount of consumed alcohol by the mother increases; in other words, it is dose related. Alcohol crosses the placenta easily. In fact, it can be smelled at delivery in the amnionic fluid of women who have been drinking before or during labor. The developing tissues of the fetus are known to be more sensitive to the toxic effects of ethanol than are adult cellular structures.

This is a preventable condition with the responsibility placed on the woman who is or is about to become pregnant. In addition to the intense study of the role of the mother's alcohol use during pregnancy, in inducing the FAS, it would be well to examine the role of the heavily drinking father prior to conception.

The reason why the medical profession has been lax in recommending abstinence from alcohol during pregnancy in the past is the residual notion that still pervades our thinking—that alcohol is not a drug.

CONCLUSION

If you drink, don't drive—or get pregnant.
If you get pregnant, drive—but don't drink.

ADDITIONAL READING

1. Hanson, J. W., *et al.* Fetal alcohol syndrome: Experience with 41 patients. JAMA. 235:1458, 1976.
2. Jones, K. L., *et al.* Pattern of malformation in offspring of chronic alcoholic mothers. Lancet. 1:1267, 1973.
3. Jones, K. L., and Smith, D. W. Recognition of the fetal alcohol syndrome in early infancy. Lancet, 2:999, 1973.
4. Jones, K. L., and Smith, D. W. The fetal alcohol syndrome. Teratology. 12:1, 1975.
5. Ouellette, E. M., *et al.* Adverse effects on offspring of maternal alcohol abuse during pregnancy. New Engl. J. Med. 297:528, 1977.
6. Shaywitz, B. A. Fetal alcohol syndrome: An ancient problem rediscovered. Drug Therapy (Hosp). 53-60 (Jan.) 1978.

IV
TREATMENT

1. Methadone Maintenance

It is 15 years since Dole began placing chronic heroin addicts on "blocking" doses of methadone. Methadone maintenance (MM) has become the most frequently used treatment for opiate addiction, with more than 80,000 patients now in such programs.

Methadone (Dolophine) is a well known synthetic narcotic used for cough, pain, and detoxification of heroin addicts. Its use for maintenance is still considered experimental, and requires FDA approval.

RATIONALE

The person on MM in moderate or high daily doses manifests two pharmacologic effects that might account for his favorable course. Methadone produces cross tolerance to other narcotics. Thus if heroin is injected, it ordinarily produces no euphoria. This has been called the blockading action. The second effect is a decreased craving for heroin. This reduction in heroin hunger is present even at low methadone dosage levels. Any narcotic could be used for maintenance purposes. Methadone had the advantages of being long-acting, effective by mouth, inexpensive, and incumbered with few side effects.

PRINCIPLES OF TREATMENT

Selection of Patients

Only those addicts who volunteer for MM are acceptable to most programs. The desire to stop using heroin must be great enough for the patient to return to the clinic daily for his drink of methadone. A candidate for MM must be currently addicted to a narcotic. A confirmed diagnosis of active opiate addiction is important. He should have failed at least one other treatment procedure (detoxification, self-help group, commitment, narcotic antagonists). Psychotic addicts do not do as well as others, but some respond to a combination of methadone and a major tranquilizer. Addicts with a substantial medical illness ought not be treated in an MM program. Pregnant addicts should be de-addicted and delivered while abstinent, if possible. Infants born of mothers in methadone programs have done well. They must be observed and treated if signs of the abstinence syndrome appear. Addicts who are also dependent upon alcohol, amphetamines, or barbiturates are poor candidates.

Juvenile addicts should be given courses of detoxification along with supportive services. Only if they relapse, is MM to be considered.

MM Procedure

The patient is switched from heroin to an approximately equivalent amount of oral methadone dissolved in a synthetic fruit juice. The dose is administered once daily. It is increased gradually to between 40-120 mg. Low dose MM is below 80 mg, high dose MM ranges between 80-160 mg. Amounts greater than 120 mg are rarely necessary. A few patients do satisfactorily on doses as low as 20 mg. The maintenance levels are continued with few changes unless side effects occur, or a greater degree of "blockade" is desired.

A history and physical examination, including a psychiatric evaluation, are done along with standard x-ray and laboratory procedures, initially and annually.

The medication is swallowed in the presence of a nurse, pharmacist, or other responsible employee after a positive identification of the patient has been made. Certified urine samples are obtained at random intervals and tested for morphine (heroin is excreted as morphine), methadone, amphetamines, cocaine, barbiturates, and quinine (a popular adulterant of heroin in some cities).

After a few months of satisfactory cooperation with the program, the patient may be allowed to take home a day's supply. As he continues to demonstrate reliability and responsibility, he may be permitted to take home a three day supply. Since the maintenance dose may be lethal for a nontolerant person, supplies taken out of the clinic require safeguards to prevent accidental ingestion. Safeguards to prevent diversion of methadone by the staff or patients must be maintained.

Some patients will do well by simply being on MM. Many will require support and assistance in restructuring their lifestyle. Counseling, family therapy, job training and finding, and physical rehabilitation may be needed. These ancillary services and others make a MM program a multidisciplinary group effort.

Evaluation

The goal of MM therapy is abstinence from all mind-altering drugs except methadone. Some addicts will sporadically try heroin during the first few months after acceptance into the program. Daily observations and the results of urine samples will determine whether or not the patient is cooperating with the goals of the program. It is expected that criminal activities will diminish or cease. Arrest records assist in making this determination. Employment or school enrollment can be objectively measured by asking that salary slips and report cards be presented as they are received.

Termination of MM

It appears that certain patients will require lifelong MM. Some patients will request discontinuance of the treatment. Others may have made so successful an adjustment that a trial of abstinence appears indicated to the staff. Young patients who have not been addicted for long periods should be reviewed periodically as candidates for termination of MM. This is accomplished by reducing the drug by 5 mg a week to avoid withdrawal symptoms. The patient is followed, and urine tests are intermittently done as long as possible. MM is reinstituted if actual or threatened relapse occurs.

REPORTS

A signed, informed consent form is obtained from each patient upon entry into treatment. This is kept in his file along with the results of examinations and progress reports. These records can legally be examined by agents of the FDA. A running inventory of methadone supplies, including amounts dispensed and remaining, is required, as with any narcotic. Progress reports on the program are submitted to the FDA annually or when program changes are to be instituted.

SIDE EFFECTS AND COMPLICATIONS

In the 15 years since MM has been employed periodic tests to detect organ damage have found no evidence of cellular changes. Certain physiologic side effects are reported including drowsiness, nausea, vomiting, dryness of the mouth, ankle edema, constipation, and increased (or decreased) libido. Tolerance develops to a number of these symptoms, others are evidence of excessive dosage.

Patients on MM who happen to take a large dose of heroin or barbiturates may sustain a respiratory arrest. Instances of fatalities are known when people other than the patient consumed the "orange juice." Children are particularly liable to drink an attractive solution from the ice box. Some programs require that doses taken home be kept in locked containers.

Concern that a painful illness may not be diagnosed in patients on MM is often expressed. Although some elevation of the pain threshold occurs, this has not proven to be a problem. Tolerance to the analgesic effects develops partially or completely. When surgery is necessary, the anesthetist and the surgeon should be aware of the methadone dose the patient is receiving. MM should be continued while in the hospital.

The treatment for methadone overdosage consists of injections of the specific narcotic antagonist. Nalline (nalorphine) or Narcan (naloxone). Since these are short-acting drugs, and methadone has a prolonged action, repeated injections are necessary for a 48 hour period. Support of cardio-respiratory functions is routinely provided.

RESULTS

Various clinics report that 50 to 60 percent of patients accepted into a MM program lose their addiction to heroin and decrease their antisocial behavior. Treatment failures are due to alcohol, barbiturate, or amphetamine dependence. Reversion to heroin addiction is frequent. A small number of patients must be discharged because of continuing criminal activities.

The above percentages do not mean that a community can rehabilitate the majority of its opiate addicts by making MM available. It is estimated that about half of the addict population will not volunteer for MM so that 25 to 40 percent of all addicts will be helped if MM were available to all those who applied.

When large numbers of addicts are successfully treated with MM, the heroin that they would have consumed remains available on the black market place. The amount of heroin in the "bag" may be increased, but some of it probably becomes available for new users. Unless MM is to become a transfer of addiction to new users, strenuous efforts to control supplies of heroin must be combined with mass MM programs.

ADVANTAGES AND DISADVANTAGES

Advantages

1. MM removes the addict from a dependence upon injecting himself many times a day with unsterile materials. He no longer needs to engage in illegal practices to obtain the money for his habit. He does not have to deal with criminals to buy his supplies or to sell stolen merchandise. He is not preoccupied during his waking hours with plans to procure his "fix."

2. Although complete abstinence from narcotics is an optimal goal, many addicts cannot remain abstinent permanently. For these, a controlled addiction to methadone is preferable to an uncontrolled addiction to heroin. MM is the only realistic mass treatment modality for the hundreds of thousands of heroin addicts.

3. It should be anticipated that the level of certain criminal activities will decrease as significant numbers of people enter MM programs. Some support for this assumption has come from a few metropolitan areas.

4. The MM patient tends to engage in constructive activities. He becomes self-supporting in many instances. He is capable of driving a car, operating heavy machinery, and performing complex psychomotor tasks.

5. MM programs are not expensive in comparison to other therapeutic efforts. Between $2,000 to $4,000 per patient-year is sufficient to maintain a well run program.

Disadvantages

1. The patient remains addicted to a narcotic. He may have to remain on methadone permanently.

2. The amount of methadone given for maintenance may be lethal if consumed by a non-tolerant individual.

3. Diversion of methadone onto the black market by patients or by a member of the staff is a problem, especially in poorly managed programs.

4. Just what happens to the heroin not used by MM patients is not known. It may be a source of supply for new addict populations.

5. *Conclusive* proof of long-term safety is not yet available.

6. The requirement to return to the clinic many times a week is an inconvenience, especially for the working patient. However, a longer acting methadone analogue (1-alpha acetylmethadol) is now under study.

SOME FREQUENT QUESTIONS ABOUT MM

1. Should MM patients who become ill be maintained? (Yes. Contact the clinic to check dosage.)

2. What about surgery while on MM? (Surgery has been performed in such cases. Remember that anesthetics and depressants are potentiated by methadone.)

3. What drugs are contraindicated in these patients? (Care should be exercised when using barbiturates, non-barbiturate sedatives, tranquilizers, narcotics, anesthetics, and the sedating antihistamines. Talwin could precipitate withdrawal symptoms.)

4. Does methadone interfere with any labatory test? (It may increase SGOT and amylase levels.)

5. How reliable is the urine test for opiates? (Fairly reliable. False positives and negatives do occur, but these can be minimized by careful urine collection and a reliable laboratory.)

6. How is a patient taken off MM? (Gradual reduction of dosage, supportive therapy, nonaddicting tranquilizers if tension is high, avoidance by patient of old heroin environment.)

SUMMARY

MM is a feasible, apparently safe, inexpensive way to treat large numbers of heroin addicts. Although it represents symptomatic treatment, the advantages far outweigh the disadvantages.

2. Methadone Maintenance and Jobs: The Beazer Decision

It is a widely accepted belief that unless the heroin addict is removed from the life situation that contributed to or reinforced his drug dependence, continued abstinence is not likely, and relapse is probable.

Needle buddies are always around to urge the person attempting to remain clean to shoot up just once. The reinforcing effects of the sights and sounds of the junkie's environment have been amply described by Wickler.(1) Even after months or years of an opiate-free existence, the addict may experience certain withdrawal symptoms on returning to the locale of his former junkie career, or upon watching others fix.

What is needed is a restructuring of the entire lifestyle, a whole new set of waking activities, different interests, and new, non-using friends. Of particular importance is work or study that will improve vocational skills. The work may be gratifying, if not, at least it occupies the time and energies of the former addict. Without work he becomes a bored, bitter and restless person. Of course, a job itself is not enough to keep a person away from heroin. A third or more addicts become addicts while employed.

The problem is that addicts have poor work habits and records, little occupational training, and a history of arrests. Some have never held a legal job. Some female addicts have never learned either homemaking or vocational skills. In addition, employers are disinclined to hire ex-addicts for a number of real and not-so-real reasons. Sometimes insurance policies are written to deter hiring these ex-offenders. There are concerns that the ex-addict will rip off the firm if he slips back into heroin usage. Insofar as methadone maintenance (MM) clients are concerned, the fact they are still taking a narcotic makes their employability an issue when alertness and psychomotor efficiency are required on the job.

It is a discouraging situation for the addict to be rid of his heroin habit for a year or two, and still be unable to find any sort of job because of his addiction history. At that point relapse is probable. Some firms have enlightened policies about hiring qualified ex-users. Others not only will not employ them but will fire them if their drug abuse history is uncovered, even if their work has been satisfactory.

THE BEAZER CASE

A recent U.S. District Court decision (Beazer, et al. vs. New York City Transit Authority, et al., 72 Civ. 5307) has required that the Transit Authority (TA) consider MM patients for positions on an individualized basis.(2) It may be an important decision for future employment of MM patients.

The Story

Carl A. Beazer is a 40-year-old black man. He had been a heroin addict since 1951. In 1960 he started work for the TA as a subway car cleaner. He was promoted to conductor in 1961 and to towerman in 1966. During May, 1971, he entered a V.A. methadone program and was a succesful participant. As is common practice, he tried a few injections of heroin early in treatment but remained drug free for the next three years.

In November, 1971, he was discharged for narcotics use when the treatment for his addiction became known to the TA. By November, 1973, Beazer was able to be removed from methadone and has remained clean since. After his discharge from the TA, Beazer worked steadily as a counselor and a supervisor in drug treatment programs and later, as a Division Chief of Wildcat Services, which employs methadone patients to do building maintenance work. Three other plaintiffs joined Beazer in the suit.

The Trial

It was brought out at the trial that Beazer had been performing his job competently when he was fired by the TA. The TA terminated him for violation of its rule against narcotic usage. The applicable regulation is 11(b) of the TA's Rules and Regulations and states:

> Employees must not use, or have in their possession, narcotics, tranquilizers, drugs of the amphetamine group or barbiturate derivatives or paraphernalia used to administer narcotics or barbiturate derivatives, except with the written permission of the Medical Director or Chief Surgeon of the System.

Under these regulations employees in methadone programs must be discharged, and applicants cannot be hired. The policy applies to operating and non-operating positions, and successful participation in a methadone program makes no difference.

The position of the TA was that: (1) methadone maintenance is a relatively new treatment procedure, (2) methadone maintenance is merely the substitution of one narcotic for another, (3) methadone maintenance fails to a significant degree in remedying the basic problems of heroin addiction, therefore such a person is still at risk, (4) even if such a person refrained from heroin use, the methadone impairs performance, (5) TA employees are in positions that require vigilance and alertness, else the public and the employee would be endangered, and (6) there is no satisfactory way to screen the reliable from the unreliable methadone patients, therefore a blanket exclusionary policy is needed.

The Findings

On August 5, 1975, Judge Griesa found as follows.

1. The TA blanket exclusionary policy is constitutionally invalid. The plaintiffs proved that substantial number of persons on methadone maintenance are as fit for employment as comparable groups.

2. Without denying the responsibilities of the TA to the millions of subway and bus riders, the exclusionary policy against those on methadone maintenance is not rationally related to safety needs.

3. The TA's policy is the result of a misunderstanding about the nature and effects of methadone maintenance. During the trial it was possible to explore, in depth, the information and misinformation about methadone maintenance.

4. From the evidence presented the following facts about methadone maintenance emerges. There are 40,000 persons in New York City on methadone maintenance and 75,000 in the entire country. As administered in these programs the physical effects of heroin can be erased and a former addict can function normally—both physically and mentally. Substantial numbers of such patients are free of antisocial behavior, do not engage in drug abuse, and are capable of being employed. The employable MM patient can be separated from the unemployable by the usual personnel selection methods.

TA's established monitoring practices of its employees can be satisfactorily used for persons on MM. If the person is ineligible for employment for valid reasons, or performs his job at a substandard level, his exclusion should be for these reasons and not because he is in a methadone treatment program.

5. The finding applies with equal or greater force to those who successfully completed a maintenance program such as in Mr. Beazer's case.

Therefore the present blanket exclusionary policy of the TA against employing, or considering for employment, any past or present methadone maintained person regardless of his individual merits is a violation of the due process and the equal protection clauses of the XIV Amendment and is unconstitutional.

Points Made During Testimony

On the ability of MM patients to work. Dr. DuPoint, Director of the National Institute of Drug Abuse, testified that "the person who is maintained on methadone performs within the range of expectation of a normal population." Dr. Dole, the founder of MM treatment program, said "some tens of thousands of MM patients who have gone to school had achieved high grades, and others have accomplished much in responsible jobs in business and elsewhere."

On drug and alcohol abuse while on MM. The witnesses agreed it was not uncommon for patients to challenge their methadone early in treatment with a few injections of heroin. Ordinarily, little effect from heroin would be noticed due to cross tolerance. Other drugs and alcohol are more serious problems with some patients. Dr. Trigg of Beth Israel Hospital stated that 75 percent of his 5,000 patients on MM for more than a year were free of illicit drug use on urine screens. Other witnesses testified that after being in an MM program for six months, about 5 percent have problems with heroin, 10 percent with other drugs, and 5 percent with alcohol.

On the employment of MM patients. From 60 to 80 percent of patients are doing useful work as employees, homemakers or students. Consolidated Edison, the New York utility, has hired 100 former addicts. The company reported that they are performing as well as other employees. Some of their jobs have been as truck drivers, drill press operators, and sheet metal workers. Other companies that have hired MM patients include Chemical Bank, Metropolitan Life, New York Telephone, and McGraw-Hill. It was also clear that certain sensitive jobs might not be suitably filled by ex-addicts.

On the identification of employable MM patients. It was pointed out that since MM patients have urine screens and interviews with their counselors, the detection of drug abuse is more likely to be uncovered than among other employees. Furthermore, supervisory personnel of TA could readily detect any improper conduct or poor work performance, as they do with other employees.

Policies of the City, State and Federal governments. The City Civil Service Commission had declared that a history of drug addiction shall not, in itself, constitute a bar to employment except in appointments to the "uniformed services." MM patients will be assisted in obtaining City jobs and each case will be judged on its individual merits. The New York State Civil Service Department provides that if an applicant has a history of drug abuse, he should be considered on his merits except in certain sensitive positions. The Drug Abuse Office and Treatment Act of 1972 provides that no person may be denied federal civilian employment or a federal professional license solely on the basis of prior drug use, except for the FBI, the CIA, and similar agencies.

Relevant Decisions

Since the issue is one of due process and equal protection, certain relevant decisions were cited. In *LaFleur v. Cleveland Board of Education* 414 U.S. 632 (1974) the Court held invalid under the due process clause of the XIV Amendment, the rules requiring teachers to take extended leaves of absence beginning with the fourth or fifth month of pregnancy. In *Sugarman v. Dougall,* supra, the Court held that the New York Civil Service Law barring noncitizens from eligibility for State employment in the "competitive class" was unconstitutional. In *Green v. Waterford Board of Education,* 473, F 2d. 629 (2d Cir. 1973) the Court asked why a pregnant teacher was treated differently from teachers having other forms of disability. The Court stated: "Why the Board should choose, by means of an inflexible rule, to manifest particular concern with the health of a pregnant woman, but not, for example, with the health of a male or female teacher recuperating from a heart attack, is nowhere explained."

Relief Granted

The TA is to re-examine the employability of the four named plaintiffs without regard to the invalid policy. The TA will submit its conclusions to the Court, which will determine whether any of the plaintiffs should be reinstated or hired, and what rights to back pay they have—if any.

It should be remembered that lower court decisions are appealable by either side.

NOTES

1. Wickler, A. Conditioning factors in opiate addiction. In: Wilner, D. G. and Kassebaum, G. G., eds. *Narcotic Addiction,* McGraw-Hill, New York, 1965.
2. Beazer v. New York City Transit Authority. National Institute on Drug Abuse, 11400 Rockville Pike, Rockville, Maryland 20852, 1975.

3. Darvon N: Its Role in Opiate Addiction

INTRODUCTION

Darvon (propoxyphene hydrochloride) (Lilly) is a widely used analgesic intermediate in action between aspirin and codeine. Darvon N (propoxyphene napsylate) is a water insoluble salt. Its absorption is therefore slower, and its duration of action is longer than Darvon. Equivalent analgesic dosages would be: Darvon 65 mg = Darvon N 100 mg.

Propoxyphene is not considered to be a narcotic. However, its structural formula does resemble that of methadone. The treatment of respiratory depression due to a propoxyphene overdose is best accomplished with a narcotic antagonist. Nevertheless, propoxyphene withdrawal effects are mild, and physical dependence is much less than with methadone.

Darvon has been used to control the symptoms of narcotic withdrawal on an occasional basis for many years. The general impression was that it was helpful for small "habits," but provided only incomplete relief of the withdrawal syndrome when a substantial amount of narcotics had been used. Two factors may have contributed to this impression: (1) the amounts used were those commonly employed for analgesia, and therefore too low, and, (2) the amount of heroin used by addicts was greater in the past than it is today.

PHARMACOLOGY

Both salts of propoxyphene are safe in average doses. There is good evidence that the napsylate is safer than the hydrochloride when large amounts are taken. Two year chronic toxicity studies with the napsylate salt in rats and dogs showed no consistent changes except with daily doses of 50 mg/kg/day in the dog and 200 mg/kg/day in the rat. At these levels liver enlargement, elevations of alkaline phosphatase, and tissue changes consistent with chronic hepatitis are found. Acute lethal doses produce convulsions and respiratory depression in these animals and in man.

A fatality from a combination of 800 mg of Darvon plus alcohol and a central nervous system depressant is recorded. On the other hand, recovery has followed the ingestion of 6,500 mg of Darvon and 9,000 mg of Darvon N alone.

When compared to codeine for analgesic activity, it is considered to be half as effective. Comparable doses would be Darvon 65 mg = codeine 32 mg. Studies that used small doses of Darvon (32 mg or less) showed it to be more effective than a placebo. A favorite combination is one of Darvon and aspirin. This is rational because experimental work has shown that the combination is better than either agent alone. Darvon has essentially no antipyretic or anti-inflammatory action. Therefore in painful febrile or infectious conditions the Darvon-aspirin combination is particularly suitable.

DARVON AS A DRUG OF ABUSE

Darvon was introduced as an analgesic 25 years ago. It has become the most frequently prescribed analgesic in the United States. Five years after its introduction the first case of addiction was reported by Elson and Domino. Since then small numbers of case reports have described oral and parenteral addiction states.

During 1973 Tennant reported on a widespread abuse of the drug among American soldiers stationed in West Germany. He estimated that 15 to 20 percent of the 180,000 soldiers had used Darvon for non-medical purposes. Its ready availability in supply rooms and medical aid kits, and liberal prescribing practices made it an easy and favorite means of getting high. He reported 13 deaths due to overdose. Dosages were not mentioned. Respiratory depression with pulmonary edema and convulsions were the commonly observed terminal events. Other apneic soldiers were revived with respiratory support and nalorphine (Nalline). Other complications included toxic psychotic reactions, addiction to the drug, and inflammatory reactions at the site of the intravenous injection. Propoxyphene apparently has a marked sclerosing effect upon veins and soft tissues. In fact, intravenous Darvon addiction is supposed to be self-limiting because of sclerosis of the superficial veins over a period of weeks or months.

Darvon N has been in use for a short time. It is known to be an item of street commerce where it is called "Yellow Footballs." It sells for about a dollar a capsule on the black market. Much of its non-medical use seems to be directed toward reducing a heroin "habit" or avoiding the withdrawal effects of heroin. Because of its insolubility in water, parenteral injection will probably never be popular, although instances of addicts injecting supended material is known. It can be predicted that individual cases of oral Darvon N dependence will be reported.

DETOXIFICATION WITH DARVON N

The rapid, stepwise removal of a drug that had been consumed to the extent that physical dependence upon it was established, is called detoxification. Detoxification from opiates is ordinarily accomplished with methadone over a period of days or a few weeks. Methadone provides complete suppression of the opiate withdrawal syndrome, therefore gradual reduction of the methadone dosage will keep the addict relatively comfortable during the detoxification process.

Many other drugs have been used for the same purpose. Sedatives and tranquilizers will reduce the excitatory symptoms of the abstinence syndrome. Opioids such as Lomotil and Paregoric, antihistamines, and anticholingeric compounds will give some relief. Present day heroin dependence is of a low order, and many of the complaints made by the detoxifying addict are related to anxiety or are manipulative efforts to obtain more drug. Detoxification without the support of drugs ("cold turkey") is frequently accomplished by addicts on the streets, in jails, or when entering therapeutic communities for long term treatment.

Tennant should be credited with reviving interest in propoxyphene. He has detoxified about 400 heroin addicts with Darvon N. He gives them 800 mg the first day, 1,400 mg the second day, 1,200 mg the third day, 800 mg the fourth day, and, finally, 600 mg the fifth day. He claims good results with abrupt withdrawal from the Darvon N with minimal production of abstinence effects. The patients remain alert and active. Sometimes a tranquilizer or a hypnotic is needed to supplement the Darvon N dosage schedule.

Darvon N has been used by List to terminate patients who wish to come off methadone maintenance therapy. Certain patients have difficulties during detoxification from methadone even when the methadone dosage is slowly decreased. Apparently, they can be switched to Darvon N and made drug free within a brief period.

DARVON N AS A MAINTENANCE AGENT

The use of Darvon N for detoxification is interesting, but it is not a significant advance since, as indicated, many chemicals can accomplish similar results. On the other hand if a safe, non-narcotic, non-addicting agent could be found to provide satisfactory maintenance for opiate addicts, this would be very helpful and important. Some addicts object to taking an addicting drug like methadone over long periods of time. Others, especially some minority members have expressed the fear that methadone is the dominant culture's genocidal weapon. In actual fact, a larger proportion of white addicts than minority group addicts are enrolled in methadone maintenance programs.

Darvon N has been used in seven programs in the Los Angeles area and by private physicians to treat heroin addiction. Maintenance doses range from 400-1600 mg a day. Constipation, which may be a problem with methadone, is not encountered with any regularity. Male impotence is supposed to be less frequent than with methadone. It is claimed that too much Darvon N is experienced as unpleasant, therefore there is less demand to increase the maintenance dosage. One further claim, which is difficult to understand, is that while on Darvon N, cigarettes, alcohol, and sedatives are sometimes unpleasant.

SIDE EFFECTS

The side effects include nausea, vomiting, and upper abdominal pain after taking large doses of Darvon N. A small number of seizure events have occurred, especially in those who continue to use heroin. Liver dysfunction in those taking large amounts over long periods of time would be a matter of concern. It should be remembered that the doses employed exceed the analgesia dose of Darvon N by far, and that neither animal nor human safety data are yet available for high dose Darvon N maintenance.

Other side effects are related to central nervous system functions. Blurred vision, dizziness, drowsiness, nervousness, and feelings of detachment are reported by patients. The seizure events mentioned above are difficult to classify. They are described as losses of consciousness without incontinence or clonic movements.

CAUTIONS

The following points should be remembered about Darvon and Darvon N.

1. Darvon must never be confused with Darvon N. Darvon may be dangerous in the amounts mentioned in this article for Darvon N.

2. The daily doses of Darvon N used for maintenance are large, and we do not know whether these amounts, used over months or years, are safe. The possibility that liver or other organ impairment might occur is raised by the animal studies.

3. The use of Darvon N for the treatment of opiate addiction repre-

sents a new use for an approved drug. For this purpose it is an investigational drug. Therefore, the patient's written, informed consent is necessary. State and federal authorities should be asked about compliance with their regulations.

4. The use of Darvon N by physicians to treat opiate dependent people may be counter-productive. Detoxification alone is almost never enough to assure prolonged abstinence. Long, bitter experience has amply demonstrated that opiate detoxification will rescue less than one in twenty. Maintenance therapy must be supplemented with ancillary services to which a physician rarely has access. After 15 years of methadone maintenance treatment programs it is clear that the drug acts simply to hold the patient in therapy. A major personality reconstruction must proceed during the maintenance period. If the physician is unable or unwilling to accomplish the reconstructive process, he should not engage the patient in treatment.

DISCUSSION

The use of Darvon N as a maintenance agent in the narcotic addictions should be seen as part of a continuing search for better, safer substances. Darvon N (in contrast to methadone) is not a narcotic, has a low dependence liability, and has a relatively mild withdrawal syndrome. It is also non-lethal to some nontolerant person who may consume a daily dose deliberately or accidentally. On the other hand, side effects do occur, the long term toxicity is unknown, and it may be prescribed too casually because it is not a highly regulated drug. Controlled studies are badly needed before it enters widespread use as a maintenance agent. These studies are underway, and their results are awaited with interest.

REFERENCES

1. Toxicology and Applied Pharmacology 19:(3) (July) 1971, has devoted its entire issue to the pharmacology of propoxyphene.
2. Fraser, J. F. and Isbell, H. Pharmacology and addiction liability of d 1 and d-propoxyphene. Bull. Narcot. 12:9, 1960.
3. Elson, A. and Domino, E. F. Dextropropoxyphene addiction: Report of a case. J.A.M.A. 183:482, 1963.
4. McCarthy, W. H. and Keenan, R. L. Propoxyphene hydrochloride poisoning. Report of the first fatality. J.A.M.A. 187:460, 1964.
5. Tennant, F. S. Complications of propoxyphene abuse. Arch. Int. Med. 132:191, 1973.

6. Tennant, F. S. Propoxyphene napsylate for heroin addiction. J.A.M.A. 226:1013, 1973.

4. Heroin Maintenance: A Solution or a Problem?

WHAT IS HEROIN?

Heroin is diacetylmorphine, a semi-synthetic alkaloid from the oriental poppy made by treating morphine with acetic anhydride. It is rapidly reconverted to morphine in the body and is excreted in the urine (and reported on lab slips) as morphine. By weight it is two to three times more potent than morphine. In general, the effects of equivalent amounts of morphine and heroin are similar. The only way that intravenous injections of morphine can be distinguished from heroin is the frequent histamine effects of morphine, noted as "pins and needles."

It should be noted that disability and death due to chronic heroin use is almost invariably due to unsterile injections or the presence of contaminants (hepatitis, pulmonary infections and fibrosis, tetanus, endocarditis). Heroin overdose is, of course, a cause of death directly related to the drug, but even most cases of overdose are supposed to be due to a hypersensitivity reaction to the adulterant. Therefore it is possible to use pure, sterile heroin for years, especially when the dose can be stabilized, without serious harmful side effects.

WHAT IS HEROIN MAINTENANCE?

Heroin maintenance (HM) consists of providing or administering supplies of heroin to long-term heroin addicts who have been failures in other treatment methods. At present no HM programs exist in the United States. Since the heroin is used intravenously, it acts over a few hours and must be injected three to five times in 24 hours. This is in contrast to methadone maintenance, which requires a single, oral daily dose.

HM means different things to different people.

To certain New York legislators it means locking end-stage addicts up in institutions or work camps indefinitely. They would then be given heroin injections by the staff. It is assumed that many hardcore addicts will gladly give up their freedom for an assured supply of good heroin.

To the Vera Institute in New York City, which has submitted such a proposal, it consists of the addict returning to a 24-hour clinic for each heroin injection over a period of a year. During his year on heroin maintenance the staff will work with the addict to persuade him to detoxify or go into a drug-free or methadone maintenance program.

Other HM proponents advocate the adoption of the "British system," which allows the user to pick up a 24-hour supply from a pharmacist and use it to inject himself.

A small number of HM supporters see no objection to the prescribing of heroin for addicts without particular controls, just as insulin is prescribed for diabetics. It is their belief that everyone has the right to take whatever drug he wishes.

These widely varying HM concepts make it difficult to make a clear case for or against the procedure. Instead, it is necessary to evaluate the consequences of each program.

THE BRITISH SYSTEM

Many misconceptions about the current British system persist. It should be understood that the original program allowed physicians to prescribe heroin for certified addicts. It failed and was replaced by a network of narcotics treatment clinics in 1968. Physicians may no longer prescribe heroin to addicts. Now the addict goes to the clinic where an offer to de-addict him is made. If this is not acceptable, a bargaining session is held in which the client attempts to obtain as much narcotic as possible and the physician tries to keep it down to the smallest amount. Nor is the narcotic used invariably heroin. Efforts are made to convert the user into an intravenous, if not an oral, methadone addict because that drug is longer acting than heroin. At present only 16 percent of new opiate addicts attending the clinics actually get heroin, the rest receive either nothing or methadone alone.

As it functions today, the British system still has a number of negative aspects according to a recent report by Dr. Reginald Smart of Canada.

1. Illicit drug use and criminality have not disappeared from the British addict population. Because of the low doses of drugs prescribed by the clinics, addicts merely supplement their clinic supplies with street supplies.

2. There is no proof that heroin use has decreased in England. All that is known is that fewer prescriptions for heroin are being written.

3. The clinics have difficulty attracting and holding clients. Half of the

clients have used heroin for at least two years before first appearing at a clinic. Overall dropout rates are about 50 percent a year.

4. Illicit sales of heroin were found to have increased after the clinics were established.

5. A substantial increase in the number of convictions for posession or trafficking of heroin has occurred since 1968.

6. The number of registered narcotic addicts in England over the past five years has remained constant at about 3,000. According to Gould the actual number of opiate addicts may be ten times as many.

7. In addition to the above points, it should be noted that the addict mortality rate in England is 27 per 1,000 per year, even higher than the American rate. This occurs despite the sterile syringes and sterile heroin that is distributed there. A good number of the deaths are caused by unsterile techniques, which addicts persist in using in spite of the instructions and demonstrations given them in the clinics.

SOME PROS AND CONS

Ever since the heroin addiction epidemic of the past ten years spread across the United States, some form of HM has been proposed for this country. The supporters of HM felt that it would reduce crime and reduce heroin addiction. Others expressed the feeling that "if those junkies want to shoot that stuff into their veins, let them." Some of the proponents of the idea had the rather simple notion that "if it worked in Britain, it will work here." Serious students of the problem provided more cogent reasons for supplying heroin to addicts. They noted that a large number, estimated at 50 percent of the addict population, will not enter any currently available treatment facility, or if they did, they would quickly fail. Therefore, hundreds of thousands of heroin dependent people will not be reached by any present treatment opportunity. They will serve as a source of spread of the addiction to new users. Furthermore, they will continue their antisocial activities to support their habits, threby underwriting the operations of the criminal narcotics syndicates.

Those who opposed the practice of HM pointed to the fact that it had been tried with morphine in this country in the 1920s and had dismally failed. They claimed that our problems were so different from the English situation that what seemed to work there, would not necessarily work here. It was believed that if heroin were offered to addicts, they would hardly be motiviated to go into therapeutic communities, methadone detoxification, or maintenance programs. These programs might be put out of business by the appeal of the free, good heroin. The deterrent to becoming a heroin addict would be eliminated, because one could always depend on a legal supply of quality heroin for the rest of one's life.

There is general agreement on both sides that HM should be reserved for the addict who has failed in other treatment programs. Those under 21 are generally excluded, and proof of addiction for at least three years is generally considered necessary. Teenagers are excluded because of the risk of fixing a heroin addiction that may not have been fully developed.

The problem of determining whether a person is, in fact, a chronic narcotic addict is not easily resolved. Some individuals will go to any lengths to become enrolled in an HM program: they will manufacture "tracks," give themselves a few injections of heroin so that they will have a positive urine and Nalline test, and provide fictitious histories of failure in other treatment programs. The importance of finding out whether or not a client is a genuine addict becomes critical in accepting anyone for HM.

The amount of heroin to be administered will provide difficult decision-making issues. It is estimated that most street habits amount to 5-25 mg a day. It should be recalled that street "bags" contain only 3 to 15 percent heroin. It is very likely that HM will furnish the addict with larger amounts of heroin than he had been using. However, because of tolerance, supplementation with street heroin will still occur in an unrestricted setting.

THE ARGUMENTS

It may be well to consider each argument for and against heroin maintenance in order to come to a sensible understanding of the issues.

Will HM Lead to a Reduction in Crime?

Large scale dispensation of heroin might reduce the need to buy heroin, and therefore "hustling" activities ought to decrease. About a third of all heroin purchases are financed by shoplifting, burglary, and robbery. It is naive to imagine that universal HM will eliminate crime, even by the clients on HM; however, we can expect some reduction in antisocial activities.

Will the Illicit Heroin Distribution System Be Eliminated by HM?

Even a universal HM program would not eliminate the traffic in heroin. Many addicts will still be on the streets. Those on HM will occasionally supplement their licit supplies. A very pertinent question will be: "What will happen to the heroin that the HM clients no longer use?" If it is used to improve the contents of the "bag," to effect a major price reduction, or if it enters new consumer markets, the results will hardly be as beneficial as the proponents assume. One reason why we cannot expect that our problem will be solved by adopting the British method is that we have a vast, existing black market. To superimpose a large legal supply of heroin upon the pool of illegal heroin is a substantially different situation than exists in Britain. Such a strategy could result in a worsening of, rather than an improvement in, our situation.

Will Diversion of Heroin From HM Programs Occur?
In addition to the usual hijackings and thefts from a legal heroin pipeline, diversion will occur if even as little as a day's supply is given to the addict. It would be most unfortunate if these supplies were used to create new addicts, but unless every injection is given by clinic personnel, this will happen.

Why Institute HM If the Heroin Epidemic Is Diminishing?
It may be that current treatment and control measures are bringing about a reduction in numbers of active addicts. If so, a widespread use of HM may not be justified at this time. This does not mean that small demonstration projects should not be undertaken.

Is There No Indication for HM?
There appears to be three possible indications for a specific kind of HM program.

1. During the last phase of a heroin epidemic, when only small numbers of addicts remain capable of spreading the condition to others, it will make good sense to treat all those remaining with HM. This should be done in a controlled setting in the hope that all the "carriers" can be made noninfectious. This is essentially the justification for the British system.

2. Small numbers of chronic, criminal heroin addicts who have failed in other treatment programs could be considered for a well supervised, custodial HM program. This would not solve our narcotic problem, but we would have an opportunity to learn much about the exact nature of heroin addiction. It would also demonstrate whether or not this procedure is a proper solution for the hard-core addict.

3. A project such as that proposed by the Vera Institute could be sup-

ported to determine whether the year on HM can be used to persuade heroin addicts to move on to a drug-free or a methadone maintenance program.

CONCLUSION

A large scale, open program of HM in this country could be catastrophic. We should not be persuaded by those who think it will solve our crime in the streets problem, or by those who think that we have the inalienable right to do and take what we please. Careful, small scale efforts to answer specific questions and to increase the treatment options seem worthy of consideration.

SELECTED REFERENCES

1. Drug Abuse Council. Heroin maintenance: The issues. 1828 L St. N.W., Washington, D.C. 20036, 1973.
2. Gould, R. E. The case for heroin maintenance therapy. Drug therapy. 2:67-71 (May) 1972.
3. Judson, H. F. The British and heroin. New Yorker. Oct. 1, 1973.
4. National Clearinghouse for Drug Abuse Information. The British Narcotic System. Series 13, No. 1, Apr., 1973.
5. Phillipson, R. The implementation of the second report of the Interdepartmental Committee on Drug Addiction. In: Phillipson, R., ed. *Drug Dependence and Alcoholism.* London, Butterworth, 1970, pp. 75-98.

5. Overdose (OD)

The patient overdosed on one of the drugs of abuse may present himself to the physician as a conscious, rational, cooperative individual who has not yet absorbed much of the toxic agent from his stomach and upper intestinal tract. At the other end of the clinical spectrum, another overdosed patient may be deeply comatose, hardly breathing, with imperceptible pulse and blood pressure, and with no reflexes whatsoever. It is the latter kind of individual who will be discussed here. A patient in this condition is one of the most immediate of medical emergencies, and active intervention is needed NOW.

Often enough, the stuporous or comatose individual will have arrived at this state as a result of the absorption of one or more central nervous system depressants: the narcotics, the sedative-hypnotics, the tranquilizers, alcohol, and certain analgesics. In the absence of a history of some specific drug intoxication, a number of general support procedures must be undertaken. At time the situation is so critical that there is hardly time to ask the necessary questions or do even the briefest of physical examinations. On other occasions, when the patient has a relatively satisfactory and stable heart rate, respiratory rate and blood pressure, the luxury of obtaining specific information, or of waiting for a call from the clinical laboratory will be available.

The differential diagnosis of coma, of course, extends well beyond those due to intoxication with central nervous system depressants. Head injuries, cerebrovascular accidents, uremia, hypoglycemia, diabetic coma, post-epileptic states, myocardial infarctions, and many other conditions will require consideration. It must also be pointed out that more than one cause of coma may co-exist. Head injuries, for example, will often occur in connection with the fall a person sustained when he "blacked out" from his OD.

The following material will be presented in the form of questions the physician would ask himself on being confronted with a patient who is evidently dying of an OD. The questions are posed in approximately the order in which they arise. The priorities for action are listed as: NOW, SOON, and LATER. Clearly, everything listed under NOW cannot be performed by one person. A trained team of about four or five people will be better able to do all the necessary work simultaneously.

ACTION SCHEDULE

I Is the Patient Breathing?

1. Is the airway obstructed?

NOW: Remove obstructing objects from the mouth and throat. Look for dentures or a tongue that has fallen back, closing the pharnyx. Position the head to avoid aspiration of material that may be vomited.

SOON: Do periodic tracheal suction with a soft catheter. Consider tracheostomy if the airway cannot be kept functional.

2. Is the patient not breathing or breathing insufficiently?

NOW: Assist air exchange by providing mouth-to-mouth (12/minute) respiration, AMBU bag, or positive pressure ventilation with compressed air. Place an endotracheal tube or call for an anesthesiologist to intubate. (To tolerate the intubation, the patient must be comatose.) Inflate the cuff to prevent aspiration of vomitus.

LATER: Listen for breath sounds over both lungs. Do arterial blood gas determination. Obtain x-ray of chest for endotracheal tube placement and areas of pneumonia or atelectasis. *Are abdominal or skull films indicated at the same time?* Give antibiotics for specific infections. Prophylactic antibiotics are not desirable. *Is the patient allergic to the antibiotic?*

II Is the Heart Beating Effectively?

NOW: Do external cardiac massage (60/minute). Obtain intravenous access with 18 gauge needle or catheter. (This is not easy in long-term heroin addicts.) Blood sample for chemistries and drugs (opiates, quinine, hypnotics, tranquilizers, alcohol). Begin drip with 5 percent glucose/water or Ringer's lacetate (slow drip if danger of pulmonary edema exists, fast if shock is present).

NOW: EKG hookup to monitor for abnormal rhythms, recent myocardial infarction, etc. *Is defibrillation needed?*

III What is the Pupil Size?

NOW: Give narcotic antagonist if pupils are contracted. (See "physical examination" below for full discussion of this issue.)

IV Is Patient in Shock?

NOW: Position patient head down. (For pulmonary edema the orthopnea position is used.) Warm (avoid overheating) if hypothermic. Increase i.v. flow. Give oxygen by nasal catheter. (Correction of hypoxia might produce apnea because of decreased CO_2 sensitivity of the respiratory center. Therefore observe respiratory rate.)

V What Do I Want to Know about the Patient and the Drug?

NOW: *Ask the accompanying person:*
What was taken?
How much?
When?
How do you know?
Do you have the bottles?
Was the patient on the drug?
Why was it taken? (Suicide?)
What serious illnesses does the patient have?

If no accompanying person is present, search clothes for identification of patient and next of kin, drugs, needles and eyedropper, etc.

SOON: Do physical examination. In addition to the usual items it should focus on:

Skin: Inspection for recent needle marks, "tracks," abcesses, scars, thromophbetitis of superficial veins, or even a needle still sticking in the skin.

Mouth: Odor of alcohol or volatile solvent. If odor of alcohol is noted, it still may not explain the whole picture.

Pupil size: Small pupils generally mean opiate overdose, but a patient in shock from a heroin overdose may not have pinpoint pupils. Further, if the coma is due to mixed opiate-hypnotic intake, the pupils may or may not be constricted.

If suspicion exists that the OD is due to an opiate, then a narcotic antagonist should be given NOW. A young, apneic, comatose patient with recent needle marks over the veins should be given one or two doses of naloxone (Narcan), 0.4 mg i.v., even when constricted pupils are not present. If the respiratory depression is not due to narcotics, no harm is done. If the patient responds, the antagonist will have to be repeated, especially if the OD is due to methadone. Methadone is very easy to find on the street, so it must be considered in opiate OD. Keep the patient under observation: he may stop breathing again.

Scalp: for trauma.

Opthalmoscopic: for evidence of hypertension or diabetes.

Lungs: for consolidations.

Heart: for arrhythmias.

Abdomen: for bowel sounds, enlarged liver.

Neurological: for pain response, corneal reflex, pupillary responsiveness to light, and deep tendon reflexes. These should be recorded and periodically repeated to determine whether or not the patient is recovering.

Vital signs: record every 15 minutes.

VI Does any of the Drug Remain in the Upper Gastrointestinal Tract?

SOON: Gastric lavage if the drug is not corrosive, the endotracheal tube is in place, and the drug was presumably ingested within the past six hours. The absence of bowel sounds might extend the amount of time when lavage might retrieve significant amounts of the drug. Use at least a size 34 French tube. Aspirate stomach contents and send for drug identification. Instill one-half to 1 pint of water or saline, leave in place for one to two minutes, then drain off slowly (by gravity). Repeat till return is completely clear. Then one to three ounces of powdered, activated charcoal suspended in six ounces of water may be instilled and left in the stomach.

VII Are the Kidneys Functioning?

SOON: Insert indwelling catheter. Send urine to lab for analysis (including specific gravity) and drug identification. Chart output hourly. Chart fluid intake.

VII What Else Can Be Done?

Analeptics and stimulants? Unnecessary.

Forced diuresis and fluids? Can be harmful.

Vasopressor drugs, plasma, or dextran for hypotension? Usually not necessary, but may be needed on occasion.

Peritoneal dialysis? Not recommended.

Hemodialysis? Usually not necessary even for gluthethimide (Doriden) poisoning.

Digitalization? Might be considered for unresponsive pulmonary edema.

Diuretics? Might be considered for unresponsive pulmonary edema.

Physostigmine? Intravenous Physostigmine is a specific antidote for atropine and other drugs with anticholinergic effects. It is being used to treat overdoses of all CNS depressants.

SUMMARY

Naturally, considerable differences of opinion exist concerning the best way to treat the patient overdosed with some depressant drug. The overriding concern of most emergency room physicians is to maintain an airway and to provide cardiopulmonary assistance so that oxygenated blood is distributed to the organs needed for survival. At present, the trend is to treat conservatively, focusing upon the maintenance of the life support systems. Antidotes (except for the narcotic antagonists) are not used as much as previously. Careful regulation of water and electrolyte balance and monitoring the blood pressure, heart rate, respirations, urine flow, and level of consciousness, is the favored method at this time. Stimulants and diuretics are hardly used at present.

Finally, it can be said that there is no merit in most of the "junkie" treatments of his overdosed acquaintances. Stimulation with cold, pain, or burning is not recommended, especially for the person in shock. Forcing fluids into an unconscious or even a conscious person's mouth is not a rational approach to retrieve drugs that had been injected. Of course, the dangers of fluid aspiration exceed any possible benefit. Intravenous injections of milk (foreign protein therapy?), salt water, sugar, or vinegar simply increase the dangers of sepsis. Actually, the best treatment of narcotic overdose available on the street would be an intravenous injection of a narcotic antagonist, but this has not yet been reported.

ADDITIONAL READING

1. Bourne, P. J. *A treatment manual for acute drug abuse emergencies.* Superintendent of Documents, U.S. Gov't. Printing Office, Washington, D. C. 20402, Stock No. 1724—00302, 1974.
2. Comstock, E. C. *Guide to management of drug overdose.* PDR, 29th edition, Medical Economics Co., Oradell, N.J., 1975.
3. Kaufman, R. E. and Levy, S. B. Overdose treatment: Addict folklore and medical reality. JAMA 227:441 (Jan. 28) 1974.
4. Kaumans, A. J. R. Treatment of acute drug intoxication. Newsletter of the Massachusetts Medical Society, 10:(5) (Oct) 1970.
5. Reference Handbook. *Reactions to drug abuse.* The Medical Letter, 56 Harrison St., New Rochelle, N.Y., 10801, 1975.
6. Smith, D. E. and Wesson, D. R. *Diagnosis and treatment of adverse reactions to sedative-hypnotics.* Superintendent of Documents, U.S. Gov't. Printing Office, Washington, D. C. 20402, 1974.

6. Heroin Versus Morphine for Pain

During recent years there has been a greater interest in the more empathic management of the dying patient, especially the terminally ill cancer patient with pain.

The concept of the hospice has been introduced here from England—a nursing home focusing on the treatment of those whose life span is counted in days or weeks. The idea of a homelike, nonhospital setting staffed by understanding people experienced in attending patients in the last stages of their disease has considerable merit.

One of the standbys in Britain for the control of pain is an elixir containing heroin, cocaine, and alcohol, accompanied by a phenothiazine. This is known as Brompton's mixture, and its composition varies according to the institution using it. It apparently is a satisfactory method of relieving pain, nausea, vomiting, depressed moods, and other noxious symptoms when it is given every four hours around the clock.

In this country a number of people, in view of the British experience, advocated using heroin for pain in those with inoperable malignancies, claiming that it is preferable to the currently available narcotics like morphine or methadone. The present legal status of heroin in the United States is that it can be used only for research purposes. It cannot be prescribed in medical practice nor stocked in pharmacies without a special Schedule 1 (no medical usefulness, high abuse potential) license.

The questions to be considered in resolving the issue are: Is heroin superior as an analgesic to the available narcotics? Should it be placed in Schedule II (high abuse potential, some medical usefulness) along with morphine and related drugs? Are there any disadvantages to this limited acceptance of heroin as a therapeutic agent?

PHARMACOLOGY

Heroin is diacetylated morphine made by treating morphine base with acetic anhydride. Its advantage over morphine consists of greater potency (about three times more potent when used parenterally), greater solubility, and a somewhat more rapid transport across the blood-brain barrier. When injected intravenously its rapid onset of action may make it distinguishable from morphine. The occasional histamine reaction when morphine is given intravenously (pins and needles sensations, urticaria, wheezing) is another cue.

Fraser and his colleagues at the Addiction Research Center in Lexington, Kentucky, gave equivalent amounts of heroin and morphine subcutaneously to abstinent heroin addicts.(1) These experienced narcotic users could not distinguish between the effects of the two drugs. They preferred heroin, however, over morphine when it was given intravenously.

In another study with postoperative patients intravenous heroin could be differentiated from morphine.(2) The doses used were 5 to 7.5 mg of heroin versus 10 to 15 mg of morphine. Heroin injections were identified as having an earlier onset of action, greater sedative effects, and less tendency to induce vomiting.

Four mg of heroin subcutaneously caused more confusion, torpor, sweating, and difficulty in concentration than 10 mg of morphine in 24 healthy male volunteers.(3) Morphine, 10 mg, of heroin, 5 mg, intravenously provided equivalent relief to patients with recent myocardial infarctions.(4)

The duration of action of morphine is slightly longer than heroin. Both drugs produce tolerance and physical dependence. Cross tolerance and cross dependence occurs between both drugs. Heroin is rapidly hydrolyzed to monoacetylmorphine and to morphine in the body and is excreted in the urine as free or conjugated morphine. Urinary excretion is 90 percent complete in 24 hours, but traces can be detected for over 48 hours. Heroin solutions deteriorate and should not be used after about two weeks.(5)

When taken orally, the liver inactivates at least half of the heroin and morphine on the first pass through the portal vein and liver. The potency differential is not appreciable, and it is assessed as about morphine 1.5 to heroin 1. Both heroin and morphine are twice as potent parenterally as orally, but analgesia can be obtained by providing larger amounts of the drugs by mouth. The advantage of a Brompton-type cocktail is that it avoids the use of needles, and it gives the patient greater independence and mobility. Some psychopharmacologists decry the use of fixed mixtures of drugs but this particular elixir seems to be a felicitous one.

The issue of addicting a terminally ill patient has no practical relevance. There is no perceptible reason why someone who is going to die in the near future should not receive relief from moderate or severe pain. Nevertheless physicians tend to prescribe too little medication, and nurses administer even less for such patients.(6)

ST. CHRISTOPHER'S HOSPICE STUDY

A partial answer to the questions mentioned earlier has been given by Twycross of St. Christopher's Hospice in London.(7) He conducted a double blind, crossover, comparison study of heroin and morphine. His elixir contained 10 mg of cocaine plus either 10 mg of heroin or 15 mg of morphine. Other drugs (phenothiazines, steroids, anxiolytics, and hypnotics) were prescribed as needed. After a stabilization period 146 patients crossed over from heroin to morphine or from morphine to heroin. The elixir was offered every four hours, except when the patient was asleep at night, in doses ranging from 2.5 to 60 mg of heroin or 3.75 to 90 mg of morphine according to the patient's need. It was assumed by the investigator that from his experience heroin would cause less nausea and constipation, would improve appetite, and would leave the patient more alert and cooperative than would morphine.

Patients who were started on heroin were comparable to those started on morphine insofar as age and survival time were concerned. The distributions of the primary sites of their tumors also were equal except for tumors of the cervix and ovary. Additional medications required were the same for both groups, with women in both groups being prescribed benzodiazepines more frequently than men.

The results were rather unexpected. The women reported no differences in rating their heroin doses compared with their morphine doses for effects on pain, mood, sleep, nausea, and appetite. Satisfactory results were obtained from both medications. The men experienced more pain (p = <0.01) and more dysphoria (p = <0.02) on heroin than on morphine. Twycross concluded that morphine is at least as effective as heroin when given by mouth in equianalgesic doses.

These findings are not surprising to pharmacologists who have been well aware of the transiency of oral heroin in the body and its rapid conversion to morphine. The unusual aspect of the heroin-morphine controversy has been the emotional push to legalize heroin for treatment of the terminally ill who are in pain. At this point it does not appear to be necessary. When taken by mouth morphine can relieve pain as well as heroin.

THE ROYAL VICTORIA HOSPITAL EXPERIENCE

Reports from the Palliative Care Unit of the Royal Victoria Hospital in Montreal do not even discuss heroin as an analgesic. They report very satisfactory pain control with oral morphine. Morphine solutions are stable for at least eight weeks and probably longer. Mount's Bromptom mixture consists of morphine at various dosage levels, cocaine 10 mg, ethyl alcohol 2.5 ml, flavoring syrup 5.0 ml, and chloroform water enough to make 20 ml.(8) They are not sure of the need for the cocaine. The mixture is always given with a phenothiazine, either 10 mg of Compazine or 10 to 25 mg of Thorazine, as an antiemetic and to potentiate the morphine effect.

Two ways of starting the medication are suggested: either to work up from 2.5 mg every four hours, or for severe pain to start with 20 to 30 mg and gradually work down to a level that avoids pain and excessive drowsiness. Even in patients requiring Brompton's mixture for months to over a year, little need was found to keep increasing the dosage. In fact, decreased doses were more frequent.

The Royal Victoria Hospital group minimizes the problem of tolerance and dependence. It believes that undertreatment of severe pain encourages craving. Overtreatment also is undesirable because of constipation and sedation. The ideal is to keep adjusting the dosage so that the patient is comfortable and alert. Once the anticipation of pain is removed, progressively smaller amounts of morphine can be given.

Surgical procedures sometimes are necessary for special pain problems. It has been found that an understanding, interested staff potentiates the effect of the analgesic medication. Only 8 of 90 patients studied with interviews and questionnaires could not obtain pain control with the Brompton's mixture.(9) One had bladder spasms, two had nerve root pain, and five patients were so upset with anguish and despair that the medication was ineffective. The mean morphine dose for the group was 12.3 mg, and 78 percent required less than 20 mg per dose.

COMMENT

Of interest is the recent action by the AMA House of Delegates at its June, 1978 meeting. It recommended against reclassification of heroin from a Schedule I to a Schedule II drug. The Council on Scientific Affairs found the claim that heroin has certain advantages over morphine is based on impressions and anecdotal reports rather than on scientific data. One of the council's concerns was that reclassification would lead to more physician office break-ins. It did recommend for patients with chronic and terminal cancer pain that the common practice of prescribing analgesics "as necessary" be changed to regular, timed administration. The problem of iatrogenic addiction was not considered as important as the relief of pain in those with terminal illness.

Studies are underway at Sloan-Kettering to test the analgesic value of heroin compared with morphine, and results are awaited with interest. Since our heroin abuse problem will not be significantly altered by reclassifying the drug, no urgent need to change its legal status exists at present.

NOTES

1. Fraser, H. F. *et al. Methods for evaluating addiction liability.* J. Pharmacol. Exp. Ther. 133:371-387, 1961.
2. Morrison, J. D. *et al. Controlled comparison of the efficacy of 14 preparation in the relief of postoperative pain.* Brit. Med. J. 3: 287-290, 1971.
3. Smith, G. M. and Beecher, H. K. *Subjective effects of heroin and morphine in normal subjects.* J. Pharmacol. Exp. Ther. 136: 47-52, 1962.
4. Scott, M. E. and Orr, R. *Effects of diamorphine, methadone, morphine and pentazacine in patients with suspected acute myocardial infarction.* Lancet. 1:1065-1067, 1969.
5. Twycross, R. G. *Diamorphine and cocaine elixir.* Pharmacol. J. 212: 153-159, 1973.
6. Marks, R. M. and Sachar, E. J. *Undertreatment of medical inpa-*

tients with narcotic analgesics. Ann. Int. Med. 78: 173-181, 1973.
7. Twycross, R. G. *Choice of strong analgesic in terminal cancer: Diamorphine or morphine?* Pain. 3: 93-104, 1977.
8. Mount, B. M. *et al. Use of Brompton mixture in treating the pain of chronic disease.* Canad. Med. Ass. J. 115: 112-124, 1976.
9. Melzack, R. *et al. The Brompton mixture: Effects on pain in cancer patients.* Canad. Med. Ass. J. 115: 125-129, 1976.

7. Alternatives to Adolescent Drug Abuse

BACKGROUND

Substance abuse can be thought of as a maladaptive response to personal and interpersonal difficulties in which drug overuse becomes a way of life preferable to the actual life situation. The life situation may really be chaotic and hopeless, or boring and meaningless, or it may be perceived to be so by the young person. At any rate, viable life goals, rewarding activities, the ability to enjoy and look ahead to a fulfilling future do not exist.

In order to provide alternative options for a lifestyle of drug dependence, the substitute activities ought to be pleasure-giving, meaningful, or significant now or in the foreseeable future. The principle of providing alternatives to drug abuse has been summarized as follows. "Major inroads on drug abuse cannot be made by stressing the undesirability of drugs. It can only be done by offering *more desirable alternative involvements*—activities, lifestyles and satisfactions which are more *rewarding* than drug experiences and incompatible with dependence on chemicals." Certain areas where appropriate substitutes for drug overusage are to be found include:

1. Those providing a deep feeling of relationship to another person or to humanity.

2. Those contributing to self-knowledge or self-reliance.

3. Those offering a satisfying experience, either physical, mental, or emotional.

Before discussing the variety of alternatives, certain realities about the abuse of drugs should be recalled. Dohner lists a number of them.

1. People usually take drugs to feel better.

2. The pleasures and rewards of drug taking is what keeps people involved, less so the pharmacologic properties of the drug.

3. Drugs do not cause behavior changes, rather the individual's personality initiates the behavior, which may be made easier by the drug's ability to lessen inhibitions.

4. Any activity or drug that gives pleasure or relieves discomfort may induce psychological dependence. When a drug does it, it is because the person cannot enjoy himself or other people while not under the influence.

5. Drug users (especially experimenters or social users) are *not necessarily* immature, immoral, irresponsible, socially disadvantaged, alienated, rebellious, or mentally ill.

6. All use of illegal or socially disapproved drugs is *not necessarily* abusive, much less addictive. In other words certain usage may produce no physical, psychological, or social harm.

7. Altered states of consciousness have been sought, with and without drugs, since the beginnings of history.

8. Young men have a need to test their manliness. Our society does not provide such rituals or challenges. Sometimes chemicals are used dangerously as a way to prove oneself.

9. Individuals do not stop using mood-altering drugs until they discover something better.

10. Alternatives to drug abuse also serve as alternatives to other self-destructive or deviant behavior.

VARIETIES OF ALTERNATIVE EXPERIENCES

Many of the alternative experiences to be discussed in this section are neither new nor unique. They have either been forgotten, ignored, misused, or underdeveloped.

Physical Awareness

One of the simplest pleasures is the sensation of a healthy body in motion. Not only is tension discharged through movement, but a positive feeling tone derives from muscular activity. Motion and emotion are intimately related.

Walking, running, dancing, gymnastics, and group sports are only a few of these activities that can be gratifying. Unfortunately, many of us have lost the awareness of movement enjoyment, but this can be regained by deliberate training. Body awareness and the movement of the body through space should be brought into consciousness until the positive sensations become automatically registered and appreciated.

Physical relaxation exercises are used to overcome chronic tension states, a condition for which drugs are often prescribed and even more frequently taken. A number of methods of autogenic training are available that teach how to relax.

Sensory Awareness

Sensory perception is dulled and dimmed in a busy, congested, urban existence. In our preoccupation with training the child to remember facts, we have ignored the training of the senses. To really see is a delight, nor is it the exclusive property of the artist or poet. A number of adolescents find that "the cleansing of the doors of perception" that accompanies some psychedelic experiences most attractive. The same purity of sensory perception can be achieved without drugs and is evidently more genuine.

Psychological Awareness

The exploration of "inner space" is one of life's most fascinating and rewarding searches. Self-understanding through reading, meditation, self-observation, a psychotherapeutic relationship, or in a self-help group has been a major pathway by which many have returned from heavy drug use to the satisfactions of self-knowledge. Knowledge must precede training, and training is needed to change aggression into assertiveness and impulsivity into spontaneity.

Interpersonal Awareness

The impossibility of relating to people, including one's family, may contribute to the excessive use of drugs. Learning to enjoy close relationships by respecting, understanding, and empathizing with others is a zestful "trip." After a measure of self-understanding is achieved, honesty and openness with others becomes possible. Surprisingly, this reverberates and evokes honesty and openness from others. Another way to learn how to reach people is in well-run sensitivity or other group sessions. But the best way to learn how to enjoy people is to be with them.

Rites of Passage

Many people who become overinvolved in drugs are found to have a low self-esteem and a low estimate of their own worth. If their self-identity could be enhanced, feelings of worthlessness might be reduced. An adolescent who lives through a dangerous or difficult experience proves to himself that he can endure and has grown up. It is difficult in our culture to know that one has become an adult since we have poor rituals for this purpose.

It has been found by a few treatment groups that drug-dependent people derive great benefit from wilderness training such as Outward Bound, sky diving, or mountain climbing. Self-confidence and survival skills are acquired. The ability to trust others, perhaps for the first time, is achieved. But most important is the feeling of having accomplished something substantial.

Work As Fun

It is gratifying to know how to repair the products of today's technology, or to learn the technique of producing hand-crafted, useful, or decorative items. Such skills may eventually become a vocation that will lead to a new way of life. Non-competitive work can be as relaxing as other physical activities, and the products of one's own labor may provide lasting pleasure and feelings of achievement.

One of the most meaningful commitments of the ex-heroin addict or ex-alcoholic is to help others in the same predicament. A career in counseling in a drug treatment clinic provides the direct gratification of contributing to the rescue of another human being who is overinvolved in drugs. The ex-addict's intimate knowledge of addict rationalizations and con games is a real help. Other altruistic work activities that afford gratification are working in programs like VISTA or ACTION.

Esthetic Appreciation

Today's youth are well into the appreciation of today's music. As they come to learn more about music, art, and literature they will hopefully even participate in its creation. The products of civilization can be savored as much as those of nature.

We are all more creative than we think. If only we could find the areas of greatest meaning to the young people we are trying to help, they would prefer developing innovative and creative ideas and activities to anything else.

Learning

Intellectual learning is not highly regarded these days. Nevertheless, for some youths, study can become as exciting as it has been for members of every generation. History, language, the sciences or other subjects will attract some, not all, young people.

Another intellectual pursuit, more attractive at present, is the study of philosophy, religion, and psychology. Answers to those eternal questions of "What am I? What does it all mean? What is the nature of existence?" will be sought after, and the search is a fruitful experience in itself.

Non-rational Experience

The current popularity of yoga, Zen, mystical Christianity, and the many other forms of mystical experience have been found to be appropriate substitutes for drug dependence by many young men and women. They may have been seeking meaning through drugs. Spiritual exercises and mystical beliefs can supplant chemical insights.

Some parents may not understand or approve the quest for meaning nor comprehend some of the, to them, esoteric responses. Still they are to be preferred to the spurious answers provided by most drug experiences. Another noteworthy trend is the return of former drug-using young people to the religion of their parents, often with greater devotion and fervor than their elders manifest.

Other forms of non-rational exposure consist of sensory deprivation experiences, biofeedback training of alpha or theta waves, or exercises in directed fantasy. These and other similar efforts all attempt to better control internal processes for better functioning, enjoyment, or self-knowledge.

Social and Political Activism

The fact that some dropouts and other drug-using students were able to "stay clean for Gene" during the presidential primaries of 1968 means that working for social change and political reform is another possible alternative to a career of drug taking. When a person feels incapable of doing anything to improve a social condition, his response may be an escape into drugs, or a violent effort to destroy everything. Allowing him to participate redirects his energies and idealism into activites that are much more constructive for him and for society.

SUMMARY

The selection of a set of alternative activities appropriate for any specific individual requires his active participation. They cannot be imposed upon him. He must be attracted to the alternatives. They must be meaningful and relevant.

The alternatives that require active participation are more likely to succeed than those that permit a passive, spectator type of involvement.

Alternative options can be used early to prevent heavy involvement in drugs as well as later to offer the person being rehabilitated a new lifestyle or new leisure opportunities.

The proposed activity should be realistic. It is not enough to point the way; a reasonable chance of obtaining access to the alternative activity is necessary. This does not mean that it must be available for instant delivery. The client could benefit from participating in the creation of the alternative activity.

RECENT REFERENCES

1. Channin, A., Understanding adolescence. Alternatives to drug use. Clinical Pediatrics. 8:6-10, 1969.
2. Cohen, A. Y., The journey beyond trips: Alternatives to drugs. J. Psychedelic Drugs. 3:16-21, 1971.
3. Cohen, A. Y., Alternatives to drug abuse: Steps toward prevention. Alcohol, Drug Abuse and Mental Health Administration, Printing and Publication Management Section, Rockville, MD., 20852, 1973.
4. Dohner, V. A., Motives for drug abuse: Adult and adolescent. Psychosomatics. 8:317-324, 1972.
5. Dohner, V. A. Alternatives to drugs—a new approach to drug education. J. Drug Education. 2:3-22, 1972.

8. Marihuana: Does It Have Medical Usefulness?

Humans and *cannabis sativa* have co-existed for many millenia. The stems of the plant served as a source of hemp fiber for rope and cloth for canvas, clothing, and paper. The seeds provided oil for food. The leaves and flowering tops have been used in many primitive societies and even today are used as a folk medicine for a wide variety of ailments.

Practically every human complaint has been treated with Indian hemp. Some of the uses mentioned from various cultures seem outlandish. On the other hand, certain of the ancient uses coincide with the results of careful studies undertaken in our modern research institutes.

A few of the common therapeutic themes merit some attention. Pain, whether it was from toothache, dysmenorrhea, or rheumatism, or anticipated pain from minor surgical operations was often managed with marihuana. Skin infections of all sorts were handled with ointments of this drug. Melancholia and hysteria were treated with cannabis, presumably because it had a sedative-euphoric property. Asthma and epilepsy as indications for cannabis are mentioned from a variety of societies in various places and times.

Until the turn of this century, extracts and fluidextracts of *cannabis sativa* were on every pharmacist's shelf. Until the 1930s the drug was found either in the United States Pharmacopeia or the National Formulary. It was occasionally used for depression, to enhance appetite, and for its sedative effect. At about this time, a series of events occurred that eliminated marihuana preparations from the list of therapeutic agents.

1) The opium alkaloids, morphine, and codeine, became readily available analgesics, and synthetic compounds such as aspirin were marketed for lesser painful conditions. The barbiturates were becoming known as more reliable than extract of cannabis for procuring sleep or as a daytime sedative.

2) Cannabis was a highly variable medical agent. It gradually lost potency when exposed to air and light at room temperatures so that by the time it was prescribed, it might be inactive.

3) There was no way to standardize the plant or its preparations. The content of the active ingredient, delta-9-tetrahydrocannabinol (THC), ranges from 0 to 5 percent, depending on its genetic and environmental history. Sometimes, the dispensed material would be completely inert. At other times it would be stronger than the prescriber anticipated.

4) When taken by mouth, the usual form of its medicinal usage, absorption from the gastrointestinal tract was delayed and unpredictable. THC is completely insoluble in water, and absorption requires emulsification in a lipid-water phase.

5) By this time news stories about the evils of this "devil's weed" brought about pasage of the Marihuana Tax of 1937 that classified it as a narcotic. However, it was hardly prescribed at all by 1937.

CURRENT RESEARCH

During the past 10 years the scientific study of cannabis has begun. Much has been learned about its chemistry, metabolism, pharmacology, and, incidentally, about its therapeutic potential. A few of the older therapeutic uses have been confirmed, and new ones are under study. A number of recent developments brought about the capability to examine cannabis scientifically in a systematic fashion.

1) The synthesis of the active principle in marihuana, THC, and the development of methods to produce sufficient amounts to supply investigators.

2) Proof that THC essentially reproduces the activity of the plant material so that a pure substance can be used for research studies.

3) The ability to assay THC and other cannabinoids in the crude plant preparations and in various body fluids.

4) A decision by the National Institute on Drug Abuse (NIDA) to fund projects designed to clarify the physiologic and psychologic effects of the drug.

5) Development of a reliable source of standardized marihuana grown by University of Mississippi researchers under a contract from NIDA. The manufacture of a standard NIDA "joint" for investigations that required the smoked material.

6) An arrangement between governmental agencies—the FDA, NIDA and DEA—that permits qualified workers to obtain supplies of cannabis or pure cannabinoids for research purposes.

During the execution of the deliberate governmental policy to learn more about the effects and side effects of cannabis, a number of possible therapeutic uses were uncovered. In addition, hints from earlier efforts to use the herb for healing purposes, and some of the medical experiences of the eighteenth and nineteenth century clinicians were followed up.

A number of the potential medical applications of marihuana were based upon its mental effects, but others were not. In the latter instance, the psychic changes were by no means enjoyed and were often considered undesirable by those receiving the drug. What follows is a summary of the various pathologic states that have been explored in which cannabis was used as a treatment.

Glaucoma

In the course of a general survey of the ocular pharmacology of marihuana, Hepler found that it reduced intraocular pressure in normal subjects. Later, the reduction of ocular hypertension was confirmed in patients with open angle glaucoma. Oral THC is also effective, and eye drops of THC have been prepared in order to avoid the systemic effects. The drops have been found effective in animal studies. It should be understood that effective glaucoma medications already exist. What the cannabinoids might offer is either potentiation of the established medications or effectiveness in those instances that are not helped by the conventional medications.

Asthma

Vachon's and Tashkin's groups concurrently found that marihuana dilated bronchioles in normal subjects. Asthmatics, precipitated into an asthmatic episode by exercise or methacholine (Mecholyl), were treated with either isoproterenol (Isuprel) or oral THC. Both drugs relieved the bronchoconstriction. Isuprel was more rapid-acting, THC was effective over a long period of time. In an effort to deliver THC directly to the site of action, aerosols have been prepared. The insolubility of THC makes development of a fine particle aerosol spray technically difficult.

Smoked marihuana with its irritating terpenes and other organic materials is a poor way to deliver THC to an asthmatic. It has a direct irritant effect upon the lungs, and heavy smoking has resulted in metaplasia of the bronchial endothelium. Furthermore, the alveolar macrophages lose their bactericidal activity when exposed to marihuana smoke, according to one study. An aerosolized, well-tolerated THC might have a contribution to make in the management of asthma.

Epilepsy

Most of the work dealing with the efficacy of the cannabinoids as an anticonvulsant has been done with animals. THC seems to have an antiseizure action comparable to diphenylhydantoin (Dilantin). However, large amounts of THC in certain seizure-prone animal species, can trigger convulsive activity. A cannabinoid, cannabidiol, which is without mental effects, performs better as an anticonvulsant than THC. Insufficient information has been reported to draw conclusions about its antiepileptic effects in humans.

Anti-tumor Activity

Preliminary studies have demonstrated some tumor growth retardation *in vitro* and in mice for certain strains of tumors. THC is less effective than the currently available cancer chemotherapeutic agents. Much more work is needed in this area before anything definitive can be said.

Antibacterial Activity

A group of Czechoslovakian scientists have studied the antibiotic activity of cannabis extracts. They are effective only when applied to the skin or mucous membranes—not when taken internally. Investigators from The Netherlands found that bactericidal activity against staphlococci and streptococci exists, but not against Gram negative bacteria.

Anti-anxiety and Hypnotic Effects

Relaxing and sedative effects are commonly reported by marihuana users. The research work thus far has not conclusively proven that it can provide effective sedative-hypnotic activity. Even if it could, it would have difficulty replacing the established drugs of this class.

Analgesia and Preanesthesia

A major use of cannabis in folk medicine past and present was for the relief of pain. It does appear to have an analgesic effect when given in full doses, although the human studies have not been invariably positive. A 10 mg THC dose seems to be equivalent to 60 mg of codeine.

A number of investigators have looked into the possibility that THC might play a role as a preanesthetic agent. The results have not been impressive. One of the problems has been the increased pulse rate regularly encountered with THC. Another problem is that, when given intravenously, anxiety is a not uncommon side effect. Combinations of THC and other preanesthetic agents appear to produce undesired hypotension and respiratory depression.

Depression

Since the euphoriant effect of marihuana is a major reason for its nonmedical use, it was assumed that antidepressant effects might be demonstrable. This possibility is still open. Regelson found that cancer patients on chemotherapy showed less depression while receiving THC. On the other hand, Kotin, in a short study in a few patients, could detect no antidepressant activity.

Nausea, Vomiting, Anorexia, and Weight Loss

A number of investigations have been performed in cancer patients receiving chemotherapy to establish whether marihuana or THC can control the nausea, vomiting and loss of appetite that these patients sustain. There is a real need in many patients to obtain relief from the upsetting chemotherapy treatments. The standard anti-emetics are only incompletely efficacious. The results thus far are encouraging, and additional studies are underway. This indication may prove to be a promising one.

Alcoholism and Drug Dependence

During the nineteenth century, a number of clinicians reported that cannabis was helpful in detoxification and longer-term treatment of the addictive states. Rosenberg has provided patients on disulfiram (Antabuse) with marihuana as a sort of inducement for them to return to the clinic. There is no incompatibility between the two drugs. Some animal work indicates that THC can partially block the morphine abstinence syndrome. Whether THC will have an advantage over the standard detoxification agents remains to be seen. A new opiate detoxification drug is not a high priority item in the total opiate addiction problem.

THE SYNTHETIC CANNABINOIDS

If some valuable use for this drug is established marihuana will not be the marketed form. Marihuana contains more than a dozen cannabinoids, some 20 terpenes, a number of sterols and other assorted materials. Most of these substances do not contribute to the therapeutic effect, and they cause certain of the adverse effects—bronchial irritation, for example, THC is preferable to work with, but it is insoluble in water and it must be stored under special conditions.

In addition, the tachycardia associated with cannabis or THC is an undesirable side effect, and the psychological changes are not always helpful. Therefore, a number of synthetic cannabinoids have been developed and are now under study. They can be designed so that certain effects are eliminated and others are intensified. Water soluble compounds now are available with or without psychic activity. At present they are being studied for anticonvulsant, tranquilizing, analgesic, and intraocular pressure lowering properties. It would seem plausible that a specially designed synthetic compound will out-perform and have fewer adverse effects than the crude plant or even THC.

THE MECHANISM OF ACTION

The precise manner by which cannabis produces the changes that are medically helpful is not definitely understood. A possibility suggested by Burstein is that it inhibits prostaglandin synthetase, an enzyme which forms certain of the prostaglandins. It also has been shown to have adrenergic effects in the eye, dilating the efferent blood vessels in the iris, draining intraocular fluid, and reducing intraocular pressure in this manner. An additional reason why cannabinoid research into its therapeutic possibilities should continue is to determine whether its basic mechanism of action is different from that of the drugs now in use.

9. The Management of Acute Alcoholic States

DIAGNOSIS

An obviously intoxicated patient brought in for emergency care often has associated conditions that require diagnosis. Due to his incoordination or belligerence he may have sustained skull or skeletal fractures, a subdural hematoma, aspiration pneumonia, or other injuries. At times a person with alcohol on his breath may be comatose from diabetic acidosis, hypoglycemia, or sudden blood loss from a perforated peptic ulcer or bleeding esophageal varices.

Mixed intoxications are becoming common these days. One author reports that over 25 percent of lethally intoxicated patients had ingested both alcohol and barbiturates.(1) Blood alcohol and barbiturate levels can be helpful in establishing a complete diagnosis. During recovery from acute intoxication or from one of the withdrawal states other serious conditions may become evident. Schizophrenics may drink excessively in a futile effort to treat their emotional disorder. Alcoholic dementia, polyneuritis, or liver insufficiency might become manifest as the acute symptoms subside.

HOSPITAL CARE

A stuporous or comatose patient requires observation and treatment in a general or psychiatric hospital. As a rule a patient does not reestablish physiological equilibrium for approximately 10 days. Occasionally, he may be safely transferred to a Recovery House or Limited Care Facility after a few days. The impending withdrawal state (tremulousness, insomnia, agitation, sweating, rapid pulse) must be evaluated for the need to hospitalize. If hallucinations in any sensory system along with fever, delusions, disorientation, or seizures appear, hospitalization is clearly indicated.

NURSING CARE

Close observation is essential until it is established that other acute medical, orthopedic, or neurosurgical conditions are not present. Heart rate, blood pressure, respiration, fluid intake and output, and level of consciousness should be monitored at 15 to 45 minute intervals until the patient regains consciousness.

Bed rails and other protective devices are prudent. However, bed rails may only increase the height of a fall that a hyperactive patient sustains. A sitter (preferably a close family member) should be available in questionable situations. The sitter will also serve to help the patient interpret reality, and constitute a familiar object in a strange environment.

The room ought to be well-lighted, without shadows or other items capable of misinterpretation. Illusions are more common in a delirium than hallucinations. Anything that can be done to eliminate ambiguous sensory stimuli should be done. For the same reason, communications should be simple and direct.

If the patient is panicky, combative, or hyperactive, chemical restraints are preferable to physical restraints. The latter may be interpreted in a paranoid manner as very threatening. In addition, certain chemical quieting agents have other actions that are beneficial (antiemetic, muscle relaxant, anticonvulsant, sedative).

MEDICATION

Alcohol is still used, although infrequently, in gradual detoxification. While some rationale for its use exists, other equally effective medications will control the withdrawal symptoms and do not prolong the tissue changes produced by alcohol. Furthermore, by completely eliminating alcohol the impression is not transmitted that alcohol is a treatment for the problem. It is possible to completely and abruptly discontinue the patient's use of alcohol, providing other sedatives or tranquilizers are given when he becomes excited or agitated. Naturally, depressants are not indicated for the stuporous or comatose patient. The parenteral route is preferred when cooperation is impaired, or nausea, or vomiting exist.

The drug of choice currently is chlordiazepoxide (Librium).(2) It produces adequate sedation with little risk of dependency. It has some anticonvulsant action and few side effects. This medication can be given in 50-100 mg doses every three to four hours as necessary. In extremely over-agitated patients the 100 mg i.m. dose may have to be repeated hourly once or twice. Care should be taken not to oversedate the patient. Under ordinary conditions chlordiazepoxide can be gradually reduced over three to five days and eventually restricted to a bedtime dose.

If chlordiazepoxide is ineffective or produces some undesirable effect, chlorpromazine (Thorazine) 50-100 mg orally or intramuscularly, or thioridaine (Mellaril) 50-100 mg orally can be given every three to four hours. Paraldehyde is quite effective in 10-20 cc doses orally, but the odor is unpleasant and may irritate the gastric mucosa. It should not be used along with disulfiram (Antabuse).

Hypnotics may not be necessary and should not be used routinely. Chloral hydrate 500 mg or flurazepam (Dalmane) 30 mg can be ordered for sleep and discontinued as soon as possible.

Recent studies indicate that acute alcoholic withdrawal states are often accompanied by overhydration, and it is best to avoid parenteral fluids.(3) Exceptions occur when vomiting, high fever, or diarrhea exist, or when dehydration is demonstrated. As soon as he can swallow, the patient can have fluids *ad lib.*

Certain symptoms of the acute withdrawal syndrome require symptomatic treatment. Severe muscle tremors can be treated with diazepam (Valium) 10 mg every three to four hours. If convulsions occur, diazepam is also helpful. Diphenylhydantoin (Dilantin) has not been definitely shown to be of value. Its onset of action is too slow to be effective in withdrawal convulsions due to alcohol. Some clinicians will administer phenobarbital prophylactically. If status epilepticus intervenes, diazepam is very useful.

Barbiturates can be used for acute alcohol withdrawal, but they should probably be avoided. They produce physical and psychological dependency, are popular agents for suicide, and are no longer necessary now that safer, less addicting drugs are available. If used, they should be discontinued within a week.

It has been fairly well established that a hypomagnesemia occurs during the acute states. Whether magnesium ameliorates the symptoms, particularly the tremors and muscle irritability, is not yet proven. The recommended dose is 2 cc of a 50 percent magnesium sulfate solution given intramuscularly every four to six hours. The other electrolytes do not show consistent changes and tend to reach equilibrium as soon as oral intake is resumed.

Vitamins, particularly the B complex, are worth prescribing during the acute and convalescent phases. Parenteral vitamins are not ordinarily necessary.

It is well for the physician to learn a standard detoxification procedure for routine use and modify it for special situations. With present day management of the acute aloholic states, the mortality rate has decreased. When delirium tremens develops, there may be a mortality of about 1 percent or less when proper care is given.

AFTERCARE

It is discouraging how often a patient who has been informed of the consequences will continue to drink after a portocaval shunt or an incapacitating polyneuritis. On the other hand, somatic disease secondary to alcohol might provide leverage for some patients to finally seek help with their drinking problem. By the time their drinking has resulted in organ damage, it is almost futile to expect that they can "cut down" and become social drinkers. The goal should be abstinence for such individuals. Whatever persuasive powers the physician has should be used to induce his patient to enter into treatment with a caregiver now.

While the patient remains in the acute treatment or convalescent hospital, a study of his past drinking patterns and the needs they served should be made. As soon as the patient can cooperate, the damage done to his health, his family, his social and economic status is evaluated, and the picture discussed honestly and without judgmental attitudes. Every patient is entitled to know the consequences of continuing to drink. Some will make a rational decision to seek help. Others will require further proof of their destructive behavior. If an ongoing alcoholism program exists in the hospital, the process of instituting treatment is much easier. The ward routines automatically compel him to attend the educational films, lectures, AA meetings, group therapy sessions and other elements of the program.

Individual contacts by the professional and paraprofessional staff need not be neglected. Every problem drinker has one or more sensitive areas through which he can be "reached," if these can be found. It may be a highly prized intelligence, the integrity of his body, a beloved child, or a wife on whom he is extremely dependent. Discussions may impel him to make the great sacrifice of relinquishing alcohol if the promise of a greater reward is made clearly visible. The search for such critical elements is an important part of the persuasion process.

The alcoholic during and immediately following the period of detoxification is more amenable to change than on any other occasion. His first episode of DTs or his first hospitalization may be a sort of "hitting bottom." An intense and coordinated effort should be made prior to discharge to ensure the patient's continuation in a therapeutic program. This can be aided by talks with the patient and spouse, a psychiatric consultation, or an introduction to an Alcholics Anonymous meeting. It is best to arrange for the patient's appointments before he leaves and rely on spouse or friend to help him keep them.

Contact with the patient and support from his physician is helpful until the program "takes." In this way the physician can transfer his rapport and his relationship to the clinic, psychiatrist, AA or other group program. The physician can then feel he has fulfilled his obligation to the patient and given him an adequate start on a recovery program.

SUMMARY

The management of pathologic intoxication, the delirium tremens, alcoholic hallucinosis, and other acute alcoholic states consists of maintenance of vital functions, prevention of injury, alertness to underlying illnesses, and a restoration of proper sleep and nutritional patterns. Gradual withdrawal is recommended to prevent recurrent, major convulsions and shock. Routine administration of parenteral fluids is not indicated. Immediately following recovery from the acute state may be a propitious time to begin the alcoholic's rehabilitation.

NOTES

1. Gupta, R. C. and Kofoed, J., Toxicological Status for Barbiturates, Other Sedatives and Tranquilizers in Ontario: A 10 Year Survey, Canad. Med. Assoc. J. 94:863-865, 1966.
2. Kaim, S. C. Klett, C. J. and Rothfeld, B., Treatment of the Acute Alcohol Withdrawal State: Comparison of Four Drugs, Amer. J. Psychiat., 125:1640-1646, 1969.
3. Knott, D. H. and Beard, J. D., Diagnosis and Therapy of Acute Withdrawal from Alcohol. In Current Psychiatric Therapies; (Ed. J. H. Masserman), Grune and Stratton, 1970.

10. Alcoholics: Can They Become Social Drinkers?

The question is an old one. Chronic alcoholics have spent lifetimes sporadically attempting to moderate their drinking. Dozens of articles have been written pro and con. Few subjects arouse stronger feelings among alcohologists.

On the abstinence side are most clinicians, Alcoholics Anonymous, the National Institute on Alcohol Abuse and Alcoholism (NIAAA), and the rest of the alcohol establishment. Those who make up the pro social drinking group are a much smaller band of treatment personnel and researchers.

THE ISSUES

Most chronic alcoholics show an intermittent drinking pattern. Some are binge drinkers who may only have one or two devastating drinking sprees a year. In between they are dry or drinking moderately.

Even the heavy daily drinker who would go into one of the withdrawal syndromes if he stops will modulate his intake for months after a bout of the DT's, the threat of job loss, or entry into a treatment situation. Such reductions in consumption represent neither recovery nor remission. They are cyclic undulations in the normal course of a chronic, life-threatening behavior. To identify these fluctuations during treatment and call them improvement is a bit naive.

One characteristic of the alcohol dependent person is a general inability to consistently drink moderately. Some are so lacking in control that one drink may mean drinking until unconscious. For others, the dyscontrol is incomplete. They drink without impairing themselves or others for shorter or longer periods of time. Then, at some point, due to some noxious mood, perhaps, their control is lost. These drinkers should seek abstinence as their goal. They have too much to lose and too little to gain from attempts at controlled drinking.

Other common characteristics of many chronic alcoholics are their enormous ability to deny the seriousness of their alcoholism, and a well-developed capacity to rationalize and minimize the consequences of their drinking behaviors. These factors not only bring them into treatment late, but justify their early withdrawal by dropping out and pronouncing themselves cured. These psychological mechanisms also allow them to employ pronouncements in the media about alcoholics becoming social drinkers as a justification to commence drinking again. However, they do not lack for other excuses equally effective.

Are there ex-chronic alcoholics who can learn to drink in moderation? Probably, but they represent a small fraction of the population at risk and they cannot be predictably identified at present. Thus, at this time with our present knowledge, abstinence is the safest goal. In addition, a person who has experienced years of excessive drinking may have a liver that is functioning marginally. For this person the amount of alcohol consumed while drinking socially is too much.

On the other hand, in a culture like ours drinking is a pervasive social custom equated with friendliness, relaxation, and good cheer. Abstinence is not easy under such conditions. Pressures to imbibe are numerous. Most abstainers have made their adjustments to "friendly" exhortations to drink up. For a few, abstinence represents an irritating social exclusion that is onerous. It is these people, maladapted to abstinence, who might benefit if they could drink moderately while retaining control. Therefore research into this issue is justified and may be productive.

THE RAND REPORT

The controversy about post-alcoholic moderate drinking resurfaced recently when a Rand report by Armor *et al* entitled *Alcoholism and Treatment* was presented to the news media. Among the conclusions drawn was the highly controversial statement that the treated alcoholics who went back to controlled drinking did as well as those who remained abstinent. The reaction was immediate and was generally very critical. Since then, a number of comments both pro and con have appeared in a number of lay and scientific publications.

The report itself deals with data collected previously from eight Alcoholism Treatment Centers funded by the NIAAA. Clients were re-interviewed at six months after intake and under special conditions, 18 months after intake. The plan called for 2,320 interviews, but only 1,340, or 58 percent, could be found. Actually, most of the statistics dealt with 597 men from the above group. After dividing the group into various subgroups, it appears that the proposition that alcoholics can return to normal drinking hinges upon the results with a small number of clients.

CRITIQUE OF THE REPORT

The long litany of criticisms of the report would fill a textbook on experimental design and methodology. Many technical points will not be included here. Only the major remarks made by those who have commented publicly are noted below.

General

1. Releasing the report to the press before it had been published in a scientific journal or government publication prevented peer review, which might have strengthened the manuscript or assisted the authors in drawing conclusions that fitted the data.

2. As a result of the media's treatment of the report, a few dry alcoholics have resumed drinking, a practice that could be dangerous for them.

3. To make a newsworthy statement to the press such as "alcoholics can learn to drink moderately," and then hedge it with disclaimers is unrealistic. Of course, the media will pick up the statement and ignore the disclaimers.

4. Some clinicians have made the flat statement that they have never seen an alcoholic who could remain a social drinker for a prolonged period of time. Inevitably, they claim, he slips back into destructive drinking.

Specific

1. An 18-month follow-up provides insufficient time to evaluate the recovery status of an alcholic. Dr. J. A. Ewing, who has done one of the controlled drinking investigations, said, "In my study, the results looked promising for the first 12 to 18 months. It was only when we did a long-term follow-up ranging from 27 to 55 months after treatment ended that we detected a universal failure to maintain controlled drinking."

2. The Rand definition of normal drinking consisted of up to three ounces of ethanol a day (Ethanol is 190 proof alcohol. Three ounces would make 6 or 7 mixed drinks.), and up to five ounces of ethanol on any given day (10 or 12 drinks). This is far above the average amount used by American adults and exceeds the established definition of social drinking (2 mixed drinks or the equivalent a day). Three ounces of ethanol is an intoxicating dose for men of average weight. If consumed in one sitting, it will produce a blood alcohol concentration of 0.1 percent, a legally intoxicating level. Typically, drinkers in the study consumed less than these amounts.

3. Using the three ounces of ethanol or less limit referred to above, then more than a third of the clients studied would have to be considered normal drinkers even before entering treatment.

4. It is well known that alcoholics will underestimate the amount they

drink when questioned. Nevertheless, the Rand researchers accepted their estimates without attempting to validate them. As much as a 50 percent error could result from this deficiency alone.

5. The use of interviewers, who also have a stake in making the Alcoholism Treatment Centers look good, is likely to produce client information biased in favor of successful outcome.

6. At the six-month interview, clients were asked about their drinking patterns for the month preceding their interview. At the 18-month interview, they were questioned about their drinking during the previous six months. It cannot be assumed, therefore, that normal drinking occurred over the entire questionnaire period.

7. The number of cases in each subgroup was too small upon which to base sweeping generalizations. The six-month study found that 12 percent were normal drinkers. This percentage would fall to 2 percent if dropouts were included, a customary biostatistical procedure. The 18-month study indicated that 22 percent were normal drinkers, but the more appropriate figure is 13 percent if dropouts are included in the failure category.

8. The study failed to inquire into drug-taking activities. A client drinking moderately but also taking sedatives is no better off and may be worse off than before treatment.

SUMMARY

The advantage of the total abstinence approach is that it is safest for most alcoholics. It provides a sharp and clear danger signal the alcoholic can detect: the taking of a drink no matter what the rationalization. It avoids re-exposure to the substance that is toxic for that individual and that may complete the damage of previously impaired cellular function. It eliminates the futile notion that any of the chemical addictions, whether they be tobacco, alcohol, heroin, or sleeping pills, can be managed over long periods of time by cutting down.

The advantages of the controlled drinking approach are that the person can feel more comfortable in social situations and that people who cannot accept abstinence may be provided an alternative form of treatment. There are alcoholics who cannot or will not make it in AA or other abstinence therapies, and they should have at least one opportunity to try a controlled drinking program, if only as a learning experience.

At our current level of ignorance about treating chronic alcoholics, it seems clear that for most clinicians abstinence is a preferable goal.

REFERENCES

1. Armor, D. J., Polich, J. M. and Stambul, H. B.: *Alcoholism and Treatment.* 1700 Main Street, Rand Corporation, Santa Monica, CA 90406, R-1739-N1AAA, June, 1976.
2. Bailey, M. B. and Stewart, J.: *Normal drinking by persons reporting previous problem drinking.* Quart. J. Alcohol., *28:*305, 1967.
3. Davies, D. L.: *The problem of normal drinking in recovered alcohol addicts.* Quart. J. Stud. Alcohol., *23:*94, 1962.
4. Drewery, J.: *Social drinking as a therapeutic goal in the treatment of alcoholism.* J. Alcoholism, *9:*43, 1974.
5. Ewing, J. A. and Rouse, B. A.: *Failure of an experimental treatment program to inculate controlled drinking in alcoholics.* Brit. J. Addiction, *71:*123, 1976.
6. Fox, R.: *Behavioral Research, Therapeutic Approaches: Alcoholism.* Springer, New York, 1967.
7. Kindall, R. E.: *Normal drinking by former alcohol addicts.* Quart. J. Stud. Alcohol, *26:*247, 1965.
8. NCA/ASMA Position Statement regarding Abstinence. National Council on Alcoholism, New York, September 16, 1974.
9. Pattison, E. M., *et al: Abstinence and normal drinking.* Quart. J. Stud. Alcohol, *29:*610, 1968.
10. Sobell, M. B. and Sobell, L. C.: *Alternatives to abstinence: Time to acknowledge reality.* Addictions, *21:*2, 1974.

11. The Treatment of Alcoholism: Does It Work?

An article was published that has troubled certain members of the alcohol treatment establishment. It concluded, with qualifications, that our usual package of treatment of alcoholism gave no better results than a minimal treatment exposure.

Administrators and directors of alcohol programs were concerned that the article might be used as an excuse for cutting treatment funds by legislators. Others, who were sure their brand of treatment was effective, could not accept the results.

The final effect of the report, however, will be salutary for a number of reasons. It will impel us to take a more critical look at the existing treatment procedures. And it will force us to look more closely at the diagnosis of alcoholism and alcohol addiction.

METHOD

The article in question appeared in the May, 1977, issue of the *Journal of Studies on Alcohol.* (1) Griffith Edwards and his associates presented a controlled trial of a one-year course of treatment as compared to a single advice-giving interview. The research involved 100 married, male, working alcoholics who, because of their serious drinking problem, were referred to the outpatient clinic of the Addiction Research Unit, Institute of Psychiatry in London. What Edwards and his colleagues did was to select those patients between 25 and 60 years of age who lived within a reasonable traveling distance of the clinic. In addition, those with serious physical or mental diseases were eliminated.

Two groups of 50 patients were formed. They were matched by occupational level and by the severity of their drinking. Assignment to the two groups was made randomly. When the *treatment* and *advice* groups were examined for the demographic variables, no significant differences could be found between them.

All of the patients and their wives were carefully assessed. The patient's history, physical and laboratory examinations, and psychiatric, psychological, and social work interviews were obtained. In a session with the patient and spouse the psychiatrist indicated that alcoholism was the problem, that total abstinence should be the goal, that work should be continued or resumed, and that they should attempt to keep the marriage viable.

Those in the *advice* group were further told that the responsibility to maintain sobriety was theirs. It was then indicated that the patient would not be offered a further appointment but that someone would visit the wife each month to obtain information about the patient's status. It was stressed that if withdrawal symptoms were to occur, a general practitioner should be contacted for help. No medication was given.

The *treatment* group, on the other hand, was offered an introduction to AA, a prescription for calcium cyanamide (an Antabuse-like drug), and medication to take in case withdrawal effects appeared. A further appointment with the psychiatrist was arranged, during which a treatment plan was developed.

The social worker arranged to see the wife on a monthly basis to deal with current problems and to obtain information on progress. Outpatient care was provided, and if that proved unsuccessful, the patient was offered hospitalization with an expected stay of six weeks. The hospital program involved detoxification, group therapy, occupational therapy, and the ward milieu. Joint sessions with husband and wife were arranged when indicated. If an appointment was missed, another was offered.

Although some *advice* group patients sought help from other sources, and some *treatment* group patients engaged in only a minimal degree of contact with the Addiction Research Unit, the overall between-group differences in exposure to treatment was substantial. For example, the time spent in a psychiatric hospital was significantly greater for the *treatment group* ($p < .01$). The *advice* group patients tended to obtain brief admissions (mean = 5.2 days) to a hospital for emergencies or detoxification. The *treatment* group patients generally were admitted for a longer period (mean = 23.9 days) and engaged in a planned alcohol treatment program.

One year after the original intake interview all couples were seen for a final estimate of the patient's status. The monthly records of the social worker and psychiatrist were evaluated for changes in drinking patterns and for success in dealing with personal and social problems.

RESULTS

When the two groups were compared at the end of a year, no changes of significance were found between them. From the reports by the wives, it was found that 37 percent of the *advice* group and 38 percent of the *treatment* group had few or no drinking problems. The wives' reports also showed that 39 percent of the *advice* group and 50 percent of the *treatment* group had moderately or distinctly improved their drinking patterns. Fifty-seven percent of the patients in the *advice* group and 65 percent of the *treatment* group reported a slight or no drinking problem. Fifty-nine percent of the *advice* group and 63 percent of the *treatment* group reported improvement in their drinking patterns. The analysis of the monthly reports of drinking behavior during the year revealed no differences between the groups. The measures of social adjustment also were not significantly different.

When the patients were asked to which factors they ascribed their improvement, 54 percent of the *advice* group and 27 percent of the *treatment* group stated that changes in external realities (work, housing) were responsible ($p < .01$). All other reasons given were non-significant. A surprisingly large number—41 percent of the *advice* group and 29 percent of the *treatment* group—said the initial clinic intake interview was a factor that assisted in their improvement.

CONCLUSIONS AND RECOMMENDATIONS

The conclusion drawn by Edwards was that minimal treatment interventions gave as good results as a conventional treatment regimen in this special population of married men. The quality of treatment offered was considered to compare favorably with those in other alcohol clinics in England and abroad.

Edwards pointed out that certain other studies have shown similar results. He also cautioned against extrapolating these data to other kinds of patients.

Recommendations derived from the study are: (1) that a comprehensive assessment for treatable medical-psychiatric problems take place at the outset, (2) that first aid and counseling be readily available for the alcoholic, (3) that inpatient care be utilized for withdrawal or other serious illnesses, (4) that new treatment techniques be devised that will provide improved results, (5) that studies be made of helpseeking behavior by patients, and (6) that preventive efforts be intensified.

CRITIQUE

This is a well-designed and executed study. A number of technical objections could be made, and some of the more pertinent will be noted, but it would be preferable to accept the general validity of the conclusions and constructively attempt to benefit from the investigation by deriving further testable concepts and strategies.

Insofar as specific criticisms of the Edwards' research is concerned, a number of points can be mentioned. A double blind study would have been helpful in avoiding observer bias, but it would have been difficult to execute. It is regrettable that the study ended after one year of treatment. A post-treatment followup may have been helpful in extracting differences between the two groups.

Matkom (2, p. 1827) points out that the assumption that the more treatment a patient obtains, the better he should respond is not correct. In an open situation the sicker patients will tend to seek more intensive care and yet will respond less favorably. He also notes that the *treatment* group may have been more seriously ill than the *advice* group. Thirty-two percent of the *treatment* group as contrasted to 22 percent of the *advice* group had reported prior inpatient treatment for alcoholism.

The *treatment* group also had averaged 16.2 weeks off work during the year preceding the study (approximately 31 percent) as compared to 12.4 percent for the *advice* group. While these figures did not achieve statistical significance, the trend favored the *advice* group.

Schuckit (2, p. 1813) states that a third to a half of all alcoholics will be abstinent or almost so at some particular time. Further, a quarter to a third of all alcoholics also can be expected to cease drinking at some time during their lives even without treatment. If these facts are not considered, they may wash out significant differences between treatment vs. non-treatment groups.

The study under consideration gives further support to the idea that alcoholism is not a single disease entity but rather a multiplicity of disorders. If this is so, then a standard treatment, however effective for certain patients, must surely fail when all alcoholics are assigned to it. The analogy with pneumonia is cited by Glaser (2, p. 1819). If penicillin were considered the usual treatment for pneumonia, then those with pneumococcal pneumonia would be helped. But many others—those with staphlococcal pneumonia, for example—would not respond at all. There are many alcoholisms just as there are many pneumonias. The vast personality differences, the variations in drinking intensity, and the dissimilar life situations make a single categorization for therapeutic purposes unjustifiable and counterproductive.

If alcoholism is a heterogeneous condition, then the "average package of help" is inappropriate treatment and will be found to be no better than minimal treatment. The small number who benefit from it will be canceled out by the majority who remain unaffected.

Glaser suggests a "matching hypothesis" for alcoholism. Alcoholism should be considered multiple diseases with multiple causes, drinking patterns, and character structures involved. If this is so, then differential treatment programs designed for each person are required for optimal management. "Does treatment work?" becomes a meaningless question. Instead, "What treatment, by whom, is most effective for this specific individual with his special problems?" becomes the proper question to study.

Assuming this diagnostic plurality to be true, then the prime needs of an effective alcohol treatment program would be (1) meticulous evaluation, (2) skillful triage or sorting, and (3) a broad variety of treatment options. Of course, the notion of "the alcoholisms" is not new, neither is the concept of matching patient to treatment. These concepts are generally acknowledged but their translation into action is not consequentially executed.

Certain other implications that derive from Edwards' provocative article can be mentioned. Perhaps more emphasis should be placed on assigning the responsibility for one's own cure on the patient. The statement about personal responsibility for one's recovery to the *advice* group may have been more therapeutic than was recognized. We also should look into the therapeutic impact of a thorough assessment procedure. The patients' comments that they benefited most from changes in their environmental situation ought to be taken seriously, and increased environmental manipulations be attempted and evaluated. Finally, effective treatments that will emerge in the future should not be incorporated into a multimodality package. Instead, they should be used for the selected minority who will benefit most from them.

SUMMARY

When a report that contradicts our strongly held ideas comes forth, it is preferable to study the new information constructively rather than pick it apart to expose its inadequacies. It becomes an opportunity to rethink or retest our position. Even if the report turns out to have certain defects, it should not be discarded or set aside.

The paper under consideration should be read in its entirety and used as a stimulus to improve our diagnosis of the alcoholisms, refine our sorting skills, and improve our treatment efforts wherever possible.

NOTES

1. Edwards, G. et al. Alcoholism: A controlled trial of "treatment" and "advice." *J. Stud. Alcohol. 38:*1004, 1977.
2. Kissen, B. et al. Alcoholism: A controlled trial of "treatment" and "advice." *J. Stud. Alcohol. 38:*1804, 1977.

ADDITIONAL READING

Emrick, C. D. A review of psychologically oriented treatment of alcoholism. II. The relative effectivness of different treatment approaches, and the effectiveness of treatment vs. no treatment. *J. Stud. Alcohol. 36:*88, 1975.

12. Rehabilitation of the Addicted

After the opiate dependent person has been detoxified and is stabilized in a methadone maintenance or some drug-free program, how can he be kept from slipping back to his drugs of abuse?

Opiate addiction has been called a chronic, relapsing illness, and some people remain very pessimistic about the possibility of long-term cure. We do have, however, thousands of people in the United States who were seriously addicted to heroin or other drugs for many years, and who have remained clean for decades. They have recovered their health, restructured their lives, and made it in straight society.

We should study how they achieved and maintained abstinence in order to apply similar techniques to others attempting to do the same. The following are some factors that seem to enhance the chances of a successful outcome.

MOTIVATION

The strong desire to remain abstinent not only encourages entry into treatment but also is a major element in achieving eventual cure. Motivation is not a static mental set. It varies from day to day, even hour to hour. The therapeutic effort should be to support and enhance the patient's desire to change his life style.

How can this be done? Among other ways, by understanding what the abusive drug use meant to him, by finding more satisfactory ways to achieve these ends. The technique of telling the patient how bad drug addiction is and how harmful it is to him does not work too well with confirmed addicts.

The quality of the motivation to change is important. If the person recognizes that he is destroying himself and his family, this is helpful but it is not sufficient to sustain the drive to do something about it. What is needed is the intellectual and emotional conviction that a drug-free existence must supersede and obliterate the addicted way of life. As one heroin addict put it: "I finally came to know that I must change—not only I knew it, but every cell in my body knew it."

Since motivation fluctuates, it is valuable for the addict to be able to identify any waning drive to remain abstinent and the rationalizations that he employs to start using again. These must be learned in the course of counseling or therapy sessions, otherwise he may slip back into his previous patterns of behavior.

Prognosis can be directly related to motivation. This is why the highly motivated do well with any type of treatment and those forced into a treatment situation do poorly—unless they can be motivated by the therapist.

WORK

One of the most favorable activities that detoxified addicts can engage in is work. If the work is gratifying, so much the better, but any work is better than none. Work is difficult to obtain for those who have little training, poor work histories, and, perhaps, a serious criminal record. Furthermore, the addict's work habits are either poor or non-existent. He will require retraining even in basics, such as how to look for and apply for a job. A job, any job, is much more helpful than the dangers of being idle for long periods of time.

The advantages of having a work routine are many. The addict may lose touch with his drug-using friends. He has an occupation that might help keep his mind off drugs for many hours of the day. He may acquire a new set of friends with more socially acceptable habits. A newly acquired confidence in oneself can result from the successful ability to stay on the job.

The ex-addicts who have done best have been those who obtained work in drug treatment agencies. They have excellent information about the personal aspects of drug abuse that can be valuable, but they need training in other aspects of such work because of lack of education. To be able to help others escape from the same chemical trap that they were in is a gratifying reinforcement of their own abstinence.

RE-EDUCATION

Drug dependence can be thought of as the learning of a sequence of maladaptive behaviors. The addict way of life must be extinguished and new, more appropriate behaviors substitued. This can be achieved through counseling by rewarding acceptable behavior and by not rewarding drug-seeking behavior.

Every movement toward normal social and vocational activities should be encouraged and reinforced. Rewarding the addict for being an addict by providing him with benefits and subsidizing his addiction is destructive both to him and to society.

Some addicts are emotionally immature and cannot endure even the ordinary frustrations of daily life. Somehow they must be taught to cope with life stress so that they will not return to their drug when existence becomes difficult—as it will.

PSYCHOSOCIAL SUPPORT

Anything that can be done to assist the drug dependent person to remain sober and abstinent should be undertaken. Individual, group or family therapies, depending on which seems most appropriate for the patient, can help him through the first difficult years.

The self-help groups after the Synanon model have performed a valuable service for those who are narcotic dependent. They have demonstrated that with sufficient motivation anyone can learn and incorporate new values, attitudes, ar.d behaviors. They have shown that not only can the drug-seeking behavior of a lifetime be set aside, but also that the ex-addict can come to enjoy and prefer his new existence.

The argument that therapeutic communities do well with the highly motivated and that the less motivated leave is true. But they have provided large numbers of outstanding graduates who are clear proof that "once an addict, always an addict" is completely untrue.

Religious groups are attractive to some addicts who feel empty and without purpose. The emotional appeal of a religious movement may be just what is needed for some, but it is repugnant to others. Sports and other forms of recreation can be important. In fact, exposure to activities such as mountain climbing and survival training have proven very helpful in bolstering the self-esteem of certain ex-users. Reconstituting the family is another possible support, although this may not be effective if any one family member is not understanding and helpful.

The recovering addict should have access to his counselor even after discharge from active treatment. He could be tempted to start using the drug that made him feel better when a new life crisis looms. With the support of a therapist he might be able to endure the critical period without relapsing. Another occasional cause of relapse is overconfidence. The ex-addict may feel so well that he comes to believe that just one injection of heroin won't restart his problem.

HABILITATION

At times, the person has become addicted at so early an age that the ordinary habits of self-care and daily living have never been acquired. In such instances, habilitation, not rehabilitation is required. If necessary, the addict should be taught health and dental hygiene, proper dietary measures, how to dress, read, write, answer the phone and maintain a conversation. The addict may also need basic instruction in maintaining living quarters, personal grooming, and proper attire.

Sometimes a physical deformity has contributed to the drive to overuse drugs. if the deformity is correctible through dental or plastic surgery, it should be considered. An improved self-image can make a significant difference.

People with disorders of personality and character are overrepresented among the addicted. This is quite understandable. They were in psychic distress and were, in effect, treating their dysphoria with street drugs. They may have a depressive personality, a minimal ability to tolerate frustration, or a schizophrenic reaction that is not completely disabling. The habilitation or rehabilitation of the psychologically impaired must be undertaken lest they relapse.

Abstinence may require that the person move away from his drug-using friends and suppliers. A part of the addictive process is the ritual of group drug usage, and repeated opportunities to indulge makes the habit more difficult to extinguish.

CONTROL OF THE END-STAGE ADDICT

In a democracy the notion of exerting external controls over a person is repugnant. Nevertheless, individuals exist who resist entering treatment or who have failed repeatedly in treatment. They may provide the foci of a new drug epidemic in the neighborhood, if efforts at dealing with the current one have been partially successful.

What should be done with these recidivists? Removing such individuals from social contacts by placing them in jail or involuntarily hospitalizing them in a narcotics institution are traditional methods. Recently, there has been talk of sequestering them in a remote narcotic farm and providing them with a drug like heroin for life. It is difficult to say what is appropriate in such instances. Perhaps we feel hopeless and grasp at simplistic measures because we do not have enough knowledge and skill to treat these end-stage addicts.

Lesser degrees of control may assist the therapeutic process. If the addict is not motivated to clean up, nothing can be done. If he is not motivated but knows that he will go to some unpleasant prison if he is caught using drugs, such coercion may help keep him abstinent or relatively abstinent.

MAKING SUPPLIES DIFFICULT TO OBTAIN

No rehabilitative measure will work if there is easy access to plentiful, inexpensive supplies of the abused drug. Or to put it in another way: When supplies of illicit drugs become scarce, many users will find it too difficult to continue the heroin career. What is needed is a balanced, joint effort at reducing supplies and providing the user an opportunity to clean up. Interdicting supplies alone or rehabilitation efforts alone do not work.

We are aware of the occasional addict who stops using without treatment after many years of addiction. Why? In some cases he becomes too tired, and too old to engage in the demanding cycle of stealing, finding a dealer, injecting, and staying out of sight of the police and the people who would steal from him. In other words, making life difficult causes some to stop using; making the addict life easy and enticing encourages new users to turn on.

SUMMARY

The rehabilitation of the drug dependent person is a personal and a social gain. Each individual rescued represents a worthwhile effort. Beyond the advantages to the ex-user and those around him, the gains to society are also worth noting.

The recovered addict becomes a focal point for preventing others from entering careers of addiction and for helping users become abstinent. If he had remained addicted, he would have been a focus for others to mimic him and his drug taking. When sufficient numbers of drug dependent people in a community are rehabilitated, it becomes possible to eliminate the spread of addictive drug use to new consumers.

V
SPECIAL GROUPS
AND SITUATIONS

1. Problem Drinking in Adolescents

The following essay was contributed by Dr. Richard V. Phillipson, National Institute on Drug Abuse.

With some regularity older generations have traditionally inveighed against the wanton, drunken comportment of the younger. Therefore, it is with a certain reticence that I report on what appears to be a significant change in youthful drinking practises during the past 25 years.

So serious has the situation of continued and ever increasing numbers of young people abusing alcohol become, that the Secretary of HEW recently announced a new program of nearly $35 million to be spent on Special Target Problems and Populations, the first priority of which was youth. In recognition of the extremely severe problem of alcohol abuse among teenagers, HEW will allocate $12.5 million for eduction, prevention, treatment, and research related to problem drinking among youth in fiscal year 1980. In addition, HEW will develop and fund five comprehensive alcoholism prevention projects, targeted at 750,000 young people, with the help of the Boy Scouts, Girl Scouts, Catholic Youth organizations, and others. In cooperation with the Department of Transportation, the national media, and the alcohol beverage industry, HEW will launch an "information campaign" focusing on auto safety and encouraging sensible attitudes toward drinking among young people.

Today, alcohol-related accidents account for more than 8,000 deaths each year in the age group 15 to 24 years and are the leading cause of death for this age bracket in the United States. In addition, more than 40,000 young people are injured every year in drinking and driving accidents—many of them crippled, paralyzed, or otherwise disabled for life.

WHY IS THIS HAPPENING?

Teenage drinking is part of a larger pattern of increasing consumption of potable spirits that has become worldwide during the past quarter century. In the United Kingdom, for example, the annual per capita consumption rose between 1949 and 1974 by 47 percent for beer, over 200 percent for distilled spirits, and 284 percent for wine. There is a strong correlation between per capita use and alcohol-related problems. For cirrhosis the correlation is as high as 0.98 in Great Britian. For 20 other countries the per capita cirrhosis correlation is 0.94. In those rare instances when the per capita consumption dropped (as during Prohibition in the United States or during the two World Wars in France), the incidence of cirrhosis also fell.

The past quarter century has generally been a period of steady economic expansion and improved living standards, although not necessarily a time of tranquility. In terms of the time worked for each unit of such beverages, the cost of beverage alcohol has been reduced by at least 50 percent, while for most foods the cost has increased considerably. A gallon of milk and a gallon of wine now can be purchased for the same price. It has also been an era of relaxation of controls over the sale of alcoholic beverages for young people.

Easy availability is, of course, only a fragment of the story. Most youth has been increasingly decultured from family influences and more responsive to peer values and behavior. Youthful disenchantment with established moral attitudes has been the hallmark of the recent past. The upsurge in drug taking of all sorts has not diminished; on the contrary, it has increased adolescent alcohol consumption. Boredom and the lack of meaningful activities contribute to the abuse of alcohol.

More excessive alcohol use by the adolescent can be understood as an adaptive effort. It is an attempt to insure friendship bonds, cope with tension and the conflicts of growing up, deal with unpleasant situations at home, in the school, or elsewhere, and solve the array of problems that confront the young person. It is a tactic of adapting to inner tumult and external difficulties. That it does not solve the problem, simply evades it, does not reduce the attractiveness of the intoxicated state.

Furthermore, we have made no significant advances in the prevention or treatment of young problem drinkers, nor are any breakthroughs perceptible in the near future.

IS THERE AN ADOLESCENT DRINKING PATTERN?

Young people tend to drink less consistently than older people, but when they do, larger amounts are consumed. Therefore, they will be involved with the consequences of acute intoxication (violence, accidents, coma, etc.) more frequently than with the long-term effects of alcoholism.

HOW CAN A PARENT TELL WHETHER A SON OR DAUGHTER IS GETTING INTO TROUBLE WITH ALCOHOL?

Warning signs are not different than those noted in adults: frequent intoxications, accident-proneness, impaired school or work performance, hangover, poor appetite, police problems, and a deterioration of personal and social habits.

WHAT ABOUT ALCOHOL-DRUG COMBINATIONS?

Multiple-drug abuse in teenagers with alcohol as the basic or as a subsidary drug is a common form of substance abuse. The combination of wine or beer with sleeping pills or tranquilizers is particulary hazardous because of the super-additive effects.

SHOULD CHILDREN BE TAUGHT SOCIAL DRINKING AT HOME?

There has been a fair amount of pressure recently to make it respectable to give drink to one's young children in order that, from an early age, they may grow up to seek drinking as part of family or group activity, to be taken for granted rather than be something special, and, in general, to demystify the whole drinking experience. In an ideal world this would be fine. Unfortunately, many parents are far too confused and guilty about their own drinking to transmit anything beyond their own ambivalence. For those parents whose own attitudes toward alcohol are reasonable, the transmittal of these values can be helpful. In homes where the parents or children prefer abstinence, such instruction, of course, is unnecessary and undesirable.

SHOULD SCHOOLS PROVIDE EDUCATIONAL INFORMATION ABOUT ALCOHOL AND ITS USE?

In order to help demythologize drinking information about alcohol can be given within the context of a general health course. The difference between social drinking and destructive drinking should be pointed out. The fact that drinking does not make a young person manly or womanly can be emphasized. Hopefully, unhealthy, irresponsible drinking practises will be avoided through exposure to factual material about our national intoxicant. It will take more than the efforts of the schools to finally demolish the fiction that excessive drinking is a pattern of prestige or that it is a necessary part of socializing. It will require a revision of the media's outworn stereotypes. Television, in particular, has much to do in this regard.

WHAT IS KNOWN ABOUT SEXUAL ACTING OUT AND VIOLENCE IN CONNECTION WITH TEENAGE INTOXICATION?

Some youngsters use alcohol to dissolve their superego, to reduce their social inhibitions and gather the "courage" to attempt sexual activities that would have been difficult to achieve while sober. In a similar manner alcohol intoxication impairs judgment, diminishes controls over behavior, increases impulsivity, and impairs skilled motor functioning. As a result violent and assaultive behavior is frequent, including gang-type aggressiveness.

WHAT CAN BE DONE?

In addition to developing effective early training, education, and prevention techniques, the most manipulative variable in dealing with adolescent alcohol abuse is to decrease availability. Alcoholic beverages are so pervasive in this society that making it more difficult to obtain seems hardly possible. In fact, there is a countertrend: the production of sweet wines and sweetened milk-based beverages with alcohol added. These are attractive to juveniles because of their taste. Nevertheless, making beverage alcohol relatively more difficult to obtain, especially among teenagers, might decrease a measure of the harmful drinking practises.

WHICH TREATMENT METHOD IS PREFERRED FOR THE YOUNG ALCOHOLIC?

Group therapies are among the most frequently used techniques with or without AA. Individual therapy may be needed when a serious emotional disorder underlies the drinking problem. Antabuse has a lesser role to play, but may be helpful until new patterns of living are established.

IS IT TRUE THAT ALCOHLIC PARENTS TEND TO HAVE ALCOHOLIC OFFSPRING? ARE THE CHILDREN OF ABSTINENT PARENTS ABSTAINERS?

Alcohol parents can lead their children into unhealthy drinking habits, but they also may serve as an example that no young person will wish to follow. Therefore, some children of alcoholic parents grow up total abstainers. A parental example of complete abstinence might be followed by the children, but can, if too strict, lead to alcohol abuse as a reaction to the overly rigid restrictions on the adolescent. A vulnerability to alcoholism appears to be an inherited trait, and young men and women who have parents with severe drinking problems should be particularly careful about their use of alcohol and alcohol's easy availability.

ARE SPECIAL TREATMENT OPPORTUNITIES AVAILABLE? HOW MANY ADOLESCENT ALCOHOLICS GO ON TO CHRONIC ADULT ALCOHOLISM?

Special AA groups have been formed for young alcoholics, and even a few adolescent alcohol detoxification centers are in existence. Cirrhosis of the liver, which takes at least ten years of heavy drinking to acquire, is increasingly seen in patients in their 20s. Since the habits of a lifetime are often formed during adolescence it is believed that many young people with a drinking problem will go on to excessive adult drinking patterns.

SUMMARY

Because of our relative prosperity and the easy availability of alcohol, adolescent alcohol abuse is a growing phenomenon. The increasing use of drink in connection with every social occasion and the requirement that young people keep up with their peers in their drinking practises inevitably lead to heavy drinking. Since all are drinking equally heavily, no one identifies himself or herself as drinking too much. It is therefore concluded that over many years the psychologic and physiologic complications of alcohol will increase.

ADDITIONAL READING

1. Alcohol and Health: *The Third Special Report to the U.S. Congress* U.S. Government Printing Office, Washington, D.C., 1979.
2. Davies, J. and Stacey, R. *Teenagers and Alcohol: A Developmental Study in Glasgow,* Vol. II, Her Majesty's Stationary Office, London, 1972.
3. Edwards, G. and Grant, M. *Alcoholism: New Knowledge and New Responses.* Croom Helm, London, 1977.
4. Edwards, G. Public health implications of liquor control. Lancet 1:424, 1971.
5. Kendall, R. E. Alcoholism: A medical or a political problem. British Medical Journal. 1:367-371, 1979.
6. Rouse, B. A. and Ewing, J. A. College drinking and other drug use. In: *Drinking-Alcohol in American Society.* Eds. J. A. Ewing and B. A. Rouse, Nelson-Hall, Chicago, 1978.

2. Teenage Drinking: The Bottle Babies

Occasional drinking until drunk and restless behavior while intoxicated have been fairly conventional youthful activities associated with growing up in America.

Adolescents have imbibed both for the effects of the ethanol and for the symbolic meaning of the act of drinking. Partaking of our national intoxicant was often an effort at self-treatment for adolescent shyness and anxiety. Drinking has the double effect of producing and of justifying disinhibited acting-out behavior. The cultural symbolism of drinking by adolescents is that it simultaneously means " being one of the boys" (or girls) and "being a man," or "being grown up."

Youthful imbibing, then, directly derives from our cultural attitudes toward drinking. Although legally forbidden, drinking by those underage tends to be condoned or at least understood by most parents and authorities.

During the past few years the established mode has changed significantly. The following trends have been well documented:

1. Drinking during and out of school has extended down to grammar school students and is more frequently encountered than in the past.

2. Girls are increasingly involved in "ever having used" and in regularly drinking. By the time they graduate from high school as many girls as boys use alcoholic beverages, but not yet as often.

3. The combined use of alcohol and other drugs is often observed. Juvenile polydrug use with alcohol as the basic intoxicant is a growing problem.

4. Not only are more youngsters trying alcoholic beverages, but large numbers are drinking heavily and consistently. Pubescent alcoholism has been diagnosed in a number of pediatric psychiatric clinics.

THE EXTENT

Most surveys agree that drinking starts earlier these days. The San Mateo school district survey, which has been taken yearly since 1968, indicates that any use of alcoholic beverages by 9-12th graders during the past year rose from 65 percent in 1968 to 86 percent in 1974. Male and female students using 10 or more times increased from 25 percent to 54 percent. For those using 50 or more times during the past year, the rate increased from 16 percent in 1970 to 29 percent in 1974. It should be pointed out that even the 1968-1970 rates were quite high when compared with student usage during the 1950s or earlier.

A national survey done in 1974 reported that 63 percent of boys and 54 percent of girls in the seventh grade have had a drink. By the time they reach the 12th grade this has increased to 93 percent of the boys and 87 percent of the girls. Drinking among school dropouts is greater than among those remaining in school. Therefore, teenage drinking is actually higher than reported from information collected from school populations.

Of course, the figures cited above do not necessarily represent excessive or problem drinking. Much of it was in a family setting taken with a meal or during special occasions. The only point that can be made from these data is that drinking has become more widespread during recent years. Abstinent young men and women are fewer in number even in sections of the country where they previously were numerous.

Because of our preoccupation with youthful drug abuse we have ignored the fact that in every survey, alcohol was the most frequently used and preferred drug. It is by far, the first mind-altering drug employed.

Young people who do not use fermented beverages tend not to use other intoxicating drugs.

It is the practice of heavy binge drinking or of a consistent consumption of substantial amounts that is a matter for concern. Admittedly, patterns of drinking may be established during youth, and these can evolve into damaging drinking habits in later life. But problem adolescent drinking is a serious issue in its own right. When a young person has definite social, family, or health difficulties caused by his drinking, he can be considered a problem drinker.

The difficulty may occur in connection with an acute bout during which he becomes involved in a major auto accident. A series of drunk and disorderly arrests would indicate poor behavioral controls. Certainly, the chronic use of large amounts that leads to physical or psychological impairment, inability to attend to school work or a job, or impaired social relationships can be considered problem drinking. Many of the physical impairments of sustained, excessive alcohol intake are delayed (brain damage, liver failure, peripheral neuritis, etc.) so that only presumptive indications of future physical or neurological disability are possible.

THE ADOLESCENT ALCOHOLIC

Reports from the National Institute of Alcoholism and Alcohol Abuse confirm the rapid increase in heavy, teenage drinking. Dr. M. E. Chafetz, ex-director of NIAAA, said that 5 percent of young Americans have a drinking problem. The estimated number of problem drinkers between the ages of 12 and 17 is 1.3 million, with 750,000 believed to be hard-core alcoholics. A Boston suburb study found that by age 18, 7 percent of the boys were problem drinkers. They had family, school, or police difficulties. If these estimates are correct, then the teenager is drinking just as unwisely as the adult, for 5 to 7 percent of adults are also in trouble with their alcohol usage.

"Drying out" centers report a staggering increase in teenage clients. One program in Houston has witnessed an increase in this age group from only 6 teenagers to 1,200 in three years. Eight- and nine-year-olds have been registered for alcohol detoxification in this and other clinics.

Alcoholics Anonymous (AA) has 27 groups for "teenagers and pre-teenagers" in Southern California alone. One report from New York City schools states that 10 percent of the junior and senior high school students are "already or potential alcoholics."

Many of the well-known signs of tissue damage by alcohol are not seen in pediatric alcoholics. These will come later. Gastritis and gastrointestinal hemorrhage, though, are present in the young and old alike.

They are the result of stimulation of hydrochloric acid production and the retardation of acid absorption from the gastroduodenal tract. Inflammatory and ulcerative changes in the mucous membrane result. At Childrens Hospital in Los Angeles patients 12 to 20 years old with alcohol-related ailments like gastritis and internal bleeding are not uncommon.

Among military personnel at the San Diego Naval Hospital, alcoholics had a death rate of 15 per 1,000 patients a year. This compares with a rate of two per 1,000 for naval and 10 per 1,000 for marine personnel. The major causes of death among the alcoholics were suicide, accidents, cirrhosis of the liver, pancreatitis and peptic ulcer. When it is recalled that diseases like pancreatitis and cirrhosis do not become manifest until after many years of steady drinking, death in the 30s means a very early onset of excessive use.

It is behavioral toxicity that dominates the picture of problem drinking by teenagers. Recurrent truancy, family disruptions, and illegal activities are the presenting signs. The stealing of beer, wine, or saleable items is well know. The suburban form of this activity is called "garaging." Rowdy group drinking parties, some of which culminate in the use of dangerous weapons, are regularly reported in the press. Intoxicated youngsters are apt to become involved in malicious mischief in schools, parks, and unoccupied dwellings. The arrest rate for intoxication in those under 18 has tripled during the past decade. Accidental death, a leading cause of lethality in this age group, is particularly frequent among adolescent imbibers. A third to a half of all accidents are associated with drinking.

ALCOHOL AND DRIVING

A considerable controversy centers on the effects of lowering the legal drinking age in some states and the incidence of car accidents. In Michigan during the first year that 18-year-olds could legally buy alcoholic beverages, the auto accident rate for those 18 to 20 years old increased by 119 percent. Arrests in New Jersey rose 60 percent.

On one side of the argument are those who say that these statistics merely reflect normal yearly increases and the differential treatment accorded young drivers by the police. Others view these figures more seriously and believe that young people will die or be injured on the highways at a rate far exceeding the worst years of the Viet Nam conflict.

Sixty percent of those killed in drunk driving accidents are in their teens. Even in a single year the jump in alcohol-related accidents is impressive. The California Highway Patrol reported that deaths in the 12 to

20 age group rose from 268 in 1973 to 375 in 1974. Traffic injuries rose from 4,499 in 1973 to 6,252 in 1974.

FACTORS CONTRIBUTING TO PROBLEM DRINKING

Earlier studies emphasized the family unit as the place where lifelong drinking practices are formed. This was probably true when families exerted a considerable influence on adolescent development. It may be somewhat less valid at present. The parent's drinking behavior remains an important predictor of the teenager's drinking habits. Drinking parents ordinarily will have drinking children with the degree of usage reflecting parental patterns. Abstinent parents are more likely to have abstinent children. Of course many exceptions exist. Some children will be so upset by a drunken parent that they will react by abstaining. Overly strict, teetotalling parents may alienate a child causing a complete rejection of the parental prohibitions. These children seem prone to use liquor intemperately.

In recent years more emphasis is being placed on the influence of peers. Heavy drinking often starts on playgrounds, street corners, and similar youth gathering areas. Drinking at school special events and athletic contests has occasionally terminated in riots and forced a cancellation of the event.

Whether a child will drink, and how he will behave if drunk, is strongly determined by the culture. It is the culture or subculture that provides cues through family, friends, or mass media and informs the youth as to what is permitted. In certain subcultures aggressiveness while drunk is considered normal behavior.

The individual's personality is also a determinant in the development of destructive drinking practices. At times it is difficult to determine whether certain personality features cause or are the result of drinking excessively. Diminished personal controls, impulsivity, and antisocial trends are supposed to be predisposing personality factors. It may be so, but it should be remembered that alcohol intoxication also releases such behavior.

Young people with personality deficits in the area of mood and ego controls do tend to seek out alcohol in order to deal with their noxious feelings and instability. If drinking dissolves their problems, then they are later inclined to use it often and in large amounts. Not all youthful problem drinkers have a major personality defect. They may be relatively intact psychologically, but might have become overinvolved because the practice happened to be a cultural or family norm.

BEVERAGE CHOICE

Beer is popular among young drinkers. Although it is a dilute alcohol solution, beer is capable of causing all the problems of stronger drink. The new sweet "pop" wines are a growing favorite. Beer cans and wine bottles have become a litter problem in some schoolyards, parking lots, and beaches frequented by youths. Another contender for favor is the vodka mixes like Orange Fling and Strawberry Fling sold in bottles that resemble soda pop bottles. When liquor is used, it is often in the form of vodka because it is cheap, blends with the mix, and is less detectable on the breath.

ALCOHOL AND OTHER DRUGS

The earlier prediction that the juvenile use of cannabis would lead to a reduction in alcohol consumption has not been realized. On the contrary, marihuana users drink more alcohol than nonmarihuana users. They are used separately and together. In the latter instance it is believed that marihuana has synergistic sedative effects with alcohol. When a inquiry is made into which mind altering drug was used first, the answer is generally the legal ones: alcohol and tobacco. Later, marihuana and other drugs are added.

It is understandable that alcoholic drinks would be the preferred intoxicants. They are less expensive, more readily available, and less illegal than others. They cover up the fact that illicit drugs were also used. Parents are, somehow, relieved to find their children have been "stoned" on alcohol rather than a nonalcoholic substance.

Ethanol is here to stay. A recent survey of 200 drug abuse agencies reported that the teenage use of alcohol and marihuana was increasing, while other abused agents were decreasing slightly or were unchanged. The combined ingestion of alcohol along with other central nervous system depressants will reinforce the depressant effect. This would be true for sedatives, hypnotics, narcotics, anesthetics, and tranquilizers. When consumed with stimulants or hallucinogens, the result will be a reduction in the stimulant effect or an aberrant, unpredictable reaction.

PREVENTION

To prevent the overindulgence of a culturally entrenched, ubiquitous substance like alcohol hardly seems possible. It is especially difficult because our pattern of usage does not condemn, and sometimes applauds, excessive drinking. This is the message our children perceive, over and over, verbally and nonverbally.

What can be done? First of all, the adolescent abstainer should be reinforced and made to feel that his decision is sensible, and even courageous because it goes counter to the popular mode. But in a society pervaded by alcohol, in which it is a symbol for hospitality, fun, sexuality, and maturity, most young people are unable to swim against the alcoholic flood.

Exhorting them to renounce drink will rarely work. Instead of proscribing alcohol intake, its use should be wisely prescribed. Children should learn responsible drinking, moderation should be stressed, and drunkenness condemned from the parents in words and deeds. An episode of drunkenness that results in the destruction of property, injury, or in passing out should be met with firm disapproval. Unfortunately, such behavior is often overtly or covertly reinforced.

TREATMENT

The management of teenage alcohol abuse is by no means easy or invariably successful. It is difficult for the youngster to identify that he is doing something harmful, or that he is sick. Many of those around him, young and old, seem to be drinking as he is. Even if he admits he has a problem, his motivation to correct it is often less than adequate. He may sample an AA meeting without committing himself. If pushed to go to a psychiatrist or other mental health worker, he tends to drop out of treatment rather quickly.

Groups of teenagers with similar problems led by an understanding therapist can be helpful for some. Teenage AA assists those who are willing to accept the program. Religious appeals will attract certain youths. Some exploratory methods show promise, including one which trains appropriate teenage counselors who, with back-up assistance, may be more acceptable to the alcoholic adolescent. At times, medical counseling and psychiatric referral is mandatory, particularly in emotionally disturbed youngsters. Behavior modification had not been tried often enough in this group to comment on it. Antabuse therapy is not indicated in young people except, perhaps, in a special military situation.

Family therapy is sometimes the treatment of choice, for example, when family pressures are laid on the young person whose drinking is in response to a pathological family situation. A foster family may be needed when one or both parents are alcoholics. It is clear that the young person cannot return to his group of heavily drinking friends should he succeed in moderating or halting his use of alcohol.

3. Lowering the Drinking Age: Effects on Auto Accidents

A move to amend the law to permit 18-year-olds to vote and enter into legal contracts started 10 years ago. It then seemed anomalous to treat 18 to 20-year-olds as adults and not permit them to drink alcoholic beverages legally.

Therefore, between 1970 and 1973 about half of the United States and all 10 of the Canadian provinces and two territories lowered the legal drinking age. Some jurisdictions lowered the age to 18, others to 19. It should be noted that the legal drinking age has been 18 in New York since 1934 and 18 in Louisiana since 1948.

The legislation was viewed as enlightened and forward-looking. It was believed that if consuming alcohol would lose the symbolic significance of being grown-up, young people might learn to drink moderately and more wisely than their elders. Furthermore, most teenagers had been drinking anyway, despite their inability to purchase alcoholic beverages.

Because of restrictions on purchase and possession the patterns of their usage may have encouraged them to drink rapidly and excessively. The hope existed that the accident rate for the under 21-year-olds might even decrease since the 18-year-old in Connecticut, for example, would not have to drive to New York to purchase and consume alcohol before driving back home.

Drivers under 21 tended to have high rates of automobile collisions even before the legal drinking age was lowered. Their driving records have been poorer than older drivers, and auto insurance rates reflect this data. Even when unimpaired by the effects of alcohol, they do not drive as safely as older drivers. Sixteen and 17-year-olds perform worse than 18 and 19-year-olds insofar as accident rates are concerned. Why this should be is not precisely known. It is suggested that less caution and prudence in driving are characteristic of some young drivers. In addition, it may take years before the reflexes for successful and safe driving are fully developed.

In attempting to explain why only young drivers as a group have a high accident involvement, Carlson points out that they are faced with two learning situations: how to drive, and how to drive after drinking.(9) These two simultaneous learning situations result in a higher crash involvement than could be explained by the amount of time they spend on the road.

The disproportionately high crash statistics correlate with night driving, which he regards as the most important variable second only to the blood alcohol concentration. The overrepresentation of youth in the group of fatally injured drivers, both with or without alcohol, is partly attributable to their life-style, which includes night driving for recreational purposes.

DRINKING AND DRIVING

The effects of lowering the drinking age on various types of car accidents have been examined in numerous studies. They were intensively studied in Michigan where police statistics were analyzed shortly after the law changed. An increase of 119 percent in alcohol-related collisions among 18 to 20-year-olds was found when prelaw and postlaw periods were compared.(1) By comparison, older drivers showed a 14 percent increase in the same time period.

In another study, the rate of alcohol-related fatal accidents was compared for those over 21 and for persons 18 to 20 years of age.(2) Those older than 21 showed a 9 percent increase for the first six months and an 8 percent increase for the second six months after the law change. The 18 to 20-year-olds showed an 88 percent increase during the first six months and a 13 percent increase during the second six months. This study provided some hope that the problem was self-limiting and merely reflected an initial reckless attitude about drinking and driving.

In fact, Zylman attributed the changes to the normal cyclic fluctuations of such data and to the pressure on the police to report alcohol involvement in younger drivers who were in collisions.(3) This does not seem to be the case, as further studies have been reported.

Reports from other states support the hypothesis that significant increases in driving accidents occur among 18 to 20-year-olds in states where the drinking age was lowered in comparison to the same age group in states that did not change their legislation.(4,5) This is especially true for single vehicle accidents involving males between the hours of 9 p.m. and 3 a.m., a pattern that is known to be associated with drinking drivers in a majority of instances. The number of alcohol-related vehicle crashes involving young women is only about 10 percent of those involving young men. Their accident rate has not risen as steeply.

In Canada the experience has been approximately the same. An Ontario study showed that drivers 16 to 19 years of age were the only group who showed a significant increase in all types of collisions during the six months after the law change compared to the half year before.(6)

Whitehead investigated police records in London, Ontario, for three years before and two years after the driving law change.(7) He gathered data on drivers involved in collisions who were from 16 to 20 and those 24 years of age. From these age groups he had a nonlegal drinking group (16 to 17), the newly legal drinking group (18 to 20), and a legal drinking young adult comparison (24) group that had not been affected by the new law.

The results showed sharp increases in alcohol-associated accidents during the postlaw period. Increases of more than 300 percent were found for the 18 and 19-year-olds and more than 150 percent for the 20-year-olds. The 24-year-olds had an increase of only 20 percent during the same period. Whitehead considered the possibility that the police were especially diligent in reporting alcohol-related accidents among young drivers, but he rejected the assumption on the basis of multiple lines of evidence. The fact that the second year record was no better than the first postlaw year indicates that the problem is not simply a transient "release from restraint" effect that subsides in time.

In an extension of the study during an additional two years, Whitehead provided longer term information.(8) He detected a "spillover effect" of the law on 16 and 17-year-olds. Whereas the incidence of alcohol-associated accidents rose immediately after the law went into effect in the 18 to 20-year-old group, the increase was delayed until the second year in the 16 to 17-year-old group. This might be explained by the extra time needed for the diffusion of the awareness of the easier access to alcoholic beverages to the younger age group. Many high school seniors are 18 years old and they are a readily available source of beverages for their younger friends.

It might be argued that an upsurge in alcohol use is occurring among youth and that regardless of lowering the legal purchase age, the increase in car accidents would have occurred anyway. This factor may account for some of the increase. The abruptness of the change, however, after passage of the alcohol-purchasing age law for the 18 to 20-year olds is persuasive that the law was an important causal factor.

DISCUSSION

It is not easy to eradicate a behavior in an individual or in a society once it has been established. The disappointing increase in car accidents among drivers under 21 after passage of legislation reducing the drinking age indicates that 20 or 21 may be a more satisfactory age than 18 or 19 for permitting purchase of alcohol-containing beverages.

Some governments recently have begun to raise their minimum age for drinking and others are considering such a course. Maine has reversed its laws and changed the drinking age from 18 to 20. Saskatchewan has raised it from 18 to 19. It is difficult to say whether the upward revision of the minimum age will reverse the accident rate. Meanwhile, other jurisdictions, including California, are going ahead with proposals to lower the age from 21 for the legal purchase of alcoholic beverages.

Other proposals to deter excessive drinking include: (1) issuance of provisional driver's licenses to the 18 to 20 age group to be withdrawn for any moving violation, (2) raising the tax on beverages to increase their cost, and (3) augmenting the spot testing of the driver's breath for alcohol quantity at the roadside to deter drinking before or during the operation of a vehicle.

It is not easy to be optimistic about reversing the current high level of automobile accidents in younger men. Secondary prevention through identification of those at high risk of dysfunctional drinking-driving and their education in the hope that they will improve their drinking or their driving has not yet been proven to be effective in the age group under consideration. Efforts such as driving under the influence (DUI) programs directed at teenage violators have not reported their followup statistics.

It is in primary prevention—education and learning by example of young children to drink moderately or not at all—that the best hopes lie. This approach is a long-term effect and cannot be expected to produce any impact until a generation or two has elapsed. It also means that adult drinking patterns will have to moderate and that will be a formidable task.

Furthermore, it means that driving motor vehilcles will have to be considered a complex operation needing the highest level of sober skill to operate safely. Such cultural value shifts are required before any fundamental changes can take place in our highway behavior.

Can such value shifts occur? They are possible, but the answer is in doubt.

NOTES

1. Hammond, R. L. Legal drinking age at 18 or 21: Does it make a difference? *J. Alcohol Drug Education. 18:*9-13, 1973.
2. MICAP RECAP. Report No. 35 Michigan Council on Alcohol Problems, Lansing, Mi. 1973.
3. Zylman, R. Fatal crashes among Michigan youth following reduction of legal drinking age. *Quart. J. Stud. Alcohol. 35:*283-286, 1974.
4. Williams, P. H., *et al.* The legal minimum drinking age and fatal motor vehicle crashes. *J. Legal Studies. 4:*219-239, 1975.

5. Cucchiario, S. *et al.* The effect of the 18 year old drinking age on auto accidents. Massachusetts Institute of Technology Operations Research Center, Cambridge, Ma. 1974.

6. Schmidt, W. and Kornaczewski, A. L'abaissement de l'age auquella loide l' Ontario permet d'absorber de l'alcool et ses effets sur les accidents de'automobile attribuales a l'alcool. *Toxicomanies.* *8:*105-116, 1975.

7. Whitehead, P. C. *et al;* Change in the drinking age: Impact on young drivers. *J. Stud. Alcohol. 36:*1209-1223, 1975.

8. Whitehead, P. C. Alcohol and young drivers. Impact and implications of lowering the drinking age. Non-Medical Use of Drugs Directorate, Department of National Health and Welfare, Monograph Series No. 1., 1977.

9. Carlson, W. L. Age exposure and alcohol involvement in night crashes. *J. Safety Research. 5:*247, 1973.

4. Geriatric Drug Abuse

The attention of the public and of the experts has been focused upon the youthful drug abuser. In fact, when we think about the addict or the drug dependent person, it is the young "junkie" or "head" who come to mind. A significant drug abuse problem also exists among the elderly. This is, in part, what the National Commission on Marihuana and Drug Abuse called "America's hidden drug problem." It is certainly more covert, less investigated, and less written about, but in certain respects it is just as worthy of serious study as the adolescent situation. The youngest may freak out in public places on alien psychochemicals. Meanwhile, the aged alcohol or drug abuser passes out quietly in his drab, furnished room or in some Skid Row alley.

The drugs of geriatric abuse are almost invariably depressants. Juveniles may seek an intensification of sensation and increased awareness from hallucinogens or stimulants although they, too, prefer "downers" these days. The use of central nervous system sedatives, hypnotics, alcohol, and tranquilizers are more and more the preferred mode of altering consciousness. When stimulants are misused by oldsters, it is in combination with sedatives or narcotics. Withdrawal from a frustrating existence and evasion of life stress is what is sought after rather than new experiences of hyperalertness.

One impressive observation is the great variability in the response of an old person to various amounts of a consciousness-changing drug. They may be hypersensitive to even average amounts of a psychochemical, barbiturates, for example. This is probably due to problems with detoxification and excretion. An impaired renal clearance or a reduced capacity to induce enzyme formation to detoxify a drug are conditions associated with the aging process. These physiologic impairments are associated with a psychological brittleness, which can produce mental confusion or a fluctuating delirium from ordinary quantities of a depressant. When recent memory and time orientation are adversely affected, supervision in the taking of prescribed drugs is needed. Otherwise, too much or too little will be self-administered.

THE NARCOTIC ADDICT

Aged opiate addicts can be sorted into at least two subgroups: surviving street addicts and medical addicts. A third group, probably disappearing, is the so-called Southern-type addict.

Street Addicts

Street addicts over 60 are not often seen. Before reaching that age most have either died from the consequences of injecting unsterile materials for decades, of overdosing; or they have been done in by the addict-associated diseases or trauma. A number tire out and no longer can keep up with their rigorous "junkie" careers of "hustling" and "copping." This phenomenon has been called "maturing out" of the drug scene. Just what the elements involved in "maturing out" consist of are not well understood. It does not appear to be a psychological maturation process in most instances, rather it is a matter of physical exhaustion.

It takes a combination of an excellent constitution, extraordinary good luck and an unusual survival ability to manage to celebrate one's 60th birthday as a street addict. By that time the old junkie has learned how to remain invisible. In order to avoid police harrassment and the neighborhood rip-off artists, he maintains the lowest of profiles. His criminal activities decrease. His lack of satisfaction with street heroin may convert him to a user of methadone, morphine, Dilaudid, or Demerol. These can be bought on the street or "conned" out of well-meaning doctors. If things get too rough he will "shoot" paregoric or drink codeine cough syrup by the four ounce bottle where these items are still available without a prescription.

Some over-sixty addicts can find refuge in methadone maintenance clinics. About a thousand of them have been counted in methadone maintenance clinics around the country. Methadone maintenance is not a bad compromise for someone who has been addicted for 40 or 50 years. For such an individual the goal need not be eventual abstinence from all narcotics, as it would be for a younger person. Rather, one would consider keeping the elderly addict on methadone indefinitely if that is as far as he wants to go.

An alternative way to manage such a person is with periodic detoxifications to reduce the size of his habit because of the gradual buildup of tolerance. Although detoxification from narcotics is futile if abstinence is the goal, if we can accept a temporarily decreased opiate "habit" as a desirable end, then two or three detoxifications a year is not really a wasted effort.

Medical Addicts

The medical, or iatrogenic addict is one who has become addicted while being treated for some painful illness, usually a malignancy that runs an unexpectedly benign course, but often enough for pancreatitis, arthritis, low back pain, or postsurgical pain. The management of chronic pain is one of the more difficult problems in medicine. Not every medical addict represents a medical error. Those who are going to die within a short time should be kept as comfortable as possible and given sufficient analgesics. When such a person happens to survive a year or years in pain, the addiction becomes a vexing problem for the patient, his family, and his physician. With considerable ingenuity and effort even these ill and hurting people can be detoxified and managed. Surely, highly addicting narcotics should not be prescribed for such recurrent, non-lethal conditions as migraine or asthma. There is good reason to believe that excellent analgesics will become available that have a lower dependency-producing potential than those now at hand.

Some medical addicts have been known to search out street heroin when legitimate supplies are denied them. Detoxification with methadone should occur in a hospital and proceed slowly. The stress of an abrupt withdrawal may be too much for a depleted, medically ill person.

Southern-type Addicts

A third category of elderly opiate addicts is repesented by the individual who became overinvolved with paregoric, codeine cough syrups, or patent medicines containing opium during the days when these medicaments were easier to obtain than at present. Since that time they may have continued to receive some narcotic from a sympathetic doctor, especially if they happened to live in a small town. This is the so-called Southern-type of addiction. It was not unusual at the turn of the century for a woman, less frequently a man, with chronic complaints to be maintained on morphine or Pantopon for years. It was predominantly a Southern rural phenomenon, but was, by no means, restricted to that area.

SEDATIVE AND TRANQUILIZER DEPENDENCE

Prescriptions for sleeping pills and minor tranquilizers are at an all-time high. Two of the most common complaints among elderly patients are insomnia and nervousness. These medications give initial relief, but as tolerance develops either more is needed or the effect wanes. When large amounts are consumed, mental confusion and physical clumsiness may develop. Old patients with a marginal mental compensation are easily pushed into a delirium. This is manifested by perplexity, an impaired ability to process information, memory and concentration disturbances, and a fluctuating loss of orientation, especially for time. Nor is sudden withdrawal of the medication likely to solve the problem. Indeed, it can be catastrophic with the oldster precipitated into the delirium tremens.

It is difficult to understand how one capsule of a sleeping medication every night can be effective over years, except as a conditioned stimulus. It has been found that insomniacs on constant doses of sleeping medication after a few months sleep no more than insomniacs not given any medication. In both instances sleep was broken, without deep sleep components (Stages III and IV), and sleep latency (falling asleep time) was prolonged. Nevertheless, both groups managed to obtain more than 5 hours of sleep during the night, the minimum requirement for people over 60.

Most sleeping pills suppress dreaming sleep. When they are discontinued or reduced, a dream time overshoot occurs resulting in vivid nightmares, which wake the sleeper. As indicated, the old person, even if he is well, has a reduced ability to detoxify ingested chemicals. Furthermore, his reduced capacity to compensate behaviorally for the drug intoxication makes him accident prone. The old person has little reserve with which to adjust to agents that alter his thinking and perception.

The repertoire of a physician's sleep procurement program need not have as its keystone the barbiturate and non-barbiturate sedatives. The bulk of complaints of geriatric insomnia are the result of either ignorance of what normal sleep patterns are in old folks, or they are due to secondary causes. In the first instance it is clear that the sleep requirement is reduced with aging, 4½ to 5½ hours being the physiologic need for those over 65. Another trick that the changing sleep pattern plays on the elderly is that Stages III and IV sleep, the deepest stages, are diminished or non-existent. Therefore, they may not have the feeling that they really slept. In addition, they may dream about being awake and claim the next day that they didn't close their eyes. All night sleep tracings of such insomniacs indicate that although they did not fall asleep quickly, woke a number of times during the night, and were awake at an early hour, they still slept more than the minimum requirement.

Nocturnal pain, itching, muscle cramps, depression, and many other conditions can cause sleeplessness. For example, the need to void three or four times a night may be incompatible with proper sleep. It makes more sense to eliminate these sleep-disrupting factors than to mask them with hypnotics. Even when the insomnia seems to have no apparent cause that can be treated, there is no need to resort to sleeping potions immediately. Instead, a program of conditioning the patient should be planned that will encourage the onset of sleep. A pre-sleep ritual must be worked out and regularly followed. It would include hot drinks, warm baths, relaxation exercises, boring reading materials, and similar activities. If chemical therapy is needed, it should not be forgotten that certain antihistamines and minor tranquilizers like diazepam are as potent and effective as any hypnotic. By using these groups of agents along with the traditional sedatives in short one or two-week courses, tolerances can be avoided. A part of the effectiveness of any sleeping pill is that it acts as a conditioning agent. Therefore, a placebo may be effective for some.

A person who tends to become dependent upon mind-altering chemicals should not be treated for his tension with drugs that have a record of being abused. Immature, rather inadequate, unstable persons with a poor tolerance for frustration are liable to become overinvolved in drugs that reduce anxiety, and distance the person from life stress, especially if the drugs happen to produce a measure of euphoria. Such an individual with a high anxiety level can be treated with small doses of the phenothiazines without risk of producing a dependency. Hydroxyzine is another drug that almost never causes habituation.

The senior citizen's nursing home problem requires separate mention. The oversedation of many nursing home members is a part of a general picture of overmedication. In part, this results from piling on drug orders without a periodic review of the chart to eliminate the unnecessary, but long forgotten items. Furthermore, eccentricity, non-conformity, even irascibility, are not indications for sedation. Our problem is that we have pills easily capable of making the crotchety compliant, the demanding dulled, and the surly sedated. Why should the busy staff put up with any disrupting influence whatsoever? One answer is that we don't want to chemically obliterate all personality features, however obstreperous. Another answer is that these drugs have side effects, which require other drugs, which have side effects.

Since the source of geriatric sedative abuse is, almost invariably, the physician's order or prescription, more enlightened prescribing practices could do a good deal to solve the problem. Large quantities of sedatives should not be available to confused, elderly patients. They will inevitably be misused. When such patients escalate their intake to the equivalent of eight 100 mg secobarbital capsules in 24 hours, hospitalization is necessary for slow detoxification, support of cardiovascular function, and the prevention of convulsions.

PROPRIETARY MEDICINE ABUSE

There is a wide range of patent medicines that can be abused by the aged. The over-the-counter sleeping potions contain an antihistamine with or without a small amount of scopolamine. The wake-up pills are usually caffeine or an ephedrine-like compound. An enormous market for analgesics exists, and aspirin, an aspirin-phenacetin-caffeine combination, or other salicylates, are widely used. These preparations can be incorrectly used, for example, to take aspirin a number of times a day to prevent headache. None of these drugs are innocuous—certainly not aspirin, and toxic effects are not rare.

Despite all the warnings about bromides, their use as tranquilizers and analgesics persists. Four patent medicines containing one or more bromide salts are available. Bromo Seltzer, Alva Tranquil, Miles Nervine, and Lanabrom Elixer. Another, Neurosine, requires a doctor's prescription. The typical person who becomes overinvolved in chronic bromide intoxication is a white female over 40. Bromism and alcoholism are often associated. A blood bromide level of over 80 mg percent ordinarily signifies that the mental confusion is bromide-related. However, a bromism is rarely considered in the differential diagnosis of delirium, and its role remains unrecognized. This is particularly true of those with cerebral arteriosclerosis, and they seem predisposed to develop a bromide psychosis.

GERIATRIC ALCOHOLISM

The most serious of all drug abuse problems involving the aged is alcoholism. Of 534 consecutive over-60 patients admitted for psychiatric observation to San Francisco General Hospital, 28 percent had a serious drinking problem. Of these, 80 percent required hospitalization for their excessive drinking. A study reported from the medical service of the Harlem Hospital Center revealed that 63 percent of the men and 35 percent of the women were alcoholics. In a large house-to-house survey in the Washington Heights section of upper Manhattan, the peak incidence of alcohol abuse was found in the 45 to 54-year-old group. It was 2.3 percent in the 65 to 74-year-old group. If these figures can be extrapolated nationwide, it would mean that about a million people over the age of 55 are alcoholics.

Geriatric alcoholics can be readily subdivided into two groups. Those in the first group have had a lifelong history of excessive and destructive drinking practices, and have managed to avoid the lethal illnesses and injuries associated with such an existence. They are the last survivors of a much larger cohort of alcoholics. The outlook for abstinence is not good, although a small number do manage to stop drinking, with or without treatment. The second group consists of those who have started drinking heavily late in life. Not infrequently this has been in response to one or more of the losses that accompany aging: losses of loved ones, loss of self-esteem, and loss of feelings of worth. For their separation anxieties and situational depressions they have come to use alcohol as a form of self-treatment. It acts as a depressant, blocking the painful input from memory and from the environment. The prognosis is more favorable for this group. New interpersonal relationships must be formed, perhaps in a resocialization program. Sometimes, antidepressant medication is needed for a while. But it is usually the formation of a close relationship with one or a few people that changes their attitudes and saves them from a life that is bottled in bondage.

5. The Psychopharmacology of Aging

Although far from a precise science or even a well-practiced art, the chemotherapy of mental disorders of the aging person is moving forward. Vast areas of doubt and debate remain, however, and numbers of inaccuracies require revision. This essay will attempt to uncover some of the misconceptions, provide some general principles, and offer a number of specific suggestions about management.

GENERAL PRINCIPLES OF GERIATRIC PSYCHOPHARMACOLOGY

The Condition May Not Be Hopeless
The elderly patient is often approached by the physician with an attitude of hopelessness because of a fixation on the irreversible organic aspects of the aging brain cells and the inevitable occlusion of their blood supply. In fact there may be a substantial reversible component to the

mental deficit, which, if engaged, could ameliorate a good share of the behavioral and emotional disorder.

Certain of the symptoms of "senile deterioration" may have little to do with impaired cerebral blood flow or senile cerebral atrophy. Memory deficits, social withdrawal, negativism, delusional thinking, and other "organic" symptoms may be due to depression or a combination of depression and cerebral insufficiency. Correct the depression and a fair segment of the disturbance recedes. The substantial correction of geriatric depression is a reasonable expectation with our current therapies.

The Mental Impairment May Be Due to Extracerebral Factors

Poor nutrition to the brain is reversible at times. I am not referring to the use of cerebral vasodilators, which will be mentioned later. Rather, I am thinking of those patients who have extracerebral reasons for their cerebral decompensation. Borderline congestive heart failure, chronic pulmonary infections, emphysema, and nutritional deficiencies that interfere with cerebral transfer or utilization of oxygen and glucose are some of the correctible causes of impaired brain nutrition. The correction of a diabetic condition, malnutrition, dehydration, or some metabolic deviation such as hypothyroidism could markedly improve mental functioning.

Suspect All Drugs That the Patient Receives As a Cause of Sudden Decrements in the Mental Condition

In someone who has recently become confused, or whose condition has suddenly deteriorated, consider the possibility that his present medications may be the cause. Because of feelings of futility, we tend to assume that the geriatric patient's downhill course is just a part of a "normal" decline. The reserpine being given for hypertension may precipitate or intensify a depression. The urinary acidifier may induce acidosis and a toxic psychosis. Steroids, antihypertensives, and anticholinergics are well-known precipitators of delirium. Almost any drug, even antibiotics, will produce an adverse psychological reaction in the person hypersensitive to it.

Certain Drugs Taken for Physical Disorders Will Interact With Some Psychoactive Agents

Drug interactions are numerous. Sometimes the effect of a drug is undesirably enhanced, at other times it is blocked. The antihypertensive effect of guanethidine may be reduced by the phenothiazines. On the other hand a combination of a thiazide like Diurel taken for high blood pressure and chlorpromazine (Thorazine) or amitriptyline (Elavil) can be intensified to produce unexpected hypotensive blood pressure levels. The butyrophenones given with warfarin (Coumadin) interfere with its anticoagulant action. Antiparkinson drugs reduce the blood levels and the effectiveness of neuroleptics. The enzyme induction stimulated by barbiturates tends to accelerate the metabolism of diphenylhydantoin (Dilantin) and phenothiazines. The antidepressant effect of the tricyclic drugs is enhanced by methylphenidate (Ritalin) and thyroid.

Paradoxical Drug Reactions are More Common in the Elderly

The expected psychopharmacological effect may not only fail to appear, but on occasion the effect may be in the opposite direction. Phenobarbital may cause insomnia and excitement. Chlorpromazine can induce unruly, agitated behavior. Chlordiazepoxide (Librium) has been known to occasionally increase anxiety and aggressiveness. Explanations for such paradoxical effects are variable. Some unusual reactions may be based upon a loss of controls over behavior similar to the disinhibiting effects of alcohol.

The Starting Dose is Not the Average Dose in Old People

In order to avoid toxicity, the starting dose of psychotropic drugs should be a half to a third of a young adult's dose. Old people become posturally hypotensive more readily because their arteries are less adaptable to sudden pressure changes. They faint under such conditions because lesser alterations of blood flow produce cerebral hypoxia. Their fall can cause more serious injuries because their long bones and skull are less calcified. They are apt to bleed more from such accidents because their blood vessels are more calcified or fragile. It is prudent to increase and decrease drug doses gradually. At times, maximal excitement must be contained, then large amounts of the psychotropic drugs are needed and should be used.

Although hypotensive reactions have been used to illustrate the sensitivity of some old people to average amounts of a drug, other side effects may also be avoided if small initial doses and small increments are employed. The extrapyramidal syndromes, some of the allergic reactions, and drowsiness also will be reduced or avoided.

Adverse Effects are More Frequent in the Elderly

Because their mechanisms for detoxifying and excreting psychotropic drugs are impaired, the risk of toxic effects is greater in old people. Drowsinesss, postural hypotension, the cardiac arrhythmias, and agranulocytosis are more frequent in this age group. Certain of the extrapyramidal syndromes (Parkinsonism and akasthisias, for example) and tardive dyskinesia occur with some prediliction in those over 60. The anticholinergic effect of the tricyclic antidepressants and the neuroleptics is apt to cause urinary retention and constipation. Constipation is a trivial side effect except in the neglected elderly where it can escalate into obturator intestinal obstruction.

Old People are Marked Placebo Reactors

Old people in distress respond intensely to the nonspecific factors associated with the administration of a drug. The additional attention that accompanies giving medication, the symbolic significance of the medicine which may represent the doctor, his concern and understanding; these are factors that produce beneficial effects well beyond the pharmacologic action of the drug. It is possible that a large component of the benefits from injectable vitamins and tonics are based upon this potent placebo reactivity. It may also be one reason why so many geriatric medications have been so difficult to evaluate scientifically.

A Periodic Review of the Oldster's Drug Program Avoids Problems

With their multiple ailments geriatric patients tend to accumulate many medications. Some of these medications may continue to be used long after the doctor has forgotten about them. A routine, periodic review of all prescription and non-prescription drugs that the patient is taking will be illuminating and it may decrease the chances of undesired drug interactions.

Drugs Alone Are Not Enough

It is too much to expect that a chemical alone will be able to reverse a complex human condition like depression or psychosis. Chemotherapy must be assisted with counseling, encouragement, reassurance, and support by the physician or some other trained person. The family must be reoriented so that, if members are not therapeutic, at least they are not destructive. The more stressful components of the patient's life should be identified and changed, if possible.

Use It or Lose It

There seems to be one rule that pervades retention of mental and physical functions into senescence. "Use it or lose it" holds true for muscular development, memory retention, sexual functioning, and mental agility, along with many other human activities. Restrict use and atrophy begins. Retain some degree of activity, and gratifying levels of effective functioning will be retained. Do not restrict the psychic and somatic activities of an old person without good cause.

SOME SPECIFIC POINTS

1. The benzodiazepines are long acting drugs. When used in very large amounts, they can cumulate in the tissue and produce a delayed intoxication. It is also unnecessary to give them three or four times daily after the first week or so.

2. When the question of which sleeping pill should be used arises, the first answer should be: "Can this old patient be trained in non-drug sleep routines?" If occasional hypnotics are needed, chloral and flurazapam (Dalmane) have advantages in the advanced age groups. Another solution to the sleep problem may be to give most or all of the daily dose of the antianxiety, antidepressant or neuroleptic drug at bedtime. Sedation can be achieved in this manner, and some of the side effect will be slept through.

3. In addition to the neuroleptics, the tricyclic antidepressants also have anticholinergic effects. The patient with prostatic hypertrophy or constipation may "shut down" completely with these drugs. Even the dry mouth can be more than annoying. It can interfere with swallowing and contribute to oral infections.

4. The ability to excrete lithium decreases with age. Smaller than average doses are indicated, and lithium blood levels should be kept somewhat lower than aimed for in younger people (0.5-.1.0 mg/100 ml).

5. Geriatric patients prefer to abuse the CNS depressants rather than the stimulants. Dependence on alcohol, minor tranquilizers, sleeping pills, and, to some extent, narcotics and analgesics is well known. When treating such dependency-prone individuals for anxiety, non-dependency producing agents such as the neuroleptics in small doses are preferred.

DRUGS USED FOR GERIATRIC PROBLEMS

Most of the drugs used to improve the function of the brain cell have not been conclusively found to produce this effect. A certain amount of evidence may exist, for certain compounds, but much of it remains contradictory. It is possible that selected patients may respond to certain of the geropharmaceuticals. The expectation that all patients will benefit from all geropharmaceutical groups is unrealistic.

Cerebral Vasodilators

These include papavarine (Pavabid), cyclandelate (Cyclospasmol), isoxuprine (Vasodilan), and nicotinyl alcohol (Riniacol.) The problem is that when cerebral vessels dilate (if they can), they must compete for blood with the rest of the body, which also participates in the vasodilation.

Ergot Alkaloids

Hydergine, a mixture of ergot alkaloids, appears to increase cerebral blood flow and oxygen utilization—perhaps due to changes in neuronal metabolism. Many of the emotional-behavioral symptoms of aging are supposed to respond to treatment over a period of weeks.

Anticoagulants

In those individuals who have sustained multiple strokes, maintenance 4-hydroxycoumarin (Dicumarol) has been used to reduce blood coagulation. For specific individuals this may prolong mental functioning and life. The incidence of serious hemorrhages in 25 percent of those on prolonged therapy restricts its wider use.

Stimulants

Small doses of stimulants have successfully helped fatigue and mild depressive states. The drugs ordinarily used include pipradrol (Meretran), methylphenidate (Ritalen), deanol (Deaner), pentylentetrazol (Metrazol), ethamivan (Emivan), and magnesium pemoline (Cylert).

Procaine

Procaine (Gerovital) is under reinvestigation to determine its efficacy in the depressions that accompany the aging process. A number of double blind studies indicate some antidepressant effect.

Miscellaneous Agents

Many hormonal (anabolic steroids, estrogens, and androgens) and vitamin products have been used in problems of aging. Anticholesterol agents tend to be either unsafe or ineffective. The administration of DNA, RNA and its precursors, lipotropic enzymes, glutamic acid, nutritional supplements, and many other substances have been used at various times.

SUMMARY

Much can be done for the disturbed old patient. A cheerful, hopeful attitude, a familiarity with the modern psychotropic drugs, a thorough search for cerebral and extra-cerebral factors that may be embarrassing the nutrition of the brain, a constant focus on the person instead of his age—these will help alter what is often anticipated—an irremedial decline into decrepitude.

6. Alcoholism and Women

Established stereotypes about excessive drinking by women are, no doubt, based upon valid observations. The suburban housewife, alone, drinking because of boredom and frustration is one such prototype. The menopausal woman whose busy life as a homemaker has suddenly become empty because the children have all left the nest is another.

Newer patterns also are emerging. The liberated young college girl may find herself too heavily into drinking. The harassed executive trying to keep ahead of her job or acting the role of "one of the boys" with her co-workers might slip into a pattern of overdrinking as time goes on.

It is evident that changes in the direction of an excessive consumption of alcohol among certain groups of women are appearing more frequently these days. For this reason a re-examination of the present relationships between women and alcohol is considered worthwhile.

HOW MANY WOMEN DRINK ALCOHOLIC BEVERAGES IN THE UNITED STATES?

As of 1969, 60 percent of American women drank some quantity of fermented beverages (as compared to 77 percent of men). It is clear that these percentages are higher at present, due, perhaps, to the large numbers of teenage girls who are counted as users of some form of alcohol.

HOW MANY ALCOHOLIC WOMEN ARE THERE?

It is claimed that more than two million women are in trouble because of their destructive drinking in this country. The male:female ratio is about 4 or 5 to 1. Chafetz, on the other hand, has reported that there are three million alcoholic and problem drinking women, and that the male:female ratio is 3 to 1.

WHAT CAN BE SAID ABOUT THE PARENTS OF THE ALCOHOLIC WOMAN?

A quarter to a half of their fathers were alcoholics and were described by them as warm and gentle. The mothers tended to be described as cold and domineering, but few of the mothers were alcoholics.

CAN WOMEN DRINK AS MUCH AS MEN?

Alcohol diffuses rapidly to all tissues, and its effects parallel body weight fairly closely. Therefore, women who tend to weigh 25 to 35 percent less than men will have higher blood alcohol concentrations and will be more affected when consuming equal quantities of alcohol. Intoxification will occur sooner, and, on chronic usage, organ damage will develop earlier in women.

HOW CAN EXCESSIVE DRINKING BE DIAGNOSED IN WOMEN WHO DO NOT GIVE SUCH A HISTORY?

In general, the signs and symptoms are similar to those in men. Sometimes, edema of the face, a fine hand tremor, or redness of the palms are seen earlier in women. Cigarette burns on the fingers or upper chest may be a hint that the patient was intoxicated and fell asleep while smoking. The possibility that the patient is alcoholic should be entertained in working up complaints of amenorrhea.

ARE THERE ANY WOMEN ON SKID ROW?

Yes, about 5 percent of the residents are women, and, even under the congested living circumstances, they tend to drink alone. They have no "bottle buddies" as the men do. Their major social interactions occur when they try to obtain drinks or money from the male residents or others transiently in the area.

IS IT TRUE THAT ALCOHOLIC WOMEN ARE PROMISCUOUS?

Promiscuity occurs in only a small fraction of all chronically alcoholic women. Schuckit says only 5 percent can be described in this manner. The rest complain of a diminished interest in sex, including frigidity and dyspareunia. Promiscuous behavior may take place during the early phase of excessive drinking with the alcohol acting to release behavior from the usual ego controls.

WHAT DIFFERENTIATES FEMALE FROM MALE ALCOHOLICS?

Considerable overlap exists, but certain differences also are apparent. Women who are more emotionally disturbed and more depressed than their male counterparts are likely to be found in surveys of unselected samples of alcohol dependent persons. Often they can relate a specific stress that precipitated their excessive drinking activity. This may have been a serious sexual problem, gynecological difficulties, a middle-age identity crisis, loss of a loved one, divorce, or some similar emotionally traumatic event.

Because of the social prejudices against excessive drinking by women, they tend to drink alone and away from other people. They begin drinking later in life than men, but this is becoming less true. Alcoholic women are divorced by their spouse much more frequently than alcoholic men. Women marry men who have drinking problems more often than men marry alcoholic women.

WHAT NEW PATTERNS OF HEAVY DRINKING ARE EMERGING IN THE MORE LIBERATED WOMAN?

For many women their traditional roles are in rapid transition and the rapidity of change constitutes a stressful condition. Although eagerly seeking equality, for some, a certain ambivalence may remain because of their early indoctrination about a woman's proper place. After achieving a managerial or other important post, the pressures to drink more heavily may increase.

If they have inner doubts about their femininity or doubts about their ability to succeed, such feelings of insecurity may encourage overindulgence. As with men, the physical and psychological pressures of a demanding and difficult job may be a factor. Then, the loss of the previously more dependent state, the loneliness of the new life, even the freedom to be able to make decisions—all these may build up and culminate in drinking as a way to cope with their problems. So it is not only the unsuccessful career woman but also the successful one who may be at risk.

Women are more apt to combine sedatives and tranquilizers with alcoholic beverages. The perils of miscalculating the potentiating effects of such combinations on some occasion is a real possibility.

AA is reporting that 17- and 18-year-old-girls with drinking problems are now attending their meetings. They had been steady drinkers for a half dozen years or more.

Some observers believe that the apparent increase in female alcoholism is not so much due to newly addicted individuals as it is that women are more open about their drinking at the present time. No doubt, greater visibility is a factor, but a real increase in alcohol addiction has been demonstrated. Women are appearing much more frequently at alcohol treatment centers. They are coming to treatment for cirrhosis of the liver in greater numbers than ever. Deaths due to cirrhosis in females is being recorded by Medical Examiners with increasing regularity during the past few years.

WHAT ARE THE EFFECTS OF MATERNAL ALCOHOLISM ON THE CHILDREN?

Statistics indicate that the battered child syndrome is much more likely to occur when one or both parents drink excessively. Physical and emotional child abuse with subsequent emotional disorders in the children are documented. As the primary parent, the mother, in particular, affects her growing offspring's development. It is very difficult for adolescents to cope with their mother's drunken comportment.

WHAT IS THE FETAL ALCOHOL SYNDROME?

Chronically alcoholic, pregnant women have a high perinatal mortality rate (17 percent vs. 2 percent in non-alcoholics). The children they give birth to may be mentally deficient, show poor growth and development, and have a variety of congenital anomalies. These include facial abnormalities with small head size, short palpebral fissures, drooping eyelids, and hypoplasia of the face. Joint anomalies, cleft palate, septal defects, hemangionas, and a long list of less frequently occurring deficiencies have been diagnosed during infancy. It is suspected that many less severely affected offspring with only mild mental and growth deficiencies escape notice and are never diagnosed.

At the 1976 meeting of the American College of Cardiology, the cardiac defects found in the fetal alcohol syndrome were scrutinized. More than half of the children with the syndrome have heart abnormalities. Tetralogy of Fallot, patent ductus arteriosus, and ventricular or atrial septal defects have been diagnosed. A number of these children have required surgery to repair the congenital cardiac anomalies.

The cause of the syndrome is not malnutrition, rather it seems to be the toxic effect of alcohol or acetaldehyde upon fetal cellular and tissue development. At birth, the cord blood alcohol has been shown to be at least as high as the mother's blood levels, and in rapidly growing and reproducing cells, levels tolerated by the adult organism may damage the embryo.

It might be wondered why such an obvious connection between heavy drinking during pregnancy and gross neonatal changes had not been detected long ago. Actually, the older literature does mention fetal anomalies occurring in pregnant alcoholic women, but the strong correlation has not been made until recently.

WHAT IS THE RELATIONSHIP BETWEEN MENSTRUAL DIFFICULTIES AND DRINKING?

In Belfer's study, 67 percent of women who had menses related their drinking to the premenstrual period. Drinking either began or increased at this time. His alcoholic patients were significantly more depressed and anxious than nonalcoholic women. The endocrine changes during the premenstrum apparently intensify the pre-existing mood disorder.

ARE THERE ANY SPECIAL PROBLEMS IN TREATING ALCOHOL DEPENDENT WOMEN?

Substantial doubts about self-worth and identity seem to be present in such women. It is worthwhile to pay particular attention to the problem of their self-concept and to support and enhance it. Role definition and clarification may be important in sorting out ambivalent feelings. The established therapies, Alcoholics Anonymous, group therapies, and Antabuse are as effective with women as with men. The fact that such women are more depressed than men may require particular attention.

WHAT COUNSELING SHOULD BE GIVEN ALCOHOLIC WOMEN WHO MAY BECOME PREGNANT?

She should be appraised that persistent, high levels of alcohol during pregnancy can give rise to serious developmental problems in 30 to 50 percent of surviving offspring. She should be encouraged to use birth control measures until alcohol intake can be discontinued. If a pregnancy occurs, detoxification and abstinence is recommended during gestation. If this is not possible, termination of the pregnancy might be considered.

DO WOMEN ALTER THEIR DRINKING HABITS DURING PREGNANCY?

One report indicates that some pregnant women may reduce or stop their intake of alcoholic beverages on the basis of an aversion for such beverages. Further study of the nature of the temporary distaste is continuing.

SUMMARY

Female drinking practices are changing. They are becoming more overt, more women are drinking socially, and more are drinking excessively. In these respects, they are adapting a "masculine" type of drinking behavior. A recently rediscovered entity, the fetal alcohol syndrome, indicates that heavy drinking during pregnancy can induce a variety of serious fetal disabilities.

REFERENCES

1. Beckman, L. J.: *Women Alcoholics,* J. Studies Alcohol., *36:*797-824, (July) 1975.
2. Belfer, M. L., Shader, R. I., and Carroll, M.: *Alcoholism in Women,* Arch. Gen. Psychiat., *25:*540-544, 1971.
2. Garrett, G. R.: *Women on Skid Row,* Quart. J. Studies Alcohol, *34:*1228-1243, 1973.
4. Hanson, J. W., James, K. L., and Smith, D. W.: Fetal Alcohol Syndrome, JAMA, *235:*1458-1460, (April 5) 1976.
5. Schuckit, M., et al.: *Alcoholism: Two types of Alcoholism in Women,* Arch. Gen. Psychiat., *20:*301-306, 1969.

7. The Drug Dependent Paraplegic

There are a number of special groups who are prone to become overinvolved in the drugs that produce dependence. One subgroup is the para- or quadraplegic, those individuals who have lost the function of their lower, and sometimes upper extremities. Most frequently the paralysis is secondary to serious injury to the spinal cord. These people tend to sustain their trauma during the early decades of their lives. Military service, auto accidents, high speed sports, and other dangerous activities generate the great majority of paraplegics.

The problems of being a more or less impotent, incontinent, permanently paralyzed, young person, perhaps in pain, are evident. Considerable anger, depression, and anxiety must be overt or covert. Many paraplegics will exist without clearly defined life goals, will have difficulty enjoying, and will have pervasive feelings of hopelessness and helplessness. The blow to their self esteem may be enormous, and their self concept is often badly disrupted. Paraplegics often see themselves as weak, dependent, ineffectual semi-persons. They are therefore vulnerable to the overuse of drugs that will change their mood, reduce their awareness and their boredom, and diminish their psychic or physical pain.

THE IATROGENIC FACTOR

These are people who are normally highly medicated by their physicians with an array of tranquilizers, sedatives, analgesics and narcotics, and who would predictably be expected to misuse them. Alcohol, of course, is the major chemical of abuse among unrehabilitated paraplegics.

A table of the commonly prescribed mood-altering drugs is offered according to their liability to produce dependency. *The table should be read separately for each class of drugs.* Drugs listed as having a high dependency-producing potential under tranquilizers will not be equivalent in dependency potential to the narcotics in the same category. In addition, within each degree of dependency potential, drugs will vary somewhat on this factor. Methadone, for example, is a little less addicting than morphine, and yet it must be rated as "high" in dependency potential. Naturally, when one can, one uses drugs of low abuse potential in the paraplegic who has a history of or a character structure which may predispose to chemical dependency. (See Table V-1 on page 348.)

PSYCHOPHYSICAL FACTORS

With the current erosion of the taboos against using mind-altering drugs for recreational purposes, many paraplegics are, or will surely become, involved in the various drugs of abuse.

All this is quite understandable. These are people in despair, despondent because they lack viable motivators often impotent, and trapped in their bodies. Why shouldn't they drown their sorrows, escape from their personal prison, if only in fantasy, or obliterate their consciousness? It is understandable that some will bedrug themselves, but it is necessary to ask whether this is their best solution? Does the price they pay exceed the satisfactions of a transient release from somber reality?

The price is high, especially for this group. These are people whose

Table V-I: Dependency Potential of Prescription Drugs

Class	High	Moderate	Low	None
Analgesics and Narcotics:	Morphine, Demerol, Dilaudid, Methadone	Talwin, Codeine Darvon		Aspirin, Tylenol
Sedatives and Hypnotics:	All rapid acting barbiturates, Methaqualone, Doriden and other nonbarbiturate hypnotics.	Phenobarbital, Chloral, Paraldehyde	Dalmane	
Tranquilizers:	Meprobamate	Librium	Valium, Serax, Tranxene	Vistaril All phenothiazenes, Haldol, Serpasil, Navane, Taractan
Stimulants, Antidepressants and Antiobesity Agents	Methedrine All Amphetamines, Preludin, Ritalin	Tenuate, Pre-Sate, Tepanil, Meretran, Ionamin	Parnate, Caffeine, Sanorex, Nardil	Deaner, All tricyclic Antidepressants

disability can be defined as a regional loss of control over their bodies. With most intoxicants the loss becomes total. The disability becomes complete, and the chances for reconstitution approach zero. If we say: "Let them have their booze (or dope), they are suffering too much," we are really saying, "We give up, too," a statement that should probably never be made when caring for a paraplegic.

The major reasons for the overindulgence in mind-altering substances by the paralyzed young person can be summarized in the following list.

1. The damage to one's self-concept.

2. A response to pain, muscle spasm, and loss of ability to ambulate.

3. A diminution or loss of sexual capability.

4. The frustrations of a life of relative inactivity.

5. The impairment of bladder and rectal function.

6. An effort to treat the dysphoria with CNS depressants.

7. An attempt to achieve euphoria by chemical suppression of sobriety.

8. A covert form of self-destruction.

What are the alternatives to allowing them to be dependent on chemicals? Obviously, it is a matter of either prevention or treatment.

PREVENTION

Prevention starts with the professional staff. They must be alert to the vulnerability of the paraplegic to drug overuse. Prescribing enormous take-home supplies of abusable drugs must somehow be avoided. The facts of tolerance and cross-tolerance must be considered when trying to deal with problems of insomnia, muscle spasm, anxiety, or pain. As mentioned, there are CNS depressant agents with a low abuse potential, and these should be employed whenever possible. When drugs with a high abuse potential are required, they must not be administered interminably.

Some paraplegics should be made aware of the threat of drug dependence to them and their cooperation sought in avoiding the addicted state. Certainly, the family of the patient requires elementary instruction in the problem, else they will become conscious or unconscious pushers or, at least, procurers. A paraplegic often needs someone's help in becoming and remaining addicted to drugs or alcohol. That someone is usually a wife or husband, a parent, a doctor or aide, or a well meaning or avaricious friend.

Prevention also means providing suitable alternatives to drugs. It is realized how difficult it is to instill hope and a sense of excitement in these patients, but somehow it must be done. There is no simple prescription for alternatives. Some are appropriate for one person, some for another. At this time only general areas in which alternative activities are to be found will be mentioned. They range from religious involvement to camping, from meditation to handcrafts, and from philosophical explorations to games. Yoga will attract some, and relaxation techniques others. Training in relaxation exercises would seem worthwhile for every paraplegic. Sensory awareness training, community service, encounter groups, appropriate athletics, carpentry, and many other activities are meaningful and rewarding for selected individuals. Self-hypnosis as a means of reducing noxious affects could be included. The list is almost endless, it is the fit between the person and the activity that is most important.

The treatment of the drug dependent paraplegic is more difficult than the non-paraplegic. Motivation is less, the realities of the situation are grimmer, and the pity offered by those around him is no help. No matter how disabled, he must cooperate in his recovery. He must accept the responsibility for cleaning himself up. In other words, his self-concept must be reconstructed. He must see himself as a person capable of mature decision-making. If this can be achieved, much might be accomplished. One of the more important factors in re-establishing the paraplegic's self-image is to bring him to the point where he can do work that is meaningful for him.

How the dependency disorder is treated does not differ too much from the conventional techniques. When detoxification is indicated, this should be accomplished. The results have not been good even with addicts capable of ambulation. When we remember how infrequently the alcohol addict is cured by "drying out" procedure, this clarifies the less than 5 percent improvement rate for detoxification from other drugs. Detoxification, however, may be the beginning of a worthwhile therapeutic relationship. If intensive counseling can be combined with detoxification, then more successes might result.

A worthwhile innovation would be the development of a therapeutic community of seriously drug and alcohol dependent paraplegics. One of the first requirements for such a venture is one or two charistmatic, recovered addict-paraplegics. Such a residential facility may not only be a powerful device for making some paraplegics abstinent, but also a possible morale booster for dealing with their physical disability.

Methadone maintenance is not a desirable procedure for the heroin addict who is also a paraplegic in pain. In general, people in chronic pain should not be placed on methadone maintenance because, after a time, tolerance to the analgesic effects of the narcotic is acquired. Other methods of dealing with chronic pain should be used. For the paraplegic without a pain problem there is no particular objection to methadone maintenance, but it is hoped that it does not go on indefinitely. Rather a program of maintenance should be set up within a definite time frame. During that period the person receives appropriate psychologic and social assistance so that by the time gradual withdrawal starts, he is able to cope with his life situation on a drug free basis.

Antabuse is useful only for the alcoholic paraplegic who really wants to stop drinking, and who feels he needs the "protection" that Antabuse provides. AA or other self-help group techniques would seem like a preferable way to handle problem drinking.

SPECIAL FACTORS

Some points about the interplay between drug or alcohol addiction and paraplegia should be noted.

Heroin Addiction Can Cause Paraplegia

A small number of cases have been reported in which a transverse myelitis developed after an injection of heroin that contained septic material.

Any Intoxication Can Result in Paraplegia

The person under the influence of a chemical is accident-prone due to mental confusion, loss of control, risk-taking behavior, or paranoid ideas of grandiosity, any of which can induce dangerous activities that might sever a spinal cord.

Differences Between the Street Addict and the Paraplegic Addict Exist

Often the paraplegic becomes overinvolved in drugs following medical use of the drug. Although he may eventually look to the street for his supplies, he only infrequently becomes involved in the street life-style. It is not easy for a paraplegic to survive on Skid Row or in Needle Park. In addition, the veteran paraplegic ordinarily has enough money both for his addiction and his living expenses. He can get additional sums, if necessary, by selling off the drugs he obtains on prescriptions from his doctors or by panhandling.

Drug and Alcohol Dependency Can Antidate the Paraplegia

A number of the paraplegics in trouble with chemical dependency problems had these problems before they became paraplegic. Clearly, for them the problem is compounded, and the prognosis is worse but not hopeless. The very same personality qualities that predispose to danger-seeking behaviors that result in serious injuries are similar to those that make a person vulnerable to excessive alcohol and drug taking. These include poor impulse control, emotional immaturity, passive aggressiveness, and a sociopathic life style.

SUMMARY

The excessive use of mind-altering drugs halts the rehabilitation process, makes the paraplegic more liable to accidental injury, and causes him to lose any desire to improve himself. It is a staff responsibility to prevent or reverse this process. Special skills and techniques may have to be devised to deal with the "para-addict."

8. Doping: Drugs in Sports

The use of drugs to enhance athletic performance is hardly a new development. During the European six-day bicycle races of a century ago certain contestants would take caffeine tablets, brandy, nitroglycerin, or even a jigger of ether to improve their staying power.

Doping is the generic term for the increase in achievement during sporting contests through the use of a variety of chemicals. This discussion is limited to human doping; animal doping is not considered at this time.

WHAT IS DOPING?

It is, according to the International Olympic Committee, either the use of substances alien to the body, or physiological substances in abnormal amounts, or drugs used by abnormal methods with the aim of attaining an unfair advantage during competition. In addition, certain psychological measures to increase one's performance in sporting contests are also regarded as doping. The treatment of an illness with medication is not considered doping, although such treatment must be reported to the committee.

It is evident that the dividing line between normal training for competitive sports and doping is a bit fuzzy. For example, training at high altitude for a sporting event that will take place at sea level will increase red cell mass. It is an acceptable procedure. However, removing a pint or two of blood from the athlete a month before the contest and transfusing it immediately before the event would constitute doping.

WHAT IS THE EXPECTED RESULT OF DOPING?

The desired effects of using various substances before an athletic competition are:

1. An increase in strength, endurance and performance.

2. An intensified drive to win and to achieve intense mental concentration.

3. A diminished sense of fatigue and exhaustion.

4. Diminished pain perception.

5. A reduction in anxiety and tremulousness.

IN WHAT KINDS OF CONTESTS MAY DOPING BE USED?

Drugs might be used to excel in the following types of sporting games:

1. Contact sports like football, especially by those players who must function at maximal tenacity and strength while ignoring exhaustion and pain.

2. Endurance sports like cycling, distance running, and swimming in which sustained energy is required and fatigue must be set aside.

3. Maximal strength sports like weight lifting or hammer throwing during which a short burst of supra-maximal energy is needed.

HOW WIDESPREAD IS DOPING?

This is difficult to determine for obvious reasons. Some writers indicate that doping is extensive in certain sports such as professional football; the authorities claim the opposite. In Olympic competition, where urine testing is mandatory, only 11 of 2,080 tests were positive (0.05 percent) during the Montreal games. The awareness that one's urine will be tested is a proven deterrent strategy to discourage doping. In a doctoral dissertation by Johnson in 1970, of 93 National Football League players from 13 teams, 60 percent admitted taking amphetamines regularly. At that time the drugs were handed out by trainers or team doctors. Since they were prohibited in 1972, the players have searched out other sources, usually street dealers. Mandell's information in 1973 indicates that of 87 professional football players, 48 used amphetamines regularly, 9 occasionally, and 30 not at all. Individual writings of ex-players (*They Call It a Game, Semi-Tough, Ball Four, North Dallas Forty*) also indicate a high frequency of use. On the other hand, these figures are denied by league commissioners and other officials who generally indicate that a drug problem does not exist in their particular sport.

WHICH DRUGS ARE INVOLVED IN DOPING?

A variety of drugs has been tried. The three drug classes that are prohibited by the International Olympic Committee are the psychomotor stimulants (including the sympathomimetic amines), the narcotic analgesics, and the anabolic steroids. Other chemical agents that have been used also will be mentioned.

The Central Stimulants

The amphetamines will be described since they are the prototypic psychomotor stimulants. Cocaine, anorexiants, and related drugs are sometimes used for doping, but the amphetamines are the most frequently employed of all substances for the purpose of improving athletic achievement.

The well-known physiologic effects of the amphetamines include increased cardiac output, respiratory flow, metabolic rate, and glycogenesis. Isometric strength, work output, and persistence at a boring or demanding task are improved, although not all controlled studies have been positive. In a classical investigation by Smith and Beecher, 75 percent of swimmers, runners, shot putters, and hammer throwers performed better on amphetamines (14mg/70kg of dextroamphetamine) than on a placebo. The Smith and Beecher studies have been challenged on methodological grounds, and a final verdict about the value of the stimulants for these purposes has not been reached. Among athletes who use them, the strengthening and energizing effect of these drugs is not questioned.

The effects of stimulant consumption result in additional psychophysiologic actions that people participating in competitive sports may find desirable. These drugs increase alertness, decrease reaction time, and intensify aggressiveness. In fact, at certain dosages, a paranoid rage response might be achieved, and this state may be advantageous in maximally competitive contact sports. Another important effect is the analgesia that may accompany moderate or larger doses. This permits continued playing despite painful injuries. Naturally, such practices may result in a worsening of the original trauma.

The professional football type of amphetamine usage consists of taking 10 to 100 mg of one of the amphetamines once a week, an hour or two before the game. It is used to improve drive, strength, and endurance and to mask pain. Defensive linemen are supposed to use stimulants more than those in other positions. Mandell makes the point that quarterbacks who must react to rapidly changing situations with quick decisions are less inclined to use amphetamines, or if they do, to consume small amounts. Euphoria is said not to occur, but after-the-game insomnia, impotence, irritability, and a Monday morning physical dependence does appear under such a drug schedule. At times amphetamines are also consumed by the players to lose weight or to counteract the effects of heavy alcohol use.

The use by football players resembles the occupational ingestion of amphetamines by truckers who must drive for long periods, or by military personnel who must remain alert for extended operations. Untoward effects have been reported from such usage in those individuals sensitive to the hallucinogenic and thought distortion effects of these drugs.

Caffeine is not considered a prohibited drug, although its effect in very large amounts would resemble a small dose of the amphetamines.

The Narcotic Analgesics

At times average doses of the narcotic drugs have been taken in connection with sporting events, mainly to allow the athlete to perform despite some painful injury. Codeine, Darvon, methadone, and other opioids have been used, but on a restricted scale. The use of opiates does not appear to be a major problem at present.

The Anabolic and Other Steroids

The male sex hormones and the anabolic steroids increase body mass. They tend to increase appetite and improve nitrogen utilization. Some authorities believe that fluid retention, not muscle hypertrophy, is the reason for the weight gain, and that physical strength may not be enhanced. Furthermore, the possibility of undesired effects like virilization, impaired liver function, diminished libido, testicular atrophy, and hypertension makes their use questionable. It is difficult (sometimes impossible) to detect the anabolic steroids in the urine since they are taken during the off season and not prior to the contest.

Sedatives, Tranquilizers and Alcohol

The sedatives have been used to counteract the jitteriness that amphetamines can induce. Tranquilizers have been taken to ameliorate excessive tension and anxiety prior to a contest. Alcohol has been ingested for this purpose and also to reduce the fine tremor of marksmen in competition. Naturally, only modest amounts of these depressants are consumed, otherwise oversedation and poorer performance would result.

Local Anesthetics

Procaine and other synthetic local anesthetics are frequently injected into painful areas to permit further participation in the contest. This is analogous to the use of cortisone injections. In fact, the two drugs often are combined to produce both short and longer term analgesia.

Other Drugs

Vasodilators have little to recommend them for performance-improving purposes. They have been found to be dangerous because of possible circulatory collapse under conditions of extreme exertion. Respiratory and cardiac stimulants are also without proven value and may even be disadvantageous in doing extended physical work.

Despite the cardiorespiratory impairment caused by chronic cigarette smoking, a number of athletes still use tobacco during the interval between sports contests.

Oxygen, Vitamins, and Special Diets

Oxygen tanks and masks are fairly routinely seen in contact sport contests. Oxygen breathing decreases the time need for recovery from the oxygen deficit that accompanies overexertion. It is not helpful to use before a game. Oxygen is also used by athletes as an aid in recovering from hungover states.

Large amounts of vitamins and minerals are routinely downed by most contestants. Vitamin C and E are in particular favor. Whether they improve psychomotor performance is completely unknown.

A typical diet for championship contestants is a high protein, alkaline ash diet—the protein in the expectation that increased muscular growth might occur, and the alkaline ash to help counteract the acidosis of severe physical activity and the consequent exhaustion.

Perhaps the oddest technique to improve one's form occurred during practice trials for an international swimming competition. Two liters of compressed air were instilled via the rectum into the large intestine of the swimmers to increase their buoyancy. Apparently the results were less than desirable, but it demonstrates the lengths to which championship athletes and their coaches will go to win.

PREVENTION

With urine detection technology well worked out, and with European soccer players and the Olympic competitors routinely checked, it is odd that similar measures are not instituted for those sports in the United States where the misuse of drugs is well known. Although doping occurs at the college level, it is in professional sports, particularly—but not exclusively—football that the most widespread misuse is reported. If the voiding of a post-game urine under observation is too intrusive, saliva tests can easily be developed. It is difficult to understand the negative attitude of league officials, owners, and players toward testing for impermissible substances. They all have a great deal to lose over the long term from doping practices.

The fans must be educated to the fact that chemically-induced ferocity is not sport, and that football can be even more enjoyable without the late hits and the deliberate maimings, suspicious indicators of drug-provoked rage.

SUMMARY

It is futile to bewail the fact that notions such as "May the best team win," or "It's not who wins that counts, but how you play the game" are obsolescent. So long as spectators demand violence and victory, drugs will be used. The players will use them if only not to give the edge to their opponents. The owners will condone them because they add to the entertainment and the gate receipts. And the league commissioners will keep the lid on. A simple, non-invasive testing procedure can eliminate amphetamine and other types of competitive drug abuse. That it is not employed is clear evidence that no one in authority really wants to stop the practice.

At one time sports were considered the "moral equivalent of war." Man's inborn hostility would be rechanneled into less destructive competitions on the playing field instead of the battlefield. Although the dressing rooms following an unusually rough football game resemble a casualty station in wartime, at least the armaments involved are less deadly.

9. Aggression: The Role of Drugs

Human aggression is a complex act. In any single incident of violence, genetic, cultural, psychological, social, and situational factors are often intermingled. Much violence occurs without drugs, but certain substances will precipitate or cause hostile acting out.

DRUG-VIOLENCE INTERACTIONS

The impact of drugs upon aggressive behavior depends upon a number of factors.

1. The drug may have specific actions, inducing belligerence and hostile acts by one or more mechanisms.

2. Drug induced aggression will vary with dosages. For example, small quantities of alcohol do not incite to violence, and enormous amounts make such behavior impossible. It is with moderate to large amounts (0.1-0.4 percent blood alcohol concentrations) that violence can emerge.

3. Aggression is more likely to occur on the ascending limb of the blood drug concentration curve than on the descending limb.

4. The set and setting can modify a drug's violence-producing potential.

5. The established cultural pattern for conduct under the influence of the drug can overwhelm the pharmacologic effect.

6. The mood and personality of the user will grossly alter the action of any consciousness-modifying drug. No drug is invariably criminogenic. Instead, the person taking the drug and the conditions under which it is used are major modulators of the subsequent behavior.

MECHANISMS OF DRUG-INDUCED VIOLENCE

There are a number of paths that drug-induced violence might take.

1. The drug might diminish ego controls over comportment, releasing submerged anger than can come forth as directed or diffuse outbursts.

2. It may impair judgment and psychomotor performance, making the individual dangerous to himself and others.

3. It might induce restlessness, irritability, and impulsivity, causing a hostile combativeness.

4. The drug could produce a paranoid thought disorder with a misreading of reality. False ideas of suspicion or persecution may bring forth assaultive acts against the imagined tormentors.

5. The craving to obtain and use the drug can result in a variety of criminal behaviors, some of them assaultive.

6. An intoxicated or delirial state may result in combativeness and outbursts of poorly directed hyperactivity and violence.

7. Drug-induced feelings of bravado or omnipotence may obliterate one's ordinary sense of caution and prudence causing harm to oneself or others.

8. An amnesic or fugue state may occur during which unpredictable and irrational assaults may take place.

THE SPECIFIC DRUGS

Alcohol
In addition to being the most widely used mind-altering substance, alcohol is also the drug most often associated with violence. Its ability to evoke aggressive acts appear to be at least as great as any other drug of abuse. Many studies attest to the positive correlation between drinking and destructive behavior. More than half of the homicides are performed with the assailants having significant blood levels of alcohol. Only a slightly smaller percentage of their victims also have demonstratable blood levels of alcohol, usually having imbibed along with their eventual murderer. Spouse beating, battering children, rape, and sexual crimes against children also are associated with heavy drinking in a majority of instances. In addition, suicides often are associated with the drunken state. One-third of the injuries and half the deaths in motor vehicle accidents are alcohol-related. Each year 18,000 people die and 10 million are injured in industrial accidents involving alcohol. Some 44 percent of the private plane accidents are caused by pilots who had been drinking. Drownings, self-incinerations, and fatal falls often are the result of alcohol intoxication.

It is during the second stage of intoxication that the imbiber can become violent in word and deed. As drinking continues, judgment and the monitoring functions are impaired, paranoid misinterpretation of the environment can develop, and even a murderous state of rage might emerge.

Pathological intoxication is a special form of alcohol-connected aggression. Only a small amount of alcohol is needed to release unprovoked violent activity, and each new drinking episode is likely to reproduce the same belligerent condition. Brain damaged people control their drinking behavior with difficulty or not at all.

Sedative-Hypnotics

The pharmacologic actions of the barbiturates, the prototypes of the sedative-hypnotics, closely resemble those of alcohol. The chronic, daytime barbiturate user is unpredictable, uncoordinated, and variably confused. It should not be assumed that the diurnal user of hypnosedatives falls asleep. On the contrary, he may be overactive, argumentative, and irritable. Some of this paradoxical behavior can be accounted for as a release from the established ego controls, an inhibition of the inhibitory neuronal network. These drugs also quench apprehension and anxiety, generating the "Dutch courage" to execute a robbery or some other criminal act. In studies of drug-using prisoners the barbiturates were overrepresented among those who have been convicted of aggravated assault, robbery, and burglary. In one investigation barbiturate users had the highest rate of violent crimes compared with other drug users. Barbiturates or alcohol or both in combination accounted for 31 of a total of 36 drug-related assaults—including 7 homicides.

Motorcycle gang members seem to prefer downers before engaging in street combat. In most studies of convicted criminal populations the sedative-hypnotics rank second after alcohol as the drug used in connection with their assaultive activities. Belligerence and nastiness are commonly described by hospital personnel who have to care for chronic hypnosedative abusers. These drugs are not ideal agents to use before a mission involving skillfully executed violence except when excessive fear or guilt feelings may interfere with one's aggressiveness. Psychomotor performance is impaired, thinking is dulled, and decision-making abilities suffer. However, the use of gross force such as the fist, club, knife, or gun at close range does not require high levels of motor precision.

The rapidly acting hypnotics have been used in emergency medical situations to quiet the raging intoxicated or psychotic individual. While the procedure may be life-saving for the patient or those in his vicinity, it should, of course, not be used in those who already are toxic from CNS depressants.

Volatile Solvents

The aerosols and commercial solvents also resemble alcohol in their behavioral effects. Whatever differences exist relate to the different routes of administration and the duration of activity. The inhalants are delivered to the brain quickly. Sleepiness or stupor are rapidly achieved, allowing less time for antisocial acts than with alcohol intoxication. The duration of action is shorter than with swallowed alcohol. Accidents due to clumsiness and occasional reports of sexual and other assaults can be found in numerous case studies.

Anxiolytics

The typical result of benzodiazepine administration is a reduction of aggressive verbal and physical activity. Paradoxical hostility, however, is also known, and its causation has been studied. Occasional patients, upon losing their anxiety, will feel more hostile, perhaps as an uncovering of unexpressed anger. When the anxiety state was reduced, then the hostile effect could be released. This unmasking of argumentative or other angry behavior can occur at therapeutic dosage ranges and is not a result of intoxication.

Narcotics

The opiate dependent person under the influence of a narcotic is not likely to become involved in violence. The effects of heroin, for example, will diminish all drives. However, the need to obtain adequate supplies of the opiate every day must result in considerable amounts of criminal procurement activities. Traditionally, this kind of illicit conduct involved nonviolent crimes such as shoplifting, prostitution, dealing, and theft.

More recently the pattern of crimes against property has changed. Armed robbery, burglary, and assaults against other people have become more frequent. Rolling drunks is a specialty of junkies in some cities. Rape is an offense only rarely reported in connection with heroin addiction. Self-inflicted violence such as accidental overdose and suicide is a cause of death in about 2 percent of the heroin-dependent population each year. The conventional idea of the passive, complacent opiate addict is quite incorrect during the early phase of withdrawal. In a desperate attempt to procure relief from increasing discomfort, the addict will try anything—including murder.

A large number of heroin addicts had a history of sustained criminal involvement before the onset of their drug-taking career. During their period of heroin use, and after recovery, they may continue their felonious activities without interruption.

Stimulants

It can be predicted that stimulants in large doses with their capacity to cause hyperactivity, paranoid suspiciousness, and impulsivity will be productive of violence. The amphetamines are more likely involved than cocaine because of their long duration of action. These drugs can cause senseless aggression or criminal acts; at other times they are consumed to deliberately produce sustained energy outbursts and directed rage reactions, as in football contests. Bizarre crimes without obvious motivation can result from the delusional thinking process, the loss of impulse control, and the stereotyped, or repetitive motor acts. Instances of interminable stabbing or clubbing of a victim long since dead are well known.

When the speedfreak flourished a decade ago, the traffic in speed was more vicious and deadly than the heroin street scene. Dealers routinely carried weapons, and the clientele was caught up in a pervasive paranoia that generated a fair number of homicides. "Speed kills" was the slogan of the day. The amphetamines killed, not only from externally directed violence, but also from overdose, hypertension causing cerebral hemorrhages, and accidents due to misperceptions of reality. Of course these problems resulted from the high doses used. In therapeutic amounts, amphetamines and related drugs can reduce the overactivity and aberrant behavior of the hyperkinetic behavioral disorders of children.

Hallucinogens

With the exception of phencyclidine, violent or criminal activities during the hallucinogenic state are infrequent. The most frequent cause of lethality during an LSD experience is accidental death. The grandiose quality of certain experiences makes the individual vulnerable to an overestimation of his capabilities or an underestimation of environmental dangers. Panic and other unthinking states can result in injury. Only isolated instances of homicide have been documented.

Suicide attempts and suicide have occurred toward the waning hours or at the termination of the experience. The reasons for self-destruction include: the inability to deal with shattering uncovered, hitherto repressed memories, an attenuation of the desire to live, or the dismal, devastating image of oneself acquired under LSD.

Phencyclidine was once called "the Peace Pill," but it has turned out to be quite the opposite. The combination of delusions of power, insensitivity to pain, amnesia for antecedent events, and poor impulse control makes for the sort of bizarre assaultiveness that generates headlines. Angel dust is another misnomer. Some of its users call it, more appropriately, rocket fuel or killer weed.

Cannabis

With the advent of more potent cannabis preparations during the past few years, more intense intoxications and more profound intoxicated states will result. The prevailing belief that marijuana is a drug producing nonviolent behavior may have to be changed. At present, the context in which marijuana is used is productive of passivity and a tendency toward withdrawal. Aggression, therefore, is not seen except during the infrequent paranoid or panic reactions. If cannabis were to be consumed for purposes of fighting, it would predictably do so. At present cannabis is not generally associated with crimes of violence when compared with other drug groups.

ADDITIONAL READING

1. Boyatzis, R. E. Alcohol and interpersonal aggression. In M. M. Gross, Ed. *Alcohol intoxication and Withdrawal.* Plenum, New York, 1977.
2. Goodwin, D. W. Alcohol in suicides and homicides. Quart J. Stud. Alcohol 34:144, 1973. *IIIb.* Plenum Press, New York, 1977.
3. Research Issues No. 17, *Drugs and Crime,* Eds.: Austin, G. A. and Lettieri, D. J., NIDA, 5600 Fishers Lane, Rockville, Md. 20857, 1976.
4. Tinklenberg, J. R. Alcohol and violence. In: P. G. Bourne and R. Fox, eds. Alcoholism: *Progress in Research and Treatment,* Academic Press, New York, 1973.
5. Tinklenberg, J. R., *et al.* Drug involvement in criminal assaults by adolescents. Arch. Gen. Psychiat., 30, 685, 1974.

10. Drugs and Sexuality

It is interesting that during the past generation, two drugs have changed sexual practices more than any development since the prehistoric discovery that males had something to do with pregnancy.

Neither of them are psychotropic drugs: one is penicillin, which reduced fears of the venereal diseases, and the second is The Pill, progesterone-containing tablets that gave women control of their ovulation.

Since ancient times drugs have been used in an effort to modulate sexual thoughts and practices. A long list of medicaments have been employed to either enhance or suppress the mental and sensory aspects of sexuality. Surprisingly, at times the same substances have served such opposite objectives. Cannabis is an example of the importance of the consumer's expectations on drug effects. In early days Indian yogis used it to eliminate distracting worldly pleasures and ruminations during their meditations. Other users have sought sensual intensification with the same material. Libido alteration is an area in which expensive placebos such as ginseng root and ground boar's testicles are quite effective.

Naturally, a number of psychotropic drugs have been tried in an effort to alter sexual performance, usually in the direction of improving it. With the recent upsurge in nonmedical drug-taking generally, a reawakened interest in sex-drug interactions has developed.

ALCOHOL

It is quite unnecessary to repeat Shakespeare's often quoted passage from Macbeth concerning the effect of drink upon masculine sexuality.(1) In the intervening centuries not much additional knowledge about the action of alcohol in these matters has been acquired. Its disinhibiting effect upon controls over speech and behavior is counterbalanced by an increased difficulty in actual performance. The recent information that plasma testosterone levels are lowered by substantial ethanol intake may help explain the performance deficit. Chronic male alcoholics often complain of impotence and its frustrations, and this may be another reason for them to increase their recourse to alcohol.

When drinkers imbibe heavily over long periods, the metabolism of the gonadal hormones is deranged. Testicular atrophy and gynecomastia can result from a combination of low testosterone levels from reduced production, and high leutinizing hormone levels from impaired metabolism in the damaged liver.

HYPNOSEDATIVES

The impact of tranquilizers and sleeping pills in large quantities resembles that of alcohol. The usual inhibitions may be dissolved at intoxicating doses, but the ability to execute might suffer. Alternatively, one might fall asleep in the process. This group includes Quaalude, which still retains an undeserved reputation in some circles as a sexual enhancer. Whatever enhancement occurs is strictly due to a relaxation of the monitoring function of the ego.

THE VOLATILE NITRITES

The first nonmedical use of isoamyl and isobutyl nitrites was for their psychosexual effects in connection with orgasm. Time appears to slow down while under the influence, and sensation seems intensified. Therefore, they are inhaled prior to climax to prolong the sensory effects. During the past few years this subjective effect has become institutionalized. Porno shops now sell isobutyl nitrite under a variety of exotic trade names for those customers who require improvement of an already superlative activity. Aliphatic nitrite vapors are now also being sniffed through the waking day for whatever non-sex related intoxicating effects they can induce. All of this experimentation takes place with a drug that has hardly been studied for any chronic adverse effects it may have.

STIMULANTS

As a part of their general arousal effects, the amphetamines and related stimulants are reported to increase libidinal drives. Ejaculation may be delayed, sometimes unpleasantly, and instances of compulsive masturbation among high dose users are known. Promiscuity and various perversions are associated with chronic usage. On the other hand, a complete antipathy for sexual activity also may be mentioned by some amphetamine consumers.

In a study at the Haight-Ashbury Free Clinic an augmented sex drive was reported by 30 of 36 speed freaks. Ten of 18 males mentioned having erections and three of 18 females reported orgasms during the intravenous injection. Cocaine acted similarly, with 10 of 20 males reporting erection during the injection. In two of these respondents a painful priapism continued over the next 24 hours. The stimulants are often taken for the sexual effects rather than their euphoriant properties. Cocaine has been particularly valued in this respect.

HALLUCINOGENS

As a rule the hallucinogens produce asexual, nonerotic experiences. In my own studies with more than a thousand LSD subjects, no sexual acting out occurred, and many reported that the experience made sex irrelevant. In the Haight-Ashbury survey 44 of 48 clients interviewed said that LSD and STP were nonsexual experiences for them. Nevertheless, when the intent and the expectation of the user is in that direction, the mind-altering changes provided by the hallucinogens can be channeled into sexual matters. LSD psychotherapy has been employed in the treatment of a variety of sexual dysfunctions, but none of these studies have been controlled, and no research in this area is under way at present. Phencyclidine use has been associated with rape attacks and beatings of sex partners.

CANNABIS

As indicated, a factor like psychological set can overwhelm the pharmacological action of the psychotropic drugs. This is especially true for marihuana whose intoxicating (stoned) properties permit a variety of behaviors depending upon the non-drug variables. Like other intoxicants it relaxes sexual inhibitions and increases suggestibility. Prolongation of subjective time and increased sensory appreciation may provide psychosexual enhancement. This was reported by 48 percent of those questioned in a national survey, and by 80 percent of the Haight-Ashbury group, the latter, admittedly, a special population.

In another study a third reported no sexual effects, 5 percent spoke of negative effects and 44 percent mentioned increased sexual pleasure. The remainder said that these effects were variable. The cannabis-sex relationships are not simple. Much depends upon what the user believes marihuana will do, the entire transaction occurring inside his skull.

The recent findings that cannabis reduces testosterone levels in male humans and animals, and reduces follicule-stimulating and leutinizing hormones in female animals adds to an already complicated situation. Do these reports explain the occasional instances of masculine impotence, low sperm counts, and gynecomastia that have been encountered? What are the consequences if these hormone levels are depressed during adolescence, a period of accelerated psychosexual development? Can the lowered testosterone be the biologic substrate of the diminished drive and loss of motivation of certain users?

OPIATES

The impact of heroin on sexual activity is biphasic. During the initial phase an increase in activity is not uncommon. This honeymoon period is, no doubt, a reflection of heroin's anti-anxiety and disinhibiting properties. With continuing use, all drives, including sexual drives, are reduced. During the period of addiction to narcotics many women will become amenorrheic and frigid, and men will be impotent. This effect is reversible on detoxification. The narcotics lower gonadal (testosterone and leutinizing) hormone levels, decreasing both libido and performance.

When a heroin addict enters a methadone maintenance program, potency may be regained if only because his general health and nutrition improves. Other methadone maintenance patients continue to complain of either frigidity or impotence until the dose has been lowered below 50 mg daily. In a study of methadone maintenance patients 76 percent stated that sexual activity increased when compared to their heroin-using period, while 14 percent said that it diminished. This group had nonaddicted partners. In the group whose wives were also addicted 32 percent reported increased and 23 percent reported decreased sexual activity.

Male and female prostitutes are occasionally addicted to heroin, and for a variety of reasons. A few are addicted by their pimps to obtain better control over them. Others support their own and their pimp's habits through prostitution. Some get entangled into dependence on heroin in an attempt to treat the unhappy aspects of prostitution. A few will use heroin in an effort to treat their underlying psychopathology. The first few intravenous injections of heroin have been equated to an orgasm centered in the abdomen. This is, by no means, a common experience, and it disappears with continued use of the drug.

SUMMARY

In a recent survey of psychotherapists about the relationship between recreational drug use and sex, some interesting opinions were expressed. Sixty-three percent of those interviewed said "Yes" to the question: "Do small amounts of alcohol (1-2 ounces) increase sexual pleasure or performance?" When the same question was asked about marihuana 52 percent believed that increased pleasure or performance occurred. The question "Do people who use drugs as sexual enhancers tend to have feelings of sexual inadequacy or an inability to relate intimately?" was answered affirmatively by 78 percent.

It might be asked whether the increased use of drugs as euphoriants has led to increased sexual activity among nonmarried young people. Admittedly, the drug-related reduction of behavioral controls may produce instances of expanded activity. It is more likely, however, that people who use drugs for recreational purposes also engage in a number of other behaviors associated with, but not caused by, their drug usage. They may have a lifestyle that includes relaxed sexual attitudes, liberal political views, avant garde art and music preferences, and alienation from the established social norms.

It is a most unusual phenomenon for the younger age groups to require sex-enhancing chemicals. Until recently, it was the middle-aged person who might be expected to seek out love potions and related devices.

The possibility exists that those who routinely use chemically-assisted methods of achieving erection or sexual gratification will find subsequent nonchemical intercourse more difficult to achieve. Furthermore, over extended periods of time, drugs used for potency tend to lose their potency.

ADDITIONAL REFERENCES

1. *Drugs and Sex.* National Institute on Drug Abuse. Research Issues #2, 5600 Fishers Lane, Rockville, MD 20857, 1974.
2. Ewing, J. A. and Rouse, B. A. *Drinking: Alcohol in American Society—Issues and Current Research.* Nelson Hall, Chicago, 1978.
3. Gay, G. and Sheppard, C. W. Sex-crazed dope fiends: Myth or reality. In: Harms, E., Ed. *Drugs and Youth: The Challenge of Today,* Pergamon Press, New York, 1973.
4. Goode, E. *Drug use and sexual activity on a college campus.* Am. J. Psychiat. 128:1272-1276, 1972.
5. Jarvik, M. E. *Psychopharmacology in the Practise of Medicine.* Appleton-Century-Crofts, New York, 1977.
6. *Sexual Survey No. 14.* Current thinking on "recreational" drugs and sex. Med. Aspects Human Sexuality. 12:80-81, 1978.
7. Signell, L. T., Kapp, F. T., Fusaro, G. A., et al. *Popping and snorting volatile nitrites: A current fad for getting high.* Am. J. Psychiat. 135:1216-1218, 1978.

NOTES

1. It is provided here, however, for anyone who has forgotten the citation: Porter: "Drink is a great provoker of three things: nose-painting, sleep and urine. Lechery, sir, it provokes and unprovokes: it provokes the desire, but it takes away the performance.

Therefore much drink may be said to be an equivocator with lechery; it makes him and it mars him: it sets him on and takes him off: it persuades him and disheartens him: makes him stand to and not stand to: in conclusion, equivocates him in a sleep, and giving him the lie, leaves him." As far as women are concerned Ogden Nash summarized it as follows: "Candy is dandy But likker is quicker."

11. The Drug Schedules

Since 1970 when the Controlled Substances Act became federal law, the psychotropic drugs have come under a new system of legal controls.

There have been a number of revisions recently in the scheduling of various drugs. The concept behind the scheduling process and the positioning of various drugs will be discussed here.

No longer are drugs controlled according to pharmacological class, instead other factors are utilized. Various state laws may modify the federal statute.

WHAT ARE THE DRUG SCHEDULES?

The schedules consist of five categories of drugs into which many, but not all, of the mood altering drugs are placed. The purpose is to permit proper medical usage while attempting to deter non-medical abuse of these drugs.

ON WHAT BASIS ARE DRUGS SCHEDULED?

The actual or potential abuse of a drug as determined by its pharmacologic properties, the pattern of abuse, and the drug's dependence-producing liability are considered prior to scheduling. Immediate precursors to a controlled drug may also be scheduled when the precursor can easily be used to manufacture the controlled drug.

WHAT ARE THE VARIOUS SCHEDULES AND WHICH DRUGS ARE IN EACH?

Schedule I

Schedule I includes those drugs that have a high potential for abuse and have no current medical use in this country. All of the other schedules contain drugs that have medical usefulness in the United States. This schedule also contains drugs that can be used to make Schedule I substances, and others that have an action so similar to Schedule I drugs that it is reasonable to believe they will also be abused if they were to become available.

These drugs can be used for research purposes under a special license. A prescription cannot be written for them and they are not available in pharmacies, except in certain research hospital pharmacies. Almost a hundred chemicals are named in I, and this number increases markedly when their salts and isomers are included.

As can be seen, these agents are either narcotics or hallucinogens. They have a variable abuse potential, but since they have no established medical utility, they must all be placed here.

Schedule II

Schedule II drugs have a high abuse potential that may lead to severe psychological or physical dependence. They have a current, accepted therapeutic use. Schedule II substances require a special prescription that must be written and signed by the doctor. It cannot be telephoned in, except in an emergency. In that instance, the written prescription must be supplied within 72 hours. Refills are not permitted and the patient must see the doctor in order to obtain a new prescription. Like Schedule I items, they must be kept in a secure, locked place.

The opiates, some stimulants, and certain hypnotics are placed in Schedule II.

Schedule III

Assignment of a drug to Schedule III requires that the drug have a potential for abuse less than those in I and II. Abuse of these drugs may lead to moderate or low physical dependence or high levels of psychic dependence. Schedule III drugs require a prescription in writing or telephoned in to the pharmacy. If it is authorized on the prescription, it can

Table V-2: Examples of Schedule I Drugs

Heroin (diacetylmorphine)	LSD (lysergic acid diethylamide)
Alphaacetylmethadol (LAAM)	Marihuana (cannabis sativa)
Ibogaine	THC (delta-9-tetrahydrocanna-
Psilocybin	binol)
Peyote (lophophora Williamsii)	DMT (dimethyltryptamine)
Mescaline	

Table V-3: Examples of Schedule II Drugs

Opium (papaver somniferum)	Eskatrol (dextroamphetamine + prochlorperazine)
Morphine	Biphetamine (amphetamine + dextroamphetamine)
Codeine	
Percodan (oxycodone)	Desbutal (methamphetamine + pentobarbital)
Pantopon (opium alkaloids)	
Dilaudid (dihydromorphinone)	Methedrine (methamphetamine)
Dolophine (methadone)	Obedrin (methamphetamine + pentobarbital + vitamins)
Demerol (meperidine)	
Seconal (secobarbital)	Amytal (amobarbital)
Cocaine	Nembutal (pentobarbital)
Benzedrine (amphetamine)	Quaalude (methaqualone)
Dexamyl (dextroamphetamine + amobarbital)	Tuinal (secobarbital + ambobar-tal)
Dexedrine (dextroamphetamine)	Preludin (phenmetrazine)
	Ritalin (methylphenidate)

be refilled up to five times within six months after the original date of the prescription.

The less abusable sedative-hypnotics and so-called Class B narcotics are found here.

Schedule IV

Drugs with a low abuse potential relative to those in III, and whose abuse leads to limited physical or psychological dependence are placed in Schedule IV. Prescription requirements are the same as for III.

Certain of the hypnosedatives, weight reducing substances, and minor tranquilizers are included here.

Schedule V

To be placed in Schedule V the drug must have a lower abuse potential than those in IV. Only a limited psychological or physical dependence might result from its abuse. A prescription is not needed for many compounds in V, but the purchaser must be at least 18 years of age. He also must offer identification and have his name entered into a special log book kept by the pharmacist.

The exempt narcotics make up Schedule V and consist of those with small amounts of opium, codeine or other narcotics in a large quantity of some vehicle.

Table V-4: Examples of Schedule III Drugs

Empirin with codeine	Nodular (methprylon)
A.S.A. with codeine	Doriden (glutethimide)
Tylenol with codeine	Butisol (butabarbital)
Hycodon (hycodan + homatro-	Fiorinal
pine)	Carbrital
Paregoric (tincture of camphor-	
ated opium)	

Table V-5: Examples of Schedule IV Drugs

Luminal (phenobarbital)	Placidyl (ethchlorvynol)
Veronal (barbital)	Valmid (ethinamate)
Noctec (chloral hydrate)	Pondimin (fenfluramine)
Paraldehyde	Dalmane (flurazepam)
Talwin (pentazocine)	Tranxene (chlorazepate)
Darvon (propoxyphene)	Miltown (meprobamate)
Valium (diazepam)	Tenuate (diethylpropion)
Librium (chlordiazepoxide)	
Serax (oxazapam)	

Table V-6: Examples of Schedule V Drugs

Cheracol with codeine	Terpin hydrate with codeine
Robitussin A-C	
Cosadein	

Table V-7: Some Examples of Unscheduled Drugs

Tylenol (acetaminophen)	Mellaril (thioridazine)
Atarax (hydroxyzine)	Stelazine (trifluoperazine)
Vistaril (hydroxyzine pamoate)	Haldol (haloperidol)
Solacen (tybamate)	Navane (thiothixene)
Thorazine (chlorpromazine)	Tofranil (imipramine)
	Elavil (amitriptyline)

ARE THERE ANY UNSCHEDULED PSYCHOTROPIC DRUGS?

None of the major tranquilizers or the antidepressants are scheduled since they have little or no abuse potential. A few minor tranquilizers do not appear in any schedule. The milder analgesics are also not controlled.

DO DRUGS EVER GET RESCHEDULED?

A number of drugs have been moved from one schedule to another or have been moved to or from an unscheduled status. These moves have been made because of actual changes in the abuse of the drugs or because of an increase in information about their potential for abuse.

WHAT ARE THE PHYSICIAN'S RESPONSIBILITIES UNDER THE DRUG CONTROL ACT?

The doctor must register with the Drug Enforcement Administration (DEA) to prescribe Schedule II to V drugs. His prescription for controlled drugs must be signed and dated and it must show his full name and address. Schedule II drugs for office use are obtainable on a DEA order form.

Supplies of controlled substances retained in the physician's office are to be kept in a locked place. Theft of controlled drugs must be reported immediately to the police or the DEA. Physicians who dispense drugs have additional responsibilities including secure storage and record keeping.

WHAT ARE THE PHARMACISTS' RESPONSIBILITIES?

Pharmacists must register with the DEA in order to dispense controlled drugs. All receipts or distribution of these substances must be recorded. Schedule II transactions are to be maintained separately from other records. Records of Schedule III, IV, and V substances must be kept separately or be in a readily retrievable form.

Complete inventories are to be computed every two years and kept for the same length of time. An exact count of Schedule II items should be at hand. Estimated counts of other controlled substances are sufficient if the container holds less than 1,000 dosage units. Schedule II substances require a DEA form for ordering. Prescriptions dispensed for all controlled drugs must contain the following warning:

Table V-8: Some Examples of Rescheduled Drugs

Drug	From	To	Year
Benzedrine (amphetamine) and related drugs	III	II	1971
Preludin (phenmetrazine)	III	II	1971
Ritalin (methylphenidate)	III	II	1971
Tenuate (diethylproprion) and certain other anorectics	Unscheduled	IV	1973
Cylert (pemoline)	Unscheduled	IV	1975
Seconal (secobarbital) and other barbiturate hypnotics	III	II	1973
Quaalude (methaqualone)	III	II	1973
Valium (diazepam) and other benzodiazepines	Unscheduled	IV	1975
Propoxyphene (Darvon)	Unscheduled	IV	1977
Pentazocine (Talwin)	Unscheduled	IV	1977
Naloxone (Narcan)	I	Unscheduled	1971
Phencyclidine (PCP)	Unscheduled	II	1978

"CAUTION: Federal law prohibits the transfer of this drug to any person other than the patient for whom it was intended."

Refills for Schedule III and IV drugs, if authorized must be recorded on the back of the prescription, including date, amount and the pharmacist's initials. Partial filling of a prescription for a drug in Schedule II is permitted, providing the remaining amount is provided within 72 hours and the doctor is notified. Partial filling of Schedule III and IV substances is permitted so long as the quantity dispensed is noted on the reverse side. Partial fillings cannot exceed the total quantity prescribed multiplied by the permitted number of refills. Prescriptions ordered orally should be written and filed by the pharmacist.

Pharmacists must keep Schedule II drugs in a strong, locked cabinet or safe. Other scheduled items must be kept in a locked cabinet or dispersed among the uncontrolled drugs in a manner that will obstruct theft. If excessive amounts of controlled substances are at hand, pharmacists should contact the regional DEA office for forms and instructions about disposal. The theft of controlled substances must be reported on BNDD Form 106 to the DEA and the local police department at the time of discovery.

WHAT ARE THE CRIMINAL PENALTIES FOR TRAFFICKING?

Unauthorized manufacturing, distribution, or possession of Schedule I and II narcotics is punishable up to 15 years in prison and a $25,000 fine. For trafficking in Schedule III drugs or in the non-narcotic Schedule I and II substances, the penalty is up to five years and a $15,000 fine. For Schedule IV drugs, the penalty is a maximum of three years' imprisonment and a $10,000 fine. Trafficking in Schedule V drugs is a misdemeanor, with up to a year in jail and a $5,000 fine. Second offenses call forth punishments double that of the first offense penalty.

Unauthorized possession of a controlled drug for one's own use is punishable by up to a year in jail and a $5,000 fine. This applies to professionals and lay persons alike.

SUMMARY

The control of abusable drugs is costly in time and money, but this is counterbalanced by the advantages derived. The existence of a record keeping system at all levels of distribution prevents or quickly detects pilferage. The patient, despite the inconvenience of limited renewal privileges, benefits by the doctor's closer supervision. The community is served because a reduced supply of abusable drugs becomes available on the black marketplace. It was the rescheduling of the amphetamines and methaqualone, bringing them under tighter controls, that markedly reduce their street availability.

12. Psychotropic Drug Interactions

The drugs that act on mental processes are no different from other pharmaceutical agents in that they are capable of affecting the absorption, metabolism, and excretion of other drugs.

At times these interactions are of no clinical importance, but on other occasions they can seriously increase or decrease the desired drug effects. Occasionally, the interaction may be desirable.

In order to systematize the available information on drug-drug interactions a number of tables have been prepared. One such table appeared in "The Barbiturates: Has Their Time Gone?" describing the impact of barbiturates on the therapeutic action of some commonly used medicinal agents.

Other drug-drug interactions are presented on pages 378-384. The first group (Table V-9) consists of the minor tranquilizers. These are CNS depressants and therefore add to the effect of other depressants.

Drugs in the second group (Table V-10) are the major tranquilizers. They are also CNS depressants and add to the effect of other classes of depressants.

The drugs used for arteriosclerotic, postencephalitic, or chemical Parkinsonism can cause problems, among which is delayed or impaired absorption of other orally-administered drugs. Their anticholinergic action is responsible for the reduction in gastric motility and delayed emptying time. (See Table V-11.)

Since the anticonvulsant, diphenylhydantion, must be taken for long periods of time, its interaction with other agents is a matter of interest. (See Table V-12.)

The tricyclic antidepressants are a group of drugs often used in combination with other drugs that interact with them. The monoamine oxidase inhibitors (MAOI) are well known as drugs that interact with many common agents. Other sedatives that have a significant involvement with the metabolism of other drugs include chloral and alcohol. (See table V-13.)

COMMENTARY

The biphasic action of alcohol usage may require clarification. During chronic alcohol intake metabolizing enzymes are induced. They inactivate other classes of drugs more rapidly than would ordinarily occur, therefore the action of certain sedatives, anticonvulsants and anticoagulants is diminished.

During a bout of heavy drinking the excess amounts of enzyme present are used by the large quantities of alcohol that must be metabolized, and the other categories of drugs using related enzymes for their metabolic breakdown have a longer than usual period of action. The resistance of drying out chronic alcoholics to sedatives and anesthetics is well known. Their additive effects during an acute episode of alcohol intake are likewise well documented.

ADDITIONAL READING

1. Ayd, F. V., *Psychotropic Drug Combinations: Good and Bad,* International Drug Therapy Newsletter, 12:13-16 (Apr.), 1972.

2. *Evaluations of Drug Interactions,* American Pharmaceutical Assn., 1973.
3. Goodman, L. S. and Gilman, A., *The Pharmacological Basis of Therapeutics,* Fifth Edition, MacMillan, New York, 1975.
4. Hansten, P. D., *Drug Interactions,* Second Edition, Lea & Ferbiger, Philadelphia, 1975.
5. *The Medical Letter on Drugs and Therapeutics Reference Handbook,* 56 Harrison St., New Rochelle, New York, 10801, 1975.

Table V-9: Minor Tranquilizers

Drug or Drug Class	Examples	When Combined With	Produces These Effects
Benzodiazepines	Valium Librium Dalmane Serax Tranxene Clonapin	Alcohol	Additive: increased CNS depression; increased plasma levels of the benzodiazepine.
Meprobamate	Equinal Miltown Deprol Pathibamate	Alcohol	Decreased sedative effect in chronic alcohol user due to enzyme induction. Increased CNS depression during acute alcohol intoxication due to reduced metabolism and additive effect.

Table V-10: Major Traquilizers

Drug or Drug Class	Examples	When Combined With	Produces These Effects
Phenothiazines	Thorazine Mellaril Compazine Stelazine Prolixin	Ismelin	Decreased antihypertensive effect by blockade of NE uptake
		Epinephrine	Blocks epinephrine effect
		Levodopa	Decreased levodopa effect due to dopa-blockade
	Serentil Trilafon Sparine Vesprin Quide Permitil Tindal	Antiparkinsonian drugs	Reduces plasma levels of phenothiazines
		Barbiturates	Reduces phenothiazine effectiveness
		Alcohol	Additive effect
		Diurel	Hypotensive episodes
		Lithium	Decreased phenothiazine plasma level
Butyrophenones	Haldol Innovar	Lithium	Increased butyrophenone toxicity
		Aldomet	Increased butyrophenone toxicity
		Alcohol	Additive effect
		Epinephrine	Blocks epinephrine effect
		Levodopa	Decreased levodopa effect due to dopa-mine blockade

Table V-11: Antiparkinsonian Agents

Drug or Drug Class	Examples	When Combined With	Produces These Effects
Antiparkinsonian Drugs	Artane Akineton Cogentin Kemadrin Pagitane	Levodopa	Impaired absorption of levodopa due to decrease in gastrointestinal motility
		Phenothiazines	Reduced phenothiazine blood levels
		Tricyclic Antidepressants	Additive anticholinergic effect
Levodopa	Dopar Larodopar Sinemet Bendopa	MAOIs	Hypertensive crisis by increased NE and DA release
		Phenothiazines Butyrophenones Dilantin	Decreased levodopa effect by inhibition DA uptake Decreased levodopa effect
		Papavarine Pyridoxine	Decreased levodopa effect Decreased levodopa effect by increase in decarboxylation
		Inderal	Increased levodopa effect; increased hypertensive effect
		Epinephrine	Increased epinephrine effect

Table V-12: Diphenylhydantoin

Drug or Drug Class	Examples	When Combined With	Produces These Effects
Diphenylhydantoin	Dilantin Phelantin Phenytoin	Barbiturates	Decreased anticonvulsant effect due to enzyme induction
		Alcohol	Decreased anticonvulsant effect in chronic alcohol abuse due to enzyme induction Increased anticonvulsant effect during acute alcohol intoxication due to decreased metabolic breakdown
		Anticoagulants	Increased diphenylhydantoin toxicity due to enzyme inhibition
		Chloromycetin	Increased diphenylhydantoin toxicity due to enzyme inhibition
		Corticosteroids	Decreased corticosteroid effect due to enzyme induction
		Oral Contraceptives	Fluid retention, increased seizures tendency
		Antabuse	Increased diphenylnydantoin intoxicity
		Hyperstat	Decreased anticonvulsant activity
		Quinidine	Increased quinidine effect
		Lidocaine I.V.	Increased cardiac depression

Table V-13: Antidepressant and Antimanic Drugs

Drug or Drug Class	Examples	When Combined With	Produces These Effects
Tricylic Antidepressants	Tofranil Elavil Norpramine Aventyl Pertofrane Sinequan Vivactil	MAOIs Thyroid Ritalen Alcohol Barbiturates Antiparkinsonian drugs Oral contraceptives Epinephrine	Hyperpyrexia, convulsions Increased antidepressant effect Increased antidepressant effect Decreased antidepressant effect Decreased antidepressant effect Addictive anticholinergic effect Decreased antidepressant effect Hypertensive crisis by inhibition of NE up-take
		Dicumarol Diurel Phenothiazines	Increased anticoagulant effect Increased antidepressant effect Increased antidepressant effect
		Ismelin Catapress Aldomet	Decreased antihypertensive effect
MAOIs	Marplan Nardil Parnate Eutonyl	Tricyclic antidepressants Antidiabetics Levodopa Demerol	Hypertensive crisis Increased hypoglycemia Hypertensive crisis Hypertension, convulsions, coma by alternate metabolic pathway to normeperidine

Drug or Drug Class	Examples	When Combined With	Produces These Effects
	[Furoxone Matulane]	Epinephrine	Hypertensive crisis
		Ritalen	Hypertensive crisis
		Tyramine in foods & beverages	Hypertensive crisis by increased NE release
		Amphetamines	Hypertensive crisis
		CNS depressants	Increased depressant effect
		Antiparkinsonian drugs	Increased anticholinergic effects
Lithium Carbonate	[Eskalith Lithane Lithronate]	Haldol	Increased Haldol toxicity
		Tricyclic antidepressants	Additive antidepressant effect
		Aldomet and other sodium depleting diuretics	Increased lithium toxicity

Drug or Drug Class	Examples	When Combined With	Produces These Effects
Chloral Hydrate	Noctec Aquachloral Beta-Chlor Felsules	Alcohol	Prolonged hypnotic effect due to synergism
		Warfarin	Increased anticoagulant effect by displacement from binding sites
		Lasix	Vasomotor instability
		Antabuse	Flush, emesis, abdominal pain, delirium due to inhibition of acetaldehyde metabolism
		Flagyl	Minor antabuse-like symptoms
		Antidiabetic Sulfonylureas	Minor antabuse-like symptoms
Alcohol (in addition to those already mentioned)		Salicylates	Increased gastrointestinal bleeding due to additive inflammatory effect
		Anticoagulants	Decreased anticoagulant effect during chronic alcohol abuse due to enzyme induction
			Increased anticoagulant effect during acute intoxication because of competition for enzymes

INDEX